The Chemistry of the Tetracycline Antibiotics

MEDICINAL RESEARCH
A Series of Monographs

1. Drugs Affecting the Peripheral Nervous System
   edited by Alfred Burger *out of print*
2. Drugs Affecting the Central Nervous System
   edited by Alfred Burger *out of print*
3. Selected Pharmacological Testing Methods
   edited by Alfred Burger *out of print*
4. Analytical Metabolic Chemistry of Drugs
   by Jean L. Hirtz *out of print*
5. Biogenic Amines and Physiological Membranes in Drug Therapy
   edited by John H. Biel and Leo G. Abood
6. Search for New Drugs
   edited by Alan A. Rubin
7. Clofibrate and Related Analogs
   by Donald T. Witiak, Howard A. I. Newman, and Dennis R. Feller
8. Quantitative Drug Design: A Critical Introduction
   by Yvonne Connolly Martin
9. The Chemistry of the Tetracycline Antibiotics
   by Lester A. Mitscher

Additional Volumes in Preparation

The Chemistry of the Tetracycline Antibiotics

Lester A. Mitscher
Department of Medicinal Chemistry
The University of Kansas
Lawrence, Kansas

MARCEL DEKKER, INC. New York and Basel

Library of Congress Cataloging in Publication Data

Mitscher, Lester A.
The chemistry of the tetracycline antibiotics.

(Medicinal research; v. 9)
Includes bibliographical references and indexes.
1. Tetracycline. I. Title. II. Series.
[DNLM: 1. Tetracyclines. W1 ME64H v. 9 / QV360
M684c]
QD377.T45M57 547'.76 78-12971
ISBN 0-8247-6716-0

MARCEL DEKKER, INC.

270 Madison Avenue, New York, New York 10016

Current printing (last digit):
10 9 8 7 6 5 4 3 2 1

PRINTED IN THE UNITED STATES OF AMERICA

Dedicated to the Memory
of my Mother

ABOUT THE SERIES

This series of monographs was conceived by the late Dr. Fred Schueler of Tulane University. His untimely death came prior to the completion of the first volumes of the series, and his friend and very able colleague, Dr. Alfred Burger of the University of Virginia, took on the task of editing the first three volumes of the series. Dr. Burger's heavy responsibilities forced him to withdraw from further active participation with the series, and the next three volumes were selected from books already under contract to Marcel Dekker, Inc., with Dr. Gary Grunewald of the University of Kansas as Consulting Editor. At this point an Editorial Advisory Board was selected and Grunewald became the Series Editor. The traditions established under the leadership of Schueler and Burger will be continued.

It is hoped that books for the series will serve a useful role in the areas of medicinal chemistry, chemical pharmacology, and biochemistry. It is the intent of the Editor and the Editorial Advisory Board that books selected for the series should be timely and fill a definite need in the general areas mentioned. We welcome suggestions for future monographs in the series.

Gary L. Grunewald

PREFACE

The tetracycline antibiotics began to appear in the late 1940's, having been discovered through highly organized, integrated research efforts carried out in industrial laboratories. Because of their wide antimicrobial and clinical spectrum, convenience of administration and relative lack of dangerous side effects, they immediately assumed a major rôle in chemotherapy and remain to this day among the most widely dispensed of all therapeutic entities.

The first decade of the tetracycline era was indisputably the era of the microbiologist, with those tetracyclines finding their way into clinical use being prepared by fermentation processes growing out of massive screening programs using soil organisms, or by the use of mutant cultures derived by random genetic manipulation of previously discovered strains. Because of the relative molecular complexity of the tetracyclines, their relative instability toward common reagents, the difficulty in separating reaction products, and the labor involved in structural analysis, the organic and medicinal chemistry of the tetracyclines was slower to develop. Soon, however, these problems were reduced to manageable proportions, and at this time several hundreds of derivatives have been reported in the literature and at least five semisynthetic analogs are in clinical use. All of the major fermentation-derived tetracyclines have now been prepared by total chemical synthesis, although not yet in economically viable yields, and new compounds which would not be accessible from fermentation sources are being prepared by chemical means.

The purpose of this volume is to bring together in one place a synopsis of the voluminous and scattered literature on the chemistry of these drugs in the hope that more chemists will be inspired to accept the challenge presented by these fascinating substances.

The magnitude of the job can be realized by considering that already by 1956 a monograph appeared on chlortetracycline which contained 4000 papers. The field has been anything but static since then. A subject so vast defies comprehensive review. I have chosen to concentrate particularly on the chemistry of the tetracyclines and apologize in advance for any errors of omission in the introductory chapters which may offend or amuse my clinical, microbiological and biochemical colleagues.

Certain aspects of the tetracycline story have resulted in various controversies such as the antitrust suits, the theft of cultures and processes, the Panalba® incident, and so on. This would provide a rich pageant for a more talented writer but has, reluctantly, been judged outside the scope of this work and is treated only briefly.

A number of my students and colleagues have read various portions of this book and their constructive comments have strengthened it considerably. The faults which remain are mine. I am most grateful to my secretary, Mrs. Carolyn Kelly, for her skill and patience in typing the various drafts and preparing the final camera-ready copy.

Lester A. Mitscher

CONTENTS

The Chemistry of the Tetracycline Antibiotics

CHAPTER 1

ORIENTING SURVEY

1.1---History and interrelationships between the clinically available members of the tetracycline family.

Chlortetracycline (CTC) was the first member of this antibiotic family to be discovered. The tetracycline saga was inaugurated by an announcement on 21 July, 1948 at a meeting of the New York Academy of Sciences.[1] CTC was uncovered through a soil screening program established at Lederle Laboratories by Benjamin J. Duggar, a retired professor of mycology from the University of Wisconsin. The producing culture was named *Streptomyces aureofaciens* and the antibiotic was characterized by a broad activity spectrum against pathogenic microorganisms, oral activity, and relative freedom from life threatening toxicity so it rapidly earned a major place in clinical medicine. Shortly thereafter, in 1949, Kane, Finlay and Sobin of the Pfizer Laboratories reported the discovery of another broad spectrum tetracycline antibiotic, oxytetracycline (OTC), in fermentation liquors of *Streptomyces rimosus*.[2]

During the course of experiments directed at elucidation of the structure of these two substances, it was discovered that hydrogenation of CTC resulted in halogenolysis and that the product, tetracycline (TC), retained the useful activity spectrum of the first two members of the family.[3] In addition, it was more stable than CTC and OTC. TC appears to represent the first clinically successful antibiotic produced by purely chemical manipulation of a preexisting antibiotic. Subsequent to these reports, TC was found to be present in fermentations of both _S. aureofaciens_ and _S. rimosus_, as well as strains named _S. viridofaciens_. TC has become the dominant member of the family in terms of utilization and, unfortunately for semantic clarity, the term "tetracycline" can mean either this specific chemical substance or the family as a whole. To avoid confusion as far as possible, the antibiotic will be referred to as "TC" in this work, and the family as "the tetracyclines".

In 1957, studies with mutant strains of _S. aureofaciens_ carried out at Lederle Laboratories in attempts to obtain higher potency, and to produce TC free from contamination with CTC, resulted in the formation of a new, highly active, antibiotic lacking the 6α-methyl group of CTC.[4] The new antibiotic 6-demethylchlortetracycline (DMCTC), was considerably more stable than its predecessors. Higher and more sustained blood levels obtained with this agent allowed the administration of smaller doses at less frequent intervals while the antimicrobial spectrum remained essentially intact. In addition to its clinical usefulness, this substance has been the raw material from which many new and interesting derivatives have been made.

In examining the chemistry of TC, it was found that the Mannich reaction with formaldehyde and a variety of secondary amines led to products of considerably enhanced water solubility.[5] These products revert rapidly to TC under physiological conditions so they serve as useful prodrugs for parenteral administration. In 1958, pyrrolidinomethyltetracycline (PMTC) was introduced, followed by lysinomethyltetracycline (LMTC). These substances were the first of the second generation tetracyclines--those not available by purely microbiological techniques--to find clinical use.

Two antibiotics were subsequently prepared by chemical transformation of OTC in the Pfizer Laboratories and introduced to the market place. In 1965, 6-methyleneoxytetracycline (MOTC), prepared by a process involving selective dehydration of a suitably protected analog of OTC, followed by removal of the protecting group, was commercialized.[6] Shortly thereafter, in 1967, one of its hydrogenation products, α6-deoxyoxytetracycline (DOOTC) was released.[7] Each of these products is more lipid soluble than OTC and the pharmacodynamic differences which result from this difference has led to a clinical vogue for these materials. DOOTC has the virtue of requiring lower doses on oral administration than its predecessors, and its slow excretion allows it, under some circumstances, to be the first "one-a-day" tetracycline.

The most recently introduced member of the tetracycline family (1972) is 7-dimethylamino-6-demethyl-6-deoxytetracycline

(DDDTC), a substance derived from the chemical transformation of DMCTC.[8] Although it is currently limited to use in treating gonorrhea, DDDTC is active in vitro against a number of strains resistant to the other tetracyclines and, thus, has the broadest spectrum of any tetracycline now in clinical use. Furthermore, against a wide variety of strains encountered in clinical practice, this antibiotic has good activity against organisms resistant to the other tetracyclines.

1.2---Nomenclature, absolute stereochemistry and numbering system.

The name tetracycline derives from the naphthacene nucleus that these antibiotics possess. Formula 1 is that of TC itself and is correct in an absolute stereochemical sense. The rings are lettered A through D from right to left and the numbers start at the bottom of ring A. TC is the parent substance of the series for nomenclatural purposes. Although several alternate canonical structures can be drawn for TC, the enolized form in formula 1 has been selected arbitrarily and is used almost exclusively in the literature.

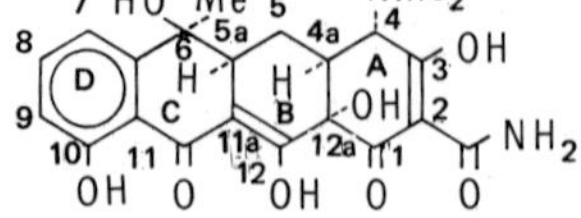

(1)

For convenience, trivial names are based on 1. For example, CTC can be unambiguously designated as 7-chlorotetracycline, OTC as 5α-oxytetracycline, and DOOTC, less clearly, as α6-deoxy-5α-oxytetracycline. The prefix "α" used in the case of DOOTC refers to one of the two isomers resulting from removal of the oxygen from C_6, for this carbon remains asymmetric on removal of the OH group and confusion could result if the prefix were not used, especially as both isomers exist.

The Chemical Abstracts formal indexing names for those antibiotics are considerably more complex and are rarely used in general writing.

CTC 2-naphthacenecarboxamide, 7-chloro-4-(dimethylamino) 1,4,4a,5,5a,6,11,12a-octahydro-3,6,10,12,12a-pentahydroxy-6-methyl-1,11-dioxo-[57-62-5] 4S-4α,4aα,6β, 12aα.

TC 2-naphthacenecarboxamide, 4-(dimethylamino)-1,4,4a, 5,5a,6,11,12a-octahydro-3,6,10,12,12a-pentahydroxy-6-methyl-1,11-dioxo-[60-54-8] 4S-4α,4aα,5aα,6β,12aα.

DMCTC 2-naphthacenecarboxamide, 7-chloro-4-(dimethylamino)-1,4,4a,5,5a,6,11,12a-octahydro-3,6,10,12,12a-pentahydroxy-1,11-dioxo-[127,33-3] 4S-4α,4aα,5aα,6β,12aα.

DDDTC 2-naphthacenecarboxamide, 4,7-bis(dimethylamino)-1, 4,4a,5,5a,6,11,12a-octahydro-3,10,12,12a-tetrahydroxy-1,11-dioxo-[10118-90-8] 4S-4α,4aα,5aα,12aα.

PMTC 2-naphthacenecarboxamide, 4-(dimethylamino)-1,4,4a, 5,5a,6,11,12a-octahydro-3,6,10,12,12a-pentahydroxy-6-

methyl-1,11-dioxo-*N*-(1-pyrrolidinylmethyl)-[751-97-3] 4*S*-4α,4aα,5aα,6β,12aα.

QTC 2-naphthacenecarboxamide, 4-(dimethylamino)-1,4,4a,5,5a,6,11,12a-octahydro-3,5,6,10,12,12a-hexahydroxy-6-methyl-1,11-dioxo-[79-57-2] 4*S*-4α,4aα,5α,5aα,6β,12aα.

MOTC 2-naphthacenecarboxamide, 4-(dimethylamino)-1,4,4a,5,5a,6,11,12a-octahydro-3,5,10,12,12a-pentahydroxy-6-methylene-1,11-dioxo-[914-00-1] 4*S*-4α,4aα,5α,5aα,12aα.

DOOTC 2-naphthacenecarboxamide, 4-(dimethylamino)-1,4,4a,5,5a,6,11,12a-octahydro-3,5,10,12,12a-pentahydroxy-1,11-dioxo-[564-25-0] 4*S*-4α,4aα,5α,5aα,6β,12aα.

1.3---Extent of utilization in medicine.

Americans are prolific consumers of drugs. In 1972, 10 billion doses of antibiotics, representing some 2,400,000 Kg of these substances, were certified for use in the United States alone by the Federal Food and Drug Administration. This is sufficient to provide 50 doses per year for every man, woman and child in the country. In 1971, 160 million prescriptions were written for antibiotics, an increase of 35% in four years.[9] Much of this usage represents tetracyclines. In a survey of 1.05 billion prescriptions carried out in 1967, antibiotics represented the single most prescribed category (12.3%). Of this, tetracyclines represented 30.5%. This was broken down as follows:[10]

TC	22%
DMCTC	5.4
MOTC	1.5
OTC	1.2
DOOTC	0.3
CTC	0.1

For purposes of comparison, the other antibiotic families ranked as follows:

Penicillins	24.6%
Aminocyclitols	10.9
Macrolides and Lincomycins	11.3
Peptides	13
Chloramphenicol	2.6
Polyenes and Griseofulvin	7
Miscellaneous	8.3

With the time that has passed since these figures were obtained, undoubtedly the relative utilization pattern has changed somewhat, but the proportions are probably not far off. Examination of Table 1-1 supports this conclusion. These data represent the relative occurrence of various antibiotics among the 200 most frequently prescribed drugs in the United States. Tetracycline is second only to ampicillin as the most frequently prescribed generic drug in the United States and has been in the top 50 since the listing began in 1966. There is, therefore, no doubt that the tetracyclines are widely used clinically and are big business for the companies that market them. It is interesting to consider that the use of TC alone exceeds that of some entire antibiotic families.

The relatively heavy utilization of TC itself reflects the current view of these substances held both by academic and practicing physicians. When it seems appropriate to prescribe a tetracycline, the prevailing opinion is that TC itself will usually accomplish the clinical result as well as

Table 1-1. Relative position of antibiotics in the top 200 drugs prescribed in The United States of America in 1975. This data emphasizes oral medication as it is taken from drug store records rather than hospital records. Data is from <u>Pharmacy Times</u>, April, 1977.

Antibiotic	Rank
Ampicillin - generic	3
TC•HCl - generic*	5
V-cillin K	9
Erythrocin	24
Keflex	28
Ilosone	29
EM - generic	35
Achromycin V*	40
Sumycin*	50
Penicillin V-K - generic	59
Gantrisin	69
Vibramycin*	74
Pen-Vee-K	76
Mycostatin	78
Neosporin	84
Macrodantin	86
Tofranil	91
Polycillin	97
Penicillin G-K - generic	98
Pentids	109
Omnipen	117
Principen	120
Amcill	125
Azo-Gantrisin	126
Mysteclin-F	135
Cleocin	137
E-Mycin	138
Pediamycin	154
Minocin*	160
Septra	168
Terramycin*	175
Pyridium	177
Garamycin	195

*Tetracycline class

will any other member of the family. When individual choice other than TC is made, it is usually made on the basis of pharmacodynamic rather than antimicrobial spectrum or potency grounds.

1.4---*In vitro* antimicrobial spectra.

It is common for antimicrobial agents which possess different ionized forms at different pH values to give different apparent potencies when the test media are buffered at a variety of pHs. The tetracyclines are generally more potent at pH about 6 than pH 7. The precise pH optimum differs slightly for each tetracycline, but the fundamental pattern holds.[3,11]

A variety of additional factors affect the apparent *in vitro* potency of tetracyclines, particularly divalent metals. It is difficult to compare potency values obtained in one laboratory with those from another, so precise comparative values obtained from different papers are subject to a degree of reservation. The most complete set of data obtained in a single laboratory is that of Blackwood and English.[11] In Table 1-2, TC has been assigned an arbitrary relative potency value of 1.0. On this basis, CTC is the most potent of the tetracyclines and OTC or TC is the least. The overall variation is not large, however.

Table 1-3 contains *in vitro* mic values for the clinically important tetracyclines against a variety of microorganisms.[12] The two *Staph. aureus* columns demonstrate that there is extensive, though not complete, cross resistance between the members of the tetracycline family. This observation appears to hold both for naturally resistant as well as for laboratory induced resistant strains. The figures for the normally sensitive organisms do not vary more than a factor of about 4. Compared to S. aureus 5, all were significantly less potent against the TC resistant strain of S. aureus. Even DDDTC shows an 8-fold resistance increment. This increment should represent a clinically achievable dose. DOOTC might also be active against this strain *in vivo*.

The tetracyclines are bacteriostatic rather than bacteriocidal unless large doses are used. This accounts for persistence of bacteria in some clinical situations, although other factors also play important roles.

Table 1-2. *In vitro* potency of the major tetracyclines compared to TC.[11]

Tetracycline	*Kl. pneumoniae*	*S. aureus* 209P
TC	1.0	1.0
CTC	2.5	3.5
OTC	1.0	0.8
DMCTC	-	3.0
DOOTC	1.4	-
MOTC	2.3	-
MMMTC	-	1.0+

Table 1-3. *In vitro* antimicrobial spectrum of the major tetracyclines.[12]

Drug	*Ps. aeruginosa*	*A. aerogenes*	*Shigella sonnei*	*S. typhosa*	*Vibrio comma*	*Kl. pneumoniae*
CTC	-	1.56	5	1.56	-	0.39
OTC	6	2.91	5	3.12	0.55	2.5
TC	10	1.66	2.5	1.56	0.58	1.56
DMCTC	3	0.15	1.4	0.55	0.17	0.55
MOTC	6.3	0.94	1.6	1.40	0.29	1.56
DOOTC	2.3	2.54	2.2	1.56	0.31	1.87
DDDTC	-	3.00	-	3.00	-	1.50

Drug	*S. aureus* 5	*S. aureus* TC resist.	*Ps. vulgaris*	*S. pyogenes*	*Ps. Morganii*	*E. coli*
CTC	0.19	100+	-	0.04	-	1.56
OTC	0.55	100+	100+	0.06	2	1.09
TC	0.21	60	100+	0.06	2	0.73
DMCTC	0.11	35	90	0.04	0.78	0.33
MOTC	0.13	50	100+	0.03	2.2	0.43
DOOTC	0.19	8.8	100+	0.04	4.4	1.74
DDDTC	0.10	0.8	-	0.02	-	3.00

1.5---*In vivo* comparison of tetracyclines in infected mice.

The data in Table 1-4 show that the efficacy of the tetracyclines given by the oral route to infected mice does not parallel closely the *in vitro* findings. The usual explanation for this discrepancy is that biopharmaceutical factors play an important role.

Generally speaking, subcutaneous ED_{50} data for the various tetracyclines given to infected mice correspond better with the *in vitro* data than the oral data of Table 1-4 do. This contrast, evident from the comparative data in Table 1-5, suggests that variable absorption from the GI tract might be the most important biopharmaceutical factor determining the variance within the group when tested by these different methods. Consistent, reliable absorption uncomplicated by chelating ions, such as Ca(II), Mg(II), or Al(III), would represent a significant improvement over most existing tetracyclines. Another area where improvement is desirable, is finding agents which lack cross resistance in the clinic with the current tetracyclines. The properties of minocycline suggest that this is quite possible.

1.6---Safety.

The tetracyclines have a safety margin which is quite satisfactory under most circumstances. The mouse acute toxicity data in Table 1-6 for TC is representative of the group.[13]

Table 1-4. *In vivo* activity of several clinical tetracyclines given orally to infected mice.[11]

Drug	Oral ED_{50} in mice (mg/kg)		
	S. pyogenes	*S. aureus* 5	*P. multocida*
CTC	8.5	7.6	19.6
OTC	8.2	7.2	18.2
TC	6.25	5.8	22.0
DMCTC	6.7	6.0	9.8
MOTC	3.9	4.5	13.0
DOOTC	1.6	2.6	6.6
DDDTC	-	3.5	-

Table 1-5. *In vivo* activity of several clinically useful tetracyclines given subcutaneously to infected mice.[11]

Tetracycline	Subcutaneous ED_{50} in mice (mg/kg)		
	S. pyogenes	*S. aureus* 5	*P. multocida*
CTC	2.1	3.0	4.5
OTC	2.3	2.6	4.1
TC	1.89	1.2	3.6
DMCTC	1.3	1.6	3.0
MOTC	0.7	1.2	2.6
DOOTC	1.0	1.0	3.9
DDDTC	-	-	-

Table 1-6. Acute toxicity of TC in mice when administered by various routes.[13]

Route of Administration	Acute Toxicity LD_{50} (mg/kg)
Oral	6300
IV	170
IP	280

For the most part the side-effects commonly encountered in clinical practice with the tetracyclines are annoying or uncomfortable rather than life-threatening.[14,15] Anorexia, nausea, vomiting, heartburn, flatulence and diarrhea apparently occur in about 10% of patients receiving 2g or more of TC daily.[14] This seems to be due to an irritation of the mucosa although bacterial flora disturbances contribute. Hemotoxic symptoms are rare. Enterocolitis, stomatitis, glossitis, pharyngitis, dysphagia and hoarseness have been reported.[15] Candidal infections with inflammation and pruritis can involve the vulva, vagina and perianal region due to suppression of the normal flora followed by suprainfection by these TC insensitive commensals. This phenomenon is usually attributed to the effect on the bowel of unabsorbed tetracyclines and these effects are less often encountered when the drugs are given parenterally. Combinations of tetracyclines and a polyene antifungal agent are given prophylactically to avoid this, even though many authorities are opposed in principle to the administration of fixed dose combinations of antimicrobial agents, preferring to give the agents singly. It is further argued that the polyene antifungal macrolides should be reserved for use in that smaller number of cases where symptoms of superinfection are actually appearing. There is, futhermore, evidence that the prophylactic use of the combination is not particularly effective in preventing G. I. symptoms in the clinic.[16]

An antibiotic-induced suprainfection resulting in staphylococcal enterocolitis with an extremely severe diarrhea, dehydration, and circulatory collapse is known. In this condition, the intestinal mucosa is necrotic and the feces contain large numbers of TC-resistant staphylococci and death may result. This, because of the enterohepatic route of excretion followed by these drugs, may even be observed on parenteral administration.[15,17]

Phototoxicity (an exaggerated response to sunlight) leading to erythema, sunburn, etc., can be encountered and DMCTC is the tetracycline most commonly implicated in this phenomenon.[18] Severe hypersensitivity and allergic reactions are uncommon and no fatalities have been reported from this cause.[19] The tetracyclines delay blood coagulation and may potentiate the effect of dicumarol. Vitamin K synthesis, especially in the elderly with marginal liver function, can contribute to prolonged clotting times.[20] High IV doses seem to be required. Tetracyclines inhibit mammalian protein biosynthesis to some extent, although, fortunately, not so strongly as microbial protein biosynthesis. This antianabolic effect can result in elevated blood levels of nonprotein nitrogen and increased urinary nitrogen excretion. If a patient has significantly impaired kidney function, excretion of TC is impaired and azotemia, hyperphosphatemia, hyperkalemia and acidosis can be experienced. Excretion of these products puts an added burden on the kidneys.[21] The level of BUN (blood urea nitrogen) will be less accurate in reflecting renal function than the serum creatinine level in these cases. It is reported that tetracyclines can cause direct kidney damage in healthy patients. DMCTC is reported to be prone to this. The phenomenon regresses when the drug is stopped.[21] Hepatotoxicity can result in death when prolonged use of high doses is prescribed for patients with impaired renal function. IV administration of more than 1g per day or coadministration of other potentially hepatotoxic drugs is a particularly poor practice. Hepatotoxicity is especially likely to occur in pregnant women in the last trimester or in post-partum patients with kidney infections.[22] Some deaths have been attributed to this.

The tetracyclines form highly insoluble complexes with Ca(II), Mg(II), Fe(II) and Al(III) ions, especially at neutral pHs in the presence of amino acids. This not only diminishes their apparent potency _in vitro_, but impedes their absorption from the GI tract on oral administration. Thus, coadministration of antacids containing the above ions in order to reduce an accompanying gastric upset, as used to be recommended, results in diminished blood levels of the antibiotic.[23] This technique should be avoided. Hematinics will also decrease absorption of tetracyclines because of their iron content.[24] In addition, the insolubility of the complexes predisposes to deposition of significant concentrations of tetracyclines in teeth and bones.[25] The tetracyclines pass the placental barrier and appear in mother's milk, so that moderate doses lead to a definite yellowing and a reversible slowing of bone growth in fetuses, infants, and young children, where the teeth and bones are undergoing rapid development. The deposition is essentially permanent and is dose related. Excessive doses of these antibiotics can lead to weakness in bone structure and teeth although it ordinarily is only a cosmetic problem when normal doses are used. Clinicians now prefer not to administer tetracyclines to children before about the age of 8.[25] A dietary incompatibility should also be mentioned. Ion-rich foods, such as milk, depress the blood levels of tetracyclines, so the drug is usually given between meals. DOOTC is said not to be subject to as much diminution in blood level as some of the earlier tetracyclines when it is given with ion-rich foods. These are generalizations and good medical practice involves attention to the effects of ions on blood levels, but it should be pointed out that many physicians feel that stomach contents protect the patient from some of the gastric upset encountered with the tetracyclines and, in mild infections some physicians prefer to obtain these lower, but usually adequate, blood levels in order to avoid patient discomfort. It is, however, important to avoid milk and antacids in any case.

As will be seen in Chapter 5, some tetracyclines can degrade to 4-epianhydrotetracyclines. Overaged TC preparations degrading to 4-epianhydroTC show a definite toxicity.[26] This acute Fanconi-like syndrome results from damage to renal tubular function and is characterized by nausea, vomiting, albuminuria, glycosuria, aminoaciduria, hypophosphatemia, hypokalemia and acidosis. Fatal reactions have been reported, although withdrawal of the drug usually causes a slow reversal of the damage. Expiration dates should, then, be respected and tetracyclines should not be stored under conditions of excess heat and humidity. In some countries, notably the British Commonwealth, the amount of 4-epianhydroTC is carefully controlled by standards published in the official compendia. Some chemicals, notably citric acid, apparently accelerate decomposition to this unwanted product and these are no longer included in formulations.

This long recitation of potential side effects is consonant with our times. The package insert of the typical medication now contains much longer lists of possible adverse effects than indications. The lay public faced with this might gain the impression that people are dropping in the streets in great numbers from the horrible side-effects of tetracyclines. While no one wishes to make light of the very real distress susceptible individuals experience, in all fairness, a balanced account requires that it be pointed out that these drugs have been doing and continue to do much more good than harm. It seems hardly probable that the enormous utilization of these substances pointed out in section 1-3 could take place despite generalized distress among patients. When used with due regard for the possible emergence of these occasional problems, these antibiotics are among the safest drugs. Nevertheless, a new tetracycline will always be welcome which lacks quantitatively or qualitatively in these potential side-effects. In particular, an agent which did not localize in bones and teeth and which gave regular, dose related, blood levels when administered orally, even in the presence of ion rich foods and other drugs containing chelating ions, would be especially useful. The tetracyclines are also quite irritating on injection, so a painless form would also find a significant place in therapy.

1.7---Mechanism of action, and bacterial resistance.

The tetracyclines are actively transported into the cells of susceptible bacteria and exert a bacteriostatic effect by inhibiting protein biosynthesis after binding to the 30S ribosomal subparticle.[27] The binding apparently results in an inhibition of translocation of amino acid-laden transfer RNA (comprising the growing peptide chain) from the donor to the acceptor site. Cessation of protein biosynthesis results and the cells stop multiplying and will eventually die. The 80S ribosomes of eukaryotes, including yeasts and man, are much less sensitive to the effect of tetracyclines. This accounts for the useful selective toxicity of these drugs.[28] The tetracyclines exert a number of other biological effects in intact cells and in subcellular fragments, but the ribosomal reactions are currently considered to be decisive. Bacteria encountered in a clinical setting develop resistance to the tetracyclines discouragingly readily. The resistant strains are found not to accumulate the antibiotic inside their cells and are therefore immune to its action since the drug cannot reach its biochemical target area.[29] This seems associated with the membrane lipid or protein composition. It is interesting to note that cell-free ribosome preparations from TC-resistant bacteria are sensitive to the antibiotic.[28] Ability to transmit resistance of this type rapidly from one bacterium to another, even to bacteria belonging to a different genus, is very troublesome in the clinic. All the more so in that this kind of resistance is often multivalent, leading to simultaneous resistance to antibiotics of unrelated structural types to which the bacterium may not have been exposed previously. In Gram-positive bacteria, notably Staphylococci, transduction of episomal elements is involved, while in Gram-negative bacteria conjugation is involved.[29] In contrast to most other antibiotic families, R-factor mediated resistance to the tetracyclines does not appear to involve attack on the drugs themselves but involves the permiability barrier mentioned above. Cross resistance within the tetracycline family is nearly complete. Still, the bioactivity of DDDTC <u>in vivo</u> against resistant Staphylococci is encouraging in that it suggests that new agents can be found which will retain their effectiveness when the other tetracyclines have lost their value against a given bacterial strain.[30] Whether the activity of DDDTC against such strains will hold up in the clinic remains to be established.

All of the current theories of the molecular mode of action of the tetracyclines are erected on a foundation of circumstantial evidence and are wholly speculative. In the absence of any truly compelling evidence, one may serve as well as the next. Smythies et al.[31] have published a theory which proposes that the tetracyclines act on a molecular level by fitting precisely into a segment of ribosomal RNA composed of GC:GC or GC:AU and that this interaction stops the transfer of AA-laden t-RNA to its normal binding site. This clever idea, however, suffers from the requirement that this base sequence be rare and occur only in ribosomal RNA and also by needing seven or more contact binding points and several other close approach points of the Van der Waal's type. This seems to be asking rather much of a drug. It may account for the activity of TC, but it fails to provide a role for chelation, does not explain why isomerization of C_4 (only 1 of Smythies 7 points of contact) should be of overriding importance, and why isotetracycline is inactive when it appears to fit his model. Further, it seems intuitively more likely that the great specificity of interaction could be explained more readily on the basis of binding to the more species specific proteins in the ribosomes.

A less sophisticated idea can be advanced for discussion which incorporates our knowledge of the solution conformation of the tetracyclines and the known structure-activity relationships to be described in later chapters. In this case, the tetracyclines are viewed as being bound to a receptor surface requiring as contact points the chelating properties of the ring BCD β-dicarbonyl function, the acid character of the C_3-OH group (pK approximately 3 because of the resonance possibilities inherent in the β-tricarbonyl system of ring A), and the basic character of the dimethylamino function at C_4. The areas to the back and the left side in formula 2a are not in contact with the bioreceptor so relatively extensive molecular modification can be performed from C_5 to C_9 without substantial interference with binding and resulting loss of activity. It is interesting to note that L-α-aminoacids would also fit this surface and glutamate would do so particularly well. The C_3 and C_{12} carbonyl groups, whose acidities are enhanced by enolization, are carboxyl surrogates in this model. It is possible that tetracyclines are false substrates in some essential biochemical process in that a primary amino group is lacking and so the compounds cannot take part in reactions requiring covalent bond formation. Reduced activity when primary amino groups are present at C_4 would be understandable and the reduced activity accompanying the substitution of the N-Me groups by larger alkyl functions would also be understandable. Epimerization would result in a complete lack of fit at the receptor. While this idea is amusing to contemplate and correlates satisfactorily a majority of the facts regarding the bioactivity of TC and its analogs, it is highly empirical and is badly deficient in leaving the molecular nature of the receptor so vague.

A working predictive model upon which to mount a rational structure modification program would certainly be welcome.

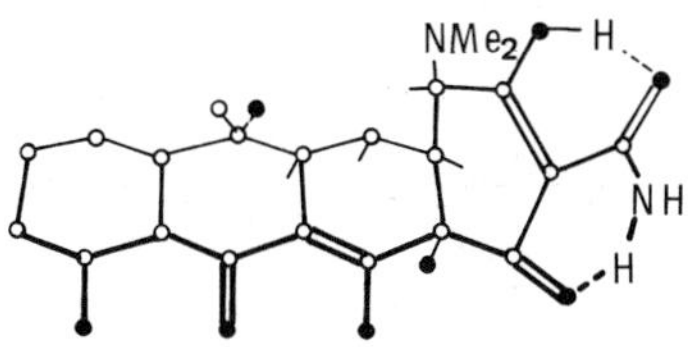

(2a)

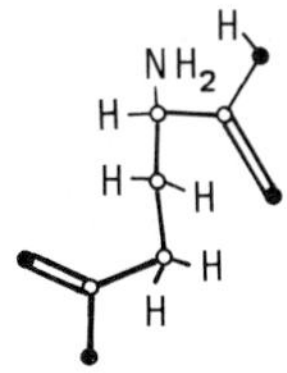

(2b)

1.8---Clinical spectrum.

Tetracyclines are frequently used for respiratory tract infections such as bacillary pneumonia, bronchitis and influenza, pertussis, mycoplasmal pneumonia, brucellosis, non-serious Staphylococcal infections, wounds and postoperative sepsis, bile infections, urinary tract infections, especially those due to sensitive strains of E. coli, cholera, various Rickettsial infections, Q-fever, relapsing fever, tularemia, bubonic plague, psittacosis, lymphogranuloma verum, trachoma, some conjunctivitis problems, actinomycosis, gas gangrene, anthrax, leptospirosis, meningitis due to H. influenzae, Meningococcal carriers, gonorrhea, non-specific urethritis, syphilis, melioidosis, acne, amoebic dysentery, malaria and sprue.

Conspicuously absent are Pseudomonas, Proteus and Salmonella infections, tuberculosis, protozoal, fungal and yeast infections.

Table 1-7 lists those conditions for which the tetracyclines are considered to be the drug of first choice.[16] This list is not extensive and the conditions listed are not common in the United States. On the other hand, the conditions are severe for the victims and the availability of reasonable and relatively safe treatment for these patients is satisfying. It is clear, however, that these indications are insufficient to account for the massive use of the tetracyclines documented in Table 1-1.

The answer lies in part in Table 1-8. This is a list of those conditions for which the tetracyclines are not the drug of first choice but are rather one of a group of drugs of second choice. These are prescribed when the drug of first choice is inappropriate by virtue of resistance, side-effects, or inconvenience, etc.[16] This list is not only long, but contains a number of relatively common ailments which are encountered in a community as well as hospital setting. Their relative cheapness, convenience of administration, breadth of spectrum and non-life-threatening side-effects conspire to make the tetracyclines used on a far larger scale than academic medicine would approve.

In all of these cases rational medicine requires the performance of the appropriate sensitivity testing.

In addition to these uses, tetracyclines are extensively utilized by dermatologists in the treatment of severe acne.[32] The mechanism of action here remains uncertain.

Table 1-7. Conditions for which tetracyclines are the drug of first choice.

Classification of the Causative Organism	Disease	Causative Organism
Gram negative Bacilli		*Bacteroides*, intestinal strains*
	Glanders	*Pseudomonas mallei***
	Melioidosis	*Pseudomonas pseudomallei****
	Brucellosis	*Brucella***
	Chancroid	*Hemophilus ducreyi*
	Granuloma Inguinale	*Calymmatobacterium granulomatis*
	Cholera	*Vibrio cholerae*
Spirochetes	Relapsing Fever	*Borrelia recurrentis*
Rickettsia	Rocky Mountain Spotted Fever; Q Fever; Endemic Typhus; Tick Bite Fever; Scrub Typhus	*Rickettsia*
Miscellaneous	Atypical Pneumonia	*Mycoplasma pneumoniae*
	Psittacosis	*Chlamydia psittaci*
	Lymphogranuloma Venereum	*Chlamydia*
	Trachoma	*Chlamydia trachomatis*
	Inclusion Conjunctivitis	*Chlamydia*

*or chloramphenicol. **with streptomycin. ***with or without a sulfonamide.

Table 1-8. Conditions for which tetracyclines are one of the drugs of second choice.

Classification of the Causative Organism	Disease	Causative Organism
Gram positive Cocci	Uncomplicated Urinary Tract Infection	Enterococcus gp. Streptococcus Anaerobic Streptococcus
Gram negative Cocci	Meningitis	Neisseria meningitidis
	Gonorrhoea	Neisseria gonorrhoeae
Gram positive Bacilli	Anthrax	Bacillus anthracis Listeria monocytogenes
	Gas Gangrene	Clostridium perfringens
	Lock Jaw	Clostridium tetani
Gram negative Bacilli		Escherichia coli Klebsiella pneumoniae Enterobacter (Aerobacter) Proteus (not mirabilis) Bacteroides
	Tularemia	Francisella tularensis
	Bubonic Plague	Yersinia pestis Pasteurella multocida
	Respiratory Infection	Haemophillis influenzae
	Meningitis	Haemophillis influenzae
	Chancroid	Haemophillis ducreyi
	Whooping Cough	Bordetella pertussis
	Vincent's Infection	Leptotrichia buccalis
	Rat Bite Fever	Spirillum minor Streptobacillus moniliformis
Spirochetes	Syphilis	Treponema pallidum
	Yaws	Treponema pertenue
	Leptospirosis	Leptospira
Actinomycetes	Actinomycoses	Actinomyces israelii
	Nocardiosis	Nocardia*
Acid Fast Bacilli		Mycobacterium marinum**

*Minocycline with a sulfonamide. **Minocycline.

1.9---Interference with the host's natural defenses.

The ideal antibiotic will not impair the host's natural defenses against microbial invasion. This is an especially important feature for an antibiotic acting by a bacteriostatic mechanism. Such antibiotics stop the fulminating phase of infection and require the normal mechanisms of the body to eradicate the remaining organisms so that normal health is restored. There is no convincing evidence that the tetracyclines are significantly immunosuppressive or suppress the other portions and components of the host's natural defense to microbial invasion.

1.10--Routes of administration, biopharmaceutical parameters and routes of excretion.

Figure 1 summarizes the absorption, distribution and excretion of TC. The tetracyclines give blood levels adequate for successful therapy on oral, intramuscular and intervenous administration. Rectal absorption from suppositories is unsatisfactory. Absorption from the stomach is minimal. Absorption from the intestines is incomplete and subject to considerable variation between individuals and is affected substantially by the contents of the GI tract. The presence of ion rich foods or medications containing Mg(II), Ca(II), Fe(II) and Al(III) depress the amount of tetracyclines which reach the blood so that relatively significant amounts of bioactive tetracyclines can be recovered from the stool. Formulations including citric acid, sodium hexametaphosphate, glucosamine and phosphate were introduced into clinical use

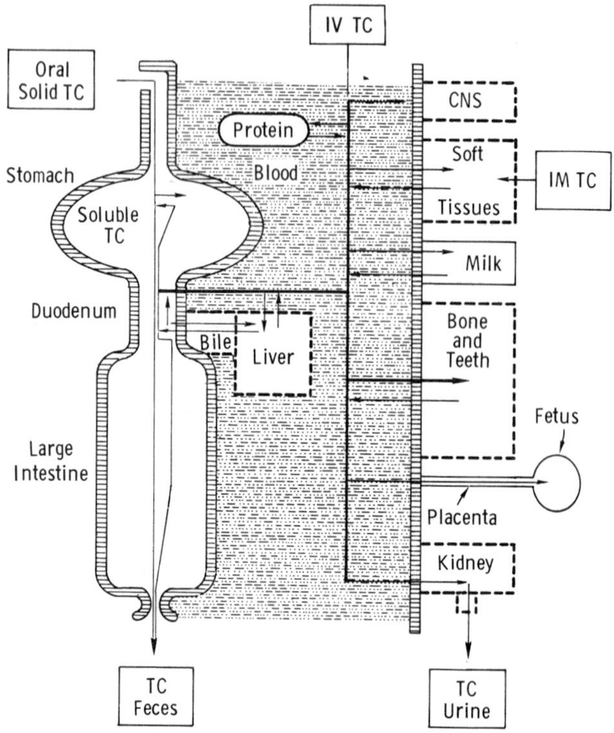

Figure 1. Schematic representation of absorption, distribution and excretion of tetracyclines.

in order to improve absorption in the presence of chelating ions, but after considerable controversy and study, it is now believed that these methods offer no significant advantage in clinical use. Some practical improvement in absorption appears, in fact, to have resulted from the exclusion of "inert" magnesium stearate or calcium carbonate from TC capsules.[33] These bioavailability considerations have recently been reviewed.[34] Dissolution of the solid drug in formulations in the stomach is necessary for adequate absorption in the duodenum and some formulations have been reported to give poor blood levels due to inappropriate particle size and dissolution rates.[34] With TC given 0.25g every 6 hours, the serum level stablizes at about 2.5mcg/ml in 24 hours. Doubling the dose leads to a peak of about 5mcg/ml and further dose increases fail to give any higher blood levels. DMCTC, DDDTC and DOOTC are better absorbed from the GI tract and this is less affected by stomach contents.

Once in the blood stream, the tetracyclines enter into the enterohepatic circulation and undergo excretion and reabsorption in the small intestine.[14,15] The tetracyclines penetrate readily, although unevenly, into most organs of the body, with particular concentrations being achieved in liver, spleen, kidney and lung. The tetracyclines form insoluble Ca(II) chelates in bone and drug taken up in this slowly metabolizing tissue remains for extended periods of time resulting in some cases in darkening (yellowing to browning) of the enamel, and in excessive doses given to quite young children, can lead to actual imperfections in the bony matrix. Tetracyclines do penetrate into the central nervous system (across the blood-brain barrier) in useful concentrations but chloramphenicol is more efficient. They do pass the placental barrier into a developing fetus and bone and tooth staining and/or imperfections can thereby occur <u>in utero</u>. Tetracyclines are also present in the milk of nursing mothers. Tetracyclines are bound reversibly to serum proteins. The extent of binding varies considerably among the tetracyclines (Table 1-9)[35,36] and the figures cited by various authorities also vary. Most authorities believe that bound drug, in

Table 1-9. Serum protein binding of the major tetracyclines.

Tetracycline	Serum Protein Binding	
TC	24%[35]	55-64%[36]
CTC	47	55
OTC	20	27-35
DMCTC	41	75-91
MOTC	79	78
DOOTC	-	82-93

general, is biologically inactive. If, as is the case with the tetracyclines, the binding is freely reversible, this binding becomes not a source of loss but rather a reservoir of the drug. The clinical meaning of such data is not clear at the moment. It seems reasonable, though, that the biological half-lives of the various tetracyclines (Table 1-10)[37] are strongly influenced by protein binding as is their tissue penetration. Table 1-11 shows what happens to the biological half-life of the tetracyclines when a repeated dosage schedule is substituted for the single dose used in assembling the data in Table 1-10.[37] The differences, which are considerable in Table 1-10, become relatively less significant when multiple dosing is used. The data in Table 1-11 are more likely to be relevant to the clinical situation where multiple dosing of patients is the standard practice. Note that the overall variation within the group, when a steady state level is present in the serum, is only 14 ± 3 Hr. This does not seem particularly significant. One infers from this data that drugs like TC which have significant tissue storage, significant protein binding, and, thus, a tendency to accumulate will give misleading results when the half-life is calculated on the basis of a single dose. The apparent persistence of DOOTC suggested by the data in Table 1-10 is rendered apparently less significant by the data in Table 1-11. What is not questionable is that less DOOTC needs be given to achieve a comparable blood level to the earlier tetracyclines. One watches the unfolding of this story with considerable interest because the clinical choice between tetracyclines is made on such biopharmaceutical factors and these kinds of data play a very significant role in drug design in structure modification programs.

The irregular absorption of the tetracyclines can be overcome by injection and this is frequently done in cases of severe infection or when the patient is unable to take medication orally. This device also results in considerable lessening of the incidence of GI upset and superinfection with its accompanying collection of side-effects. Parenteral use is,

Table 1-10. Apparent mean serum half-life in hours of various tetracyclines when given in a single oral dose.

Tetracycline	Apparent Mean Serum Half-Life (Hours)
CTC	5.5
TC	8.5
OTC	9.5
MOTC	15
DMCTC	17
DOOTC	19.5
DDDTC	17.5

Table 1-11. Apparent mean serum half-life in hours of various tetracyclines when given orally in divided doses.

Tetracycline	Apparent Mean Serum Half-Life (Hours)
TC	10.8
DMCTC	13.6
MOTC	14.3
DOOTC	16.6

however, inconvenient and usually painful. PMTC and LMTC are much more water soluble than their parent drug, TC, and are useful prodrugs for parenteral use. Of the remaining tetracyclines, OTC is considered to be the least painful on injection. For stability and solubility reasons, tetracyclines for injection are prepared in acidic (about pH 5) solution which accounts for some of the irritation. Magnesium ion is also commonly included to counteract in part the sequestration of Ca(II) which would otherwise occur adjacent to the site of injection.

The tetracyclines are excreted in therapeutically useful concentrations in the urine following oral administration and can be used for urinary tract infections.[38] Because of their lipid solubility at neutral pHs and the operation of an enterohepatic circulation, the concentration in bile may reach 10 to 20 times that of blood.[39] In cases of pyelonephritis and kidney shutdown, the incidence of liver toxicity increases due to the increased load on biliary excretion. In these conditions tetracyclines, except for CTC and DOOTC, accumulate.

It has been shown that those drugs primarily secreted by tubular secretion, such as the penicillins, have biological half-times which are remarkably insensitive to the extent of protein binding. Conversely, the tetracyclines appear to be secreted in the urine by glomerular filtration, for their half-values are strongly dependent upon the extent of protein binding. OTC, which is bound only to about 22%, is foremost, and DOOTC, which is protein bound to about 82%, is least.[37] The latter finding indicates that DOOTC may be the tetracycline of choice for treating infections when the urinary tract is not functioning properly.

Finally, Figure 2 compares the time course of the blood levels of TC and DOOTC after a single oral dose.

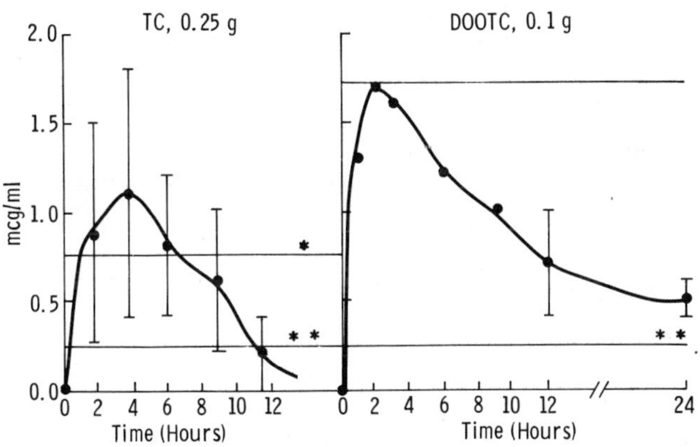

Figure 2. Blood levels as a function of time following a single oral dose of 250 mg TC or 100 mg DOOTC.

* *In vitro* mic value against *E. coli*.[12]

** *In vitro* mic value against *S. aureus 5*.[12]

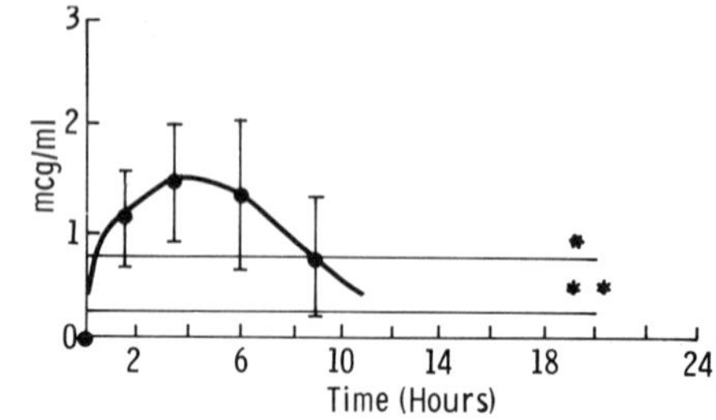

Figure 3. Blood levels as a function of time following a single IM dose of 100 mg TC.

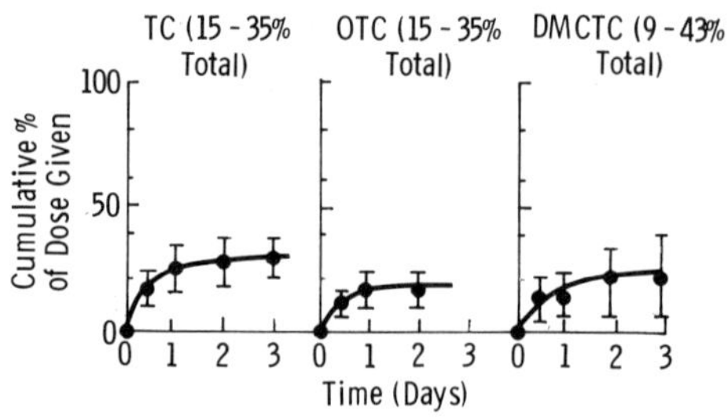

Figure 4. Urinary excretion of TC, OTC and DMCTC as a function of time following a single oral dose.

Figure 3 shows the time course of the blood levels of TC after a single IM injection. Figure 4 shows the time course of urinary excretion of TC, OTC and DMCTC after a single oral dose.

1.11--Agricultural and non-clinical uses of tetracyclines.

It has been estimated that as much as 50% of field crops spoil before they reach the table. Much of this is due to bacterial action and antibiotics are effective in treating those conditions. Tetracyclines have, for example, been reported to be active against a number of such conditions.[40]

Some quite recent reports on this subject include the control of legume little leaf disease,[41] citrus greening pathogen,[42] lethal yellowing of coconut palm,[43] pear decline,[44] elm phloem necrosis,[45] and the like. Some activity against insect pests has also been reported.[46] The presence of perceptible amounts of antibiotic residue in consumable products is, however, felt to be deleterious to health and this practice has been discontinued in the United States.

A far more substantial use is that of a feed supplement in animal husbandry. In 1969 alone, 11,000 tons of antibiotics ($90,600,000) were added to animal feed and a considerable proportion of this was CTC and OTC.[40,47] The antibiotic supplementation at subtherapeutic levels results in a demonstrable increase in weight gain over controls thus allowing animals to reach marketable weight in shorter time and with less feed. The mechanism by which this takes place is not entirely certain, but it is often considered to result from the suppression of intestinal bacteria which might divert part of the animal's energy from growth to the combat of infection and its by-products even when overt symptoms of infection may not be observable. This wholly desirable aim has resulted in the enormous utilization cited. There exists, on the other hand, a finite possibility of residues in the meat leading to human toxification and hypersensitivity and, recently, much attention has been paid to the possibility that these animals might become reservoirs of multiply antibiotic resistant organisms which could subsequently infect man. Warnings regarding R-factor carrying bacteria were published in the Swan report,[48] and subsequently led to a banning in England of feed supplementation with antibiotics either used or cross-resistant with those currently used in human therapy. Similar proposals in the United States[49] have yet to be acted on and a vigorous counter campaign is underway.[50] The last word in this controversy remains to be said. The evidence, however, supports the existence of an increased insensitivity to tetracyclines in the GI flora of animals so fed.[51]

On the other hand, antibiotics in general and tetracyclines in particular are effective remedies for many clinical infections in animals and are widely used for this purpose. Such use is not under attack in the R-factor controversy and will doubtless continue to provide a useful economic return to the farmer, the consumer and the tetracycline manufacturers.

REFERENCES

1. R. W. Broschard, A. C. Dornbush, S. Gordon, B. L. Hutchings A. R. Kohler, G. Krupka, S. Kushner, D. V. Lefemine and C. Pidacks, Science, 109, 199(1949); B. M. Duggar, Ann. N. Y. Acad. Sci., 51, 177(1948).
2. A. C. Finlay, G. L. Hobby, S. Y. P'an, P. P. Regna, J. B. Routien, D. B. Seeley, G. M. Shull, B. A. Sobin, I. A. Solomons, J. W. Vinson and J. H. Kane, Science, 111, 85(1950); P. P. Regna, I. A. Solomons, K. Murai, A. E.

Timreck, K. J. Brunings and W. A. Lazier, J. Am. Chem. Soc., 73, 4211(1951).

3. J. H. Boothe, J. Morton, J. P. Petisi, G. R. Wilkinson and J. H. Williams, J. Am. Chem. Soc., 75, 4621(1953); L. H. Conover, W. T. Moreland, A. R. English, C. R. Stephens and F. J. Pilgrim, J. Am. Chem. Soc., 75, 4622(1953); P. P. Minieri, M. C. Firman, A. G. Mistretta, A. Abbey, C. E. Bricker, N. E. Rigler and H. Sokol, Antibiotics Ann., 81(1953-54).
4. J. R. D. McCormick, N. O. Sjolander, U. Hirsch, E. R. Jensen and A. P. Doerschuk, J. Am. Chem. Soc., 79, 4561(1957).
5. W. Seidel, A. Soder and F. Linder, Munchen Med. Wochenschrift, 17, 661(1958).
6. R. K. Blackwood, J. J. Beereboom, H. H. Rennhard, M. Schach von Wittenau and C. R. Stephens, J. Am. Chem. Soc., 85, 3943(1963).
7. C. R. Stephens, J. J. Beereboom, H. H. Rennhard, P. N. Gordon, K. Murai, R. K. Blackwood and M. Schach von Wittenau, J. Am. Chem. Soc., 85, 2643(1963).
8. M. J. Martel, Jr. and J. H. Boothe, J. Med. Chem., 10, 44(1967).
9. Charles C. Edwards, M. D., Commissioner of Food and Drugs, letter to William Roemer, Secretary, American Pharmaceutical Association, dated 5 Dec., 1972.
10. N. Farnsworth in Phytochemistry, Vol. 3, L. P. Miller, Ed., Van Nostrand, New York (1973).

11. R. K. Blackwood and A. R. English, Advances in Applied Microbiology, 13, 237(1970).

12. A. R. English, Proc. Soc. Exptl. Biol. Med., 122, 1107 (1966).

13. G. S. Redin, Antimicrobial Agts. Chemother., 371(1966).

14. A. M. A. Drug Evaluations, 2nd. Ed., Publishing Sciences Group, Inc., Acton, Mass. (1973).

15. A. M. Walter, L. Heilmeyer, H. Otten and M. Plimpel, Antibiotika-Fibel, 3rd Ed., G. Thieme, Stuttgart (1969); L. E. Schindel, Antibiotica et Chemother., 13, 300(1965); S. L. Gorbach and J. G. Bartlett, New Engl. J. Med., 290, 1289(1974).

16. Anon., Brit. Med. J., 4, 402(1968); The Medical Letter, Handbook of Antimicrobial Therapy, (1976); J. Moeller and C. Kaya, Med. Klin., 62, 686(1967); R. S. W. Middleton, Brit. J. Clin. Pract., 21, 179(1967); J. Malecki, Rev. Laryng. (Bordeaux), 89, 289(1968).

17. E. H. Thaysen and K. R. Eriksen, Antibiot. Ann, 867(1956); P. Lundsgaard-Hansen, A. Senn, B. Roos and U. Waller, J. A. M. A., 173, 1008(1960); F. R. Fekety, J. A. M. A., 203, 144(1968).

18. E. M. Ory, Med. Clin. North America, 54, 1173(1970); H. Blank, S. I. Cullen and P. M. Catalano, Arch. Derm, 97, 1(1968); J. Meyer-Rohn, Med. Welt, 13, 837(1968); Y. Kotani, Acta Derm (Kyoto), 62, 55(1967); J. D. Stratigos and I. A. Magnus, Brit. J. Derm., 80, 391 (1968); P. Frost, G. D. Weinstein and E. C. Gomer, J. A. M. A., 216, 326(1971).

19. M. J. Fellner and R. L. Baer, J. A. M. A., 192, 997(1965); W. W. Furey and C. Tan, Ann. Internal Med., 70, 357(1969); I. J. Cooperman, Lancet, 2, 619(1967); R. B. Coles, J. Phillips and J. B. Nuttall, Brit. Med. J., 2, 313(1967); L. Businco, D. Lendval and E. Cardi, Acta Paediat. Lat., 21, 834(1968); J. Zelger and V. Seidl, Dermatologica, 139, 365(1969); W. B. Shelley and C. L. Heaton, J. A. M. A., 224, 125(1973).

20. R. L. Searcy, N. M. Simms, J. A. Foreman and L. M. Bergquist, Antimicrob. Agts. Chemother., 179(1964).

21. Shils, M. E., Ann. Intern. Med., 58, 389(1963); C. Van Ypersele de Strihou, Lancet, 2, 208(1970); H. Roth, K. L. Becker, R. J. Shalhoub and S. Katz, Arch. Intern. Med., 120, 433(1967); J. B. Eastwood, R. R. Bailey, J. R. Curtis P. E. Gower and H. E. DeWardener, Lancet, 2, 39, 262(1970); J. Moeller and C. Kaya, Med. Klin., 62, 686(1967); I. Perkash, P. N. Kataria and O. P. Khanna, J. Urol., 102, 102(1969); O. M. Edwards, E. C. Huskisson and R. T. Taylor, Brit. Med. J., 1, 26(1970); M. E. Phillips, J. B. Eastwood, J. R. Curtis, P. E. Gower and H. E. de Wardner, Brit. Med. J., 2, 149(1974); H. T. Lew and S. W. French, Arch. Intern. Med., 118, 123(1966); I. Singer and D. Rotenberg, Am. Intern. Med., 79, 679(1973).

22. M. H. Lepper, C. K. Wolfe, H. J. Zimmerman, E. R. Caldwell, Jr., H. W. Spies, and H. F. Dowling, Arch. Intern. Med., 88, 271(1951); J. C. Schultz, J. S. Adamson, Jr., W. W. Workman and T. D. Norman, New Eng. J. Med., 269, 999(1963); P. J. Whalley, R. H. Adams and B. Combes, J. A. M. A.,

189, 357(1964); H. F. Dowling and M. H. Lepper, J. A. M. A., 188, 307(1964); C. T. Kunelis, J. L. Peters and H. A. Edmondson, Amer. J. Med., 38, 359(1965); I. Damjanov, R. Arnold and M. Faqur, J. A. M. A., 204, 934(1968); G. C. Hanson, Postgr. Med., 44, 870(1968); H. T. Lew and S. W. French, Arch. Intern. Med., 118, 123(1966); M. Lewis, S. Schenker and B. Combes, Am. J. Dig. Dis, 12, 429(1967); W. V. Zussman, Anat. Rec., 162, 301(1968); J. D. Lloyd-Still, R. J. Grand and G. F. Vawter, J. Pediatrics, 84, 366(1974).

23. K. E. Price, Z. Zolli, Jr., J. C. Atkinson and H. G. Luther, Antibiot. and Chemother., 7, 672(1957); F. E. DiGangi and C. H. Rogers, J. Amer. Pharm. Ass., Sci. Ed., 38, 646(1949); J. Scheiner and W. A. Altemeir, Surgery, 114, 9(1962); J. E. Rosenblatt, J. E. Barrett, J. L. Brodie and W. M. M. Kirby, Antimicrob. Agts. Chemother., 134(1966); M. Schach von Wittenau and T. M. Twomey, Chemotherapy, 16, 217(1971); R. E. Notari, J. Pharm. Sci., 62, 865 (1973); A. Forsgren and H. Gnarpe, Nature New Biol., 244, 82(1973).

24. P. J. Neuvonen, G. Gothoni, R. Hackman and K. Bjorksten, Brit. Med. J., 4, 532(1970); Anon., Brit. Med. J., 4, 509 (1970).

25. K. H. Ibsen, M. R. Urist, R. E. Sognnaes and J. Keen, J. Pediat., 67, 459(1965); A. H. Kline, R. J. Blattner and M. Lunin, J. A. M. A., 188, 178(1964); H. Schwachman and A. Schuster, Ped. Clinics N. Amer., 3, 295(1956); I. S. Wallman and H. B. Hilton, Lancet, 1, 827(1962);

C. J. Witkop, Jr. and R. O. Wolf, J. A. M. A., 185, 100 (1963); P. J. Porter, E. A. Sweeney, H. Golan and E. H. Kass, Antimicrob. Agts. Chemother., 668(1966); J. Weyman, Brit. Dent. J., 118, 289(1965); L. J. Brearley, A. A. Stragis and E. Storey, Med. J. Austr., 2., 653(1968); L. J. Brearley and E. Storey, Med. J. Austr., 2, 714 (1968); K. L. Baker and E. Storey, Med. J. Austr., 1, 109(1970); I. C. Bennet, J. Oral. Ther. Pharmacol, 3, 232 (1966); C. G. Lofgren, K. A. Omnell and M. U. Nylen, Calc. Tiss. Res., 2, 145(1968); H. K. Iwamoto and W. R. Brennan, Toxicol. Appl. Pharmacol, 14, 33(1969); D. J. Stewart, Brit. Dent. J., 124, 318(1968); J. M. Conchie, J. D. Munroe and D. O. Anderson, Can. Med. Ass. J., 103, 351(1970); J. N. Swallow, J. DeHaller and W. F. Young, Arch. Dis. Child., 42, 311(1967); G. Weinmann and W. Braun, Kinderarztl. Prax., 37, 105(1969); B. Schutt, E. D. Berger, and E. Gugler, Chir. Praxis, 14, 283(1970); D. J. Stewart, Brit. Med. J., 3, 329(1973); S. Q. Cohlan, G. Berclander and T. Tiamsik, Am. J. Dis. Child., 105, 453(1963).

26. F. X. Fellers and R. Lindquist, Fed. Proc., 23, 575(1964); S. W. Frimpter, J. A. M. A., 184, 111(1958); J. M. Gross, Ann. Intern. Med., 58, 523(1963); F. Mavromatis, J. A. M. A., 193, 191(1965); L. C. Wegienka and J. M. Weller, Arch. Intern. Med., 114, 232(1964); M. J. Zimmerman and Z. L. Werther, J. Mt. Sinai Hosp., 31, 38(1964); K. F. Benitz and H. F. Diermeier, Proc. Soc. Exp. Biol. Med., 115, 930(1964); J. Brodehl, K. Gellissen, W. Hagge and H. Schumacher, Helv. Paediat. Acta, 23, 373(1968).

27. T. J. Franklin and G. A. Snow, The Biochemistry of Antimicrobial Activity, Academic Press, New York, p. 99ff (1971); W. B. Pratt, Fundamentals of Chemotherapy, Oxford University Press, New York, p. 68ff(1973); A. I. Laskin in Antibiotics, Vol. I, D. Gottlieb and P. D. Shaw, Eds., Springer Verlag, New York, p. 331ff(1967); E. F. Gale and E. Cundliffe, P. E. Reynolds, M. H. Richmond and M. J. Waring, The Molecular Basis of Antibiotic Action, J. Wiley and Sons, New York, p. 315ff(1972); H. Eagel and A. K. Saz, Ann. Rev. Microbiol., 9, 173(1955); N. A. Kuck and M. Forbes, Antimicrob. Agts. Chemother., 4, 237(1973); T. J. Franklin and A. Godfrey, Biochem. J., 94, 54(1965); A. I. Laskin and W. M. Chan, Biochem. Biophys. Res. Commun., 14, 137(1964).

28. R. Rendi and S. Ochoa, J. Biol. Chem., 237, 3711(1962); R. Rendi and S. Ochoa, Science, 133, 1367(1961); T. J. Franklin, Biochem. J., 87, 449(1963); T. J. Franklin and A. Godfrey, Biochem. J., 94, 54(1965); S. Okamoto and D. Mizuno, J. Gen. Microbiol. Japan, 35, 125(1964); A. I. Laskin and W. M. Chan, Biochem. Biophys. Res. Commun., 14, 137(1964); N. S. Beard, Jr., S. A. Armentrant and A. S. Weisberger, Pharmacol. Revs., 21, 213(1969).

29. S. Mitsuhashi, Transferable Drug Resistance Factor R, University Park Press, Baltimore (1971); J. Davies, Ann. Repts. in Med. Chem., 7, 217(1972); R. C. Clowes, Sci. Amer., 228, 18(1973); E. F. Gale, E. Cundliffe, P. E. Reynolds, M. H. Richmond and M. J. Waring, The Molecular Basis of Antibiotic Action, J. Wiley and Sons, New York,

p. 380ff(1972); W. Ritzerfeld, Muchen Med. Wochenschr., 115, 1641(1973); G. Lebek, Deut. Med. J., 23, 469(1972); R. Benveniste and J. Davies, Ann. Revs. Biochem., 42, 471(1973); T. J. Franklin, C. R. C. Critical Revs. Microbiol., 263(1973); A. M. Reynard and L. F. Nellis, Biochem. Biophys. Res. Commun., 48, 1129(1972); A. M. Reynard, L. F. Nellis and M. E. Beck, Appl. Microbiol., 21, 71(1971); D. Sompolinsky, Y. Zaidenzaig, R. Ziegler-Schlomowitz and N. Abramova, J. Gen. Microbiol., 62, 351 (1970); P. S. Ringrose and J. E. Higgins, J. Antibiotics, 27, 833(1974); F. E. Norrington and A. M. James, Biochem., Biophys. Acta, 218, 269(1970); T. J. Franklin and B. Higginson, Biochem. J., 116, 287(1970); A. Wojdani, R. R. Artalion and D. Sompolinsky, Antimicrob. Agts. Chemother., 9, 526(1976).

30. M. J. Martell, Jr. and J. H. Boothe, J. Med. Chem., 10, 44(1967); N. A. Kuck and M. Forbes, Antimicrob. Agts. Chemother., 3, 662(1973); E. C. R. Reeve and J. M. Robertson, J. Gen. Microbiol., 16, 73(1972).

31. J. R. Smythies, F. Bennington and R. D. Morin, Experientia, 28, 1235(1972).

32. R. K. Freinkel, J. S. Strauss, S. Y. Yip and P. E. Pochi, New Engl. J. Med., 273, 850(1965); J. A. Witkowski and H. M. Simons, J. A. M. A., 196, 397(1966).

33. W. P. Boger and J. J. Gavin, New Engl. J. Med., 261, 872(1959); M. Finland, Antibiotic Med., 5, 359(1958); C. M. Kunin, W. F. Jones and M. Finland, New Engl. J. Med., 259, 147(1958); E. D. Weinberg, Bact. Rev., 21, 46(1957).

34. T. D. Sokoloski, A. E. Staubus, M. R. Blum. L. J. Leeson and K. S. Lin, J. Am. Pharm. Assn., NS15, 709(1975); W. G. Crouthamel, J. W. Poole and T. Sokoloski, ibid., 461(1975); G. W. Brice and H. F. Hammer, J. A. M. A., 208, 1189(1969); D. C. Blair, R. W. Barnes, E. L. Wildner and W. J. Murray, J. A. M. A., 215, 251(1971).

35. C. M. Kunin, Ann. Intern. Med., 67, 151(1967).

36. J. E. Rosenblatt, J. E. Barrett, J. L. Brodie and W. M. M. Kirby, Antimicrob. Agts. Chemother., 6, 134(1966); M. Schach von Wittenau and J. Chiaini, Chemotherapy, suppl. 13, 41(1968); G. M. Williamson, Bull. Chem. Therap., 1, 53(1969); J. Krieglstein, Arzneimittelforsch., 23, 1527(1973); M. Schach von Wittenau and R. Yeary, J. Pharmacol. Exptl. Ther., 140, 258(1963); W. Scholtan, Arzneimittelforsch, 13, 347(1963); 18, 505(1968); G. Powis, J. Pharm. Pharmacol., 26, 113(1974); J. K. H. Ma, H. W. Jun and L. A. Luzzi, J. Pharm. Sci., 62, 1261(1973).

37. R. E. Notari, J. Pharm. Sci., 62, 865(1973).

38. C. M. Kunin, The Tetracyclines, in Antimicrobial Therapy, B. M. Kagan, ed., W. B. Saunders, Philadelphia, p. 51ff (1970).

39. J. H. Wiendl, Med. Klin., 61, 1005(1966); C. M. Kunin and M. Finland, New Engl. J. Med., 261, 1069(1959); H. F. vonElmendorf and T. Dimmling, Med. Klin., 60, 1459(1965); A. L. DeMaynard, J. C. Andriola and A. Prigot, Antibiot. Ann., 54, 102(1953).

40. H. S. Goldberg, Advan. Appl. Microbiol., 6, 91(1964); R. N. Goodman, Antimicrob. Agts. Chemother., 747(1966).

41. J. W. Boyer and J. G. Atherton, Austr. J. of Biol. Sci., 25, 43(1972).

42. T. K. Nariani, S. P. Raychandhuri and S. M. Viswanath, Current Sci., 40, 552(1971).

43. R. E. McCoy, Plant Disease Reporter, 57, 341(1973).

44. G. Nyland and W. J. Moller, Plant Disease Reporter, 57, 634(1973).

45. T. H. Filler, Plant Disease Reporter, 57, 341(1973).

46. P. O. Lal and T. P. S. Teotia, J. Antibiotics, 28, 993 (1975).

47. C. Vezina, Pure and Appl. Chem., 28, No. 4(1971).

48. M. Swan, K. L. Blaxter, H. I. Field, J. W. Howie, I. A. M. Lucas, E. L. M. Millar, J. C. Murdoch, J. H. Parsons and E. G. White, Report of the Joint Committee on the Use of Antibiotics in Animal Husbandry and Veterinary Medicine, Her Majesty's Stationery Office: London, September, 1969.

49. C. D. Van Honweling, F. D. A. Papers, 21, (1969); H. C. Hopkins, ibid., 14(1972).

50. U. S. Animal Health Association, Pharmaceutical Committee Report, October, 1969.

51. D. Siegel, W. G. Huher and F. Enloe, AAC, 6, 697(1974).

CHAPTER 2

FERMENTATION AND ISOLATION

2.1---Introduction.

All of the tetracyclines of commercial significance are either fermentation products themselves or are derived therefrom. Because of their economic value, there are relatively few accounts of their fermentative production and isolation in the open scientific literature. There is, however, a rich patent literature available. Subject to the usual reservations about the complete reliability of patents, the following selective account is perforce mostly derived from this source. There are two photocopy compilations of these patents available to make reference to these sources more convenient.[1,2] An appendix has also been prepared in which United States patents dealing with tetracyclines are listed (*q. v.*).

2.2---Fermentation.

The primary tetracyclines, TC, OTC, CTC and DMCTC, are all produced by submerged fermentation of various *Streptomyces* species isolated in soil screening programs and then nutritionally and genetically manipulated to optimize yields. The fermentations are done on a very large scale commercially 20,000 to 50,000 gallons. The organism and strain chosen not only determine maximal yields but also the identity of the antibiotic(s) formed. Although a fermentation is usually (Table 2-1) reported as producing a single agent of interest, usually small amounts of related antibiotics are present. For example, CTC fermentations frequently have up to 10% of TC present. Likewise, OTC fermentations frequently contain some TC. The "wild" strains isolated directly from soil seldom produce commercially useful quantities. Mycologists expose such cultures to nutritional studies and, particularly, to the action of mutagenic agents. Antibiotics are secondary metabolites whose production is not essential to the vigor of the producing organism. Genetic manipulation involves deleting other non-essential pathways so that the genome remaining allows the organism to thrive and whatever energy and metabolic precursors are not essential for primary metabolism can then be devoted to producing high titers of the desired antibiotic. Such specialized mutants may be genetically unstable so great care must be taken in preservation and use of such cultures. The optimal medium must be chosen to fit the requirements of the particular mutant strains and must not only give high yields but contain cheap ingredients. Annoyingly, different brands and occasionally different batches of the same brand often make a significant difference in yields. Controlling these variables is a constant job involving much experience

Table 2-1. Some cultures reported* to produce the major fermentation-derived tetracyclines.

Principal Antibiotic	Culture	Reference	
		Patent or Other	Chemical Abstracts
CTC	*Streptomyces aureofaciens*	U.S. 2,482,055 (1949)	44: 8604f (1950)
TC	*Streptomyces aureofaciens*	U.S. 2,734,018 (1956)	44: 8604f (1950)
TC	*S. viridifaciens*	U.S. 2,712,517 (1955)	44: 8604f (1950)
DMCTC	*S. aureofaciens*	U.S. 2,878,289 (1959)	44: 8604f (1950)
OTC	*Streptomyces rimosus*	U.S. 2,516,080 (1950)	
CTC	*S. sayamaensis*	*Meiji Seika Kenkyer Nempo*, 66 (1959)	54: 25025b (1960)
TC	*S. sayamaensis*	Jap. Pat. 9497 (1959)	54: 10247a (1960)
CTC	*S. rimosus*	*Fermentnaya i Spirt. Prom.*, 30, 32 (1964)	61: 7653f (1964)
OTC	*S. rimosus*	*Med. Doswiaderalna i Mikrobiol.*, 7, 125 (1955)	49: 11088c (1955)
TC	*S. rimosus*	*J. Bacteriol.*, 80, 419 (1960)	54: 25033a (1960)
CTC	*S. viridifaciens*	*Biochem. Biophys. Acta*, 58, 635 (1962)	57: 6412c (1962)
TC	*S. viridifaciens*	*Biochem. Biophys. Acta*, 58, 635 (1962)	57: 6412c (1962)
DMCTC	*S. viridifaciens*	*Biochem. Biophys. Acta*, 58, 635 (1962)	57: 6412c (1962)

CTC	*S. lusitanus*	Brit. Pat. [illegible] (1963)	[illegible]
TC	*S. lusitanus*	Belg. Pat. 658,387 (1965)	*64*: 7328f (1966)
OTC	*S. armillatus*	*Ann. Inst. Pasteur*, *87*, 580 (1954)	*49*: 4779g (1955)
OTC	*S. rimosus* mixed with *Saccharomyces fragilis*	Czech. Pat. 87,520 (1957)	*55*: 12764e (1961)
OTC	*Actinomyces varsoviensis*	Ger. Pat. 1,213,568 (1966)	*65*: 1346b (1966)
OTC	*Streptomyces henetus*	Belg. Pat. 660,294 (1965) U.S. Pat. 3,408,258 (1968)	*65*: 1346a (1966)
OTC	*S. alboflavus*	Belg. Pat. 638,881 (1964)	*62*: 8355c (1965)
OTC	*S. capuensis*	Neth. Appl. 6,400,925 (1964)	*62*: 5856a (1965)
OTC	*S. ticinensis*	Belg. Pat. 632,332 (1963)	*61*: 7664d (1964)
TC	*S. psammoticus*	*Il Farmaco, Ed. sci.*, *15*, 164 (1960)	*54*: 14567b (1960)
TC	*S. subterraneus*	Neth. Appl. 6,509,680 (1966)	*65*: 1346d (1966)
TC	*Streptomyces mediolanum*	Belg. Pat. 649,539 (1964)	*64*: 11824b (1966)
TC	*S. avellaneus*	S. African Pat. 6,705,025 (1968)	*70*: 56295n (1969)
TC	*S. phenaethylicus*	Brit. Pat. 1,286,929 (1972)	*77*: 124767g (1972)

*There is an active dispute between mycological taxonomists as to what constitutes a new species. Some prefer to create many species whereas their more conservative colleagues believe many of the new species so created should be regarded as strains. The organic chemist is unable to take sides on a rational basis in this dispute between authorities.

and as much art as science. A wide variety of media have been employed for tetracycline production.

Fermentation starts with a tube of lyophilized culture which must be opened aseptically and transferred to agar slants for incubation. The cell population is then built up in stages. First, the slants are transferred to Erhlenmeyer flasks containing sterile liquid medium on a shaker platform and after appropriate incubation the contents are aseptically transferred to 18-liter bottle fermenters and thence to small and then to large tanks. The tanks contain steam sterilized liquid media and the production fermentation proceeds for 1-4 days until optimal yields are present. The tanks are stirred and agitated with a large volume per minute of sterile air. This necessitates inclusion of an anti-foaming agent such as sterile lard oil, silicones or mineral oil. The pH of the fermentation is generally closely controlled between 6 and 7 by the periodic addition of base, usually, solid $CaCO_3$, and the temperature is maintained between 25° and 30°C. This may require warming at first and then cooling when the fermentation is proceeding vigorously.

Many energy or carbon sources have been employed including starch, dextrin, maltose, glucose, lactose, glycerol and mannitol. Nitrogen sources include amino acids, bacto-peptone, casein, corn steep liquor, meat extracts, molasses, fish solubles, seed meal from which the oils have been extracted, urea, nitrates and ammonium salts. A variety of inorganic ions must be present and calcium carbonate is specially noteworthy as it stabilizes the tetracyclines formed and may help increase yields by precipitating the antibiotics as they are formed so as to decrease their autotoxic effect on the producing organism. In addition to these more general additives, a number of specific agents are added for specialized purposes, such as use of cosynthetic factor,[3] riboflavin,[4] copper,*[5] 5-fluorouracil,*[6] bromide and thiocyanate ions,**[7] sulfonamides,***[25] etc. In fact, the removal of chlorine from the medium[8] or decreasing chlorine incorporation with a wide variety of chlorination inhibitors is technically quite important in order to facilitate processing without the need of expensive chromatographic steps as otherwise undesirable quantities of CTC are coproduced along with TC. The inhibitors are believed to work by binding copper ions needed as part of the chlorinating enzyme or by some undefined less direct route.[9] Of these agents, patents involving the use of thiocarbazates and thiocarbamates,[10] 3,6-pyridazines,[11] 2-benzoxazoylthio-N-methylcarbamate,[12] 2-chlorobenzoxazole or 2-chlorobenzothiazole,[13] 2,6-dimercapto-benzdiazole,[14] 1,3-bis(2-benzothiazolylmercaptomethyl)urea,[15]

---

* In CTC fermentations, these additives decrease the amount of TC formed concomitantly.

** In TC fermentations, these additives decrease the amount of CTC formed.

*** In DMCTC fermentations, this decreases the amount of CTC formed.

N-cyclohexyl-2-benzothiazolsulfenamide,[16] thioureas,[17] thionalide,[18] 2-mercapto-4,5-dimethylthiazole,[19] dechlorinated corn steep liquor with Ag ion,[20] multiple chlorination inhibitors,[21] diazoles,[22] 1,2,4-triazines,[23] and 2,4-dichloropyrimidines[24] have appeared.

There are an enormous number of colateral patents dealing with the fermentative production of tetracyclines and which, if any, of these contains a commercial process cannot be readily established because this is, of course, a jealously guarded secret. Selections of such patents are available for consultation for those seeking more detail.[1,2,appendix]

The yields of tetracyclines reported in these various patents are impressive. Some patents claim yields approaching 10,000 mcg/ml (10 g/liter)![26] What yields are actually encountered in production cannot be established except by guess.

2.3---Isolation - general.

There are a variety of procedures which have been employed for isolating the various tetracyclines from high-yielding fermentations. The processes are almost exclusively described in patents and their commercial status is unclear. The processes in use are dictated to a major extent by the physical and chemical properties of the antibiotics and by economic factors. The tetracyclines are amphoteric with an isoelectric point between 4 and 6. TC, for example, has an i.e.p. at 4.8[27] and its water solubility near neutrality is about 1 mg/ml. At the pH extremes, higher water solubility is seen.[28] In fact, the aqueous solubility of TC is about ten times greater at pH 1-3 than at pH 5-6.[29] The solubility/pH profile for OTC is given in Table 2-2. More recent work of relevance to gastric absorption indicates that some of the tetracyclines, notably CTC, DMCTC and MOTC, behave in a more complex manner in that the solubility in simulated gastric juice rises, as expected, when the solutions are more acidic, but then solubility decreases again in quite acidic solutions.[30] For example, CTC shows a peak of solubility at pH 3 (5 mg/ml) with the solubility at pH 2 approximately equivalent to that at pH 5 (2 mg/ml). At neutral pH's, in the presence of Ca++, Mg++ and Al+++ ions, tetracyclines show an enhanced tendency to precipitate from aqueous solutions and a correspondingly greater solubility in lower alcohols. The tetracyclines show relatively little tendency to extract at any pH into common water immiscible

Table 2-2. Water solubility of OTC as a function of pH.[28]

pH	Water Solubility in mcg/ml.
1.2	31,400
2.0	4,600
3.0	1,400
4.0	850
5.0	500
6.0	700
7.0	1,100
8.0	28,000
9.0	38,600

Table 2-3. Solubility of various tetracyclines in a variety of solvents at 28°. Data are in mg/ml.[31]

	TC•HCl	TC	OTC•HCl	CTC•HCl
Water	10.9	1.7	6.9	8.6
Methanol	20+	20+	16.4	17.4
Ethanol	7.9	20+	12.0	1.7
Benzene	0.3	1.0	0.03	0.1
Petroleum Ether	0.0	0.005	0.01	0.01
Carbon Tetrachloride	0.1	0.3	0.07	0.13
Ethyl Acetate	0.8	17.3	2.0	0.35
Acetone	0.8	17.4	10.8	0.12
Ether	0.6	3.7	0.1	0.09
Ethylene Chloride	0.8	11.3	0.4	0.25
Dioxane	7.7	14.6	6.3	1.45
Chloroform	2.9	13.8	0.4	0.02
Pyridine	20+	20+	20+	20+
Benzylalcohol	10.8	14.4	20+	1.8

organic solvents such as ether and chloroform, but solvents such as n-butanol and methylisobutylketone are useable. Table 2-3 gives a more extensive listing of the solubility properties of the tetracyclines.

The tetracyclines are stable in neutral or mildly acidic solutions. At pH extremes, especially at elevated temperatures, bioactivity is progressively lost. Table 2-4 gives relevant stability data for the major fermentation derived tetracyclines. Table 2-5 gives the stability/pH profile for OTC at 200 mcg/ml. A discussion of the chemistry involved under these conditions will be deferred to Chapter 5, Sections 5.2 and 5.3.

Table 2-4. Stability data for the major fermentation-derived tetracyclines.

Antibiotic	Half-Life	Conditions	Reference
Acid			
CTC	8.2 min	0.2N H_2SO_4/100°	32
	2.1 min	1.0N H_2SO_4/100°	33
	7.3 hr	1.0N H_2SO_4/50°	34
TC	< 2 min	0.2N H_2SO_4/100°	32
	< 1 min	1.0N H_2SO_4/100°	33
	15.5 hr	1.0N H_2SO_4/25°	34
OTC	4.5 min	1.0N H_2SO_4/100°	33
	6.3 hr	1.0N H_2SO_4/50°	34
DMCTC	7.4 hr	1.0N H_2SO_4/100°	33
Base			
CTC	< 0.3 min	0.1N NaOH/100°	33
	18.6 min	pH 10 buffer/22°	35
	53 min	pH 8.8 buffer/29°	34
TC	6.8 min	0.1N NaOH/100°	33
	>11 hr	pH 10 buffer/22°	32
	101 min	0.1N NaOH/60°	34
	12 hr	pH 8.8 buffer/24°	35
OTC	2.2 min	0.1N NaOH/100°	33
	33 hr	pH 8.5 buffer/37°	32
	10.9 hr	0.1N NaOH/23°	34
DMCTC	40 min	0.1N NaOH/100°	33

Table 2-5. Stability of OTC at 200 mcg/ml in aqueous solutions of various pH when kept at 37°C.[28]

pH	T½ (hour)
1.0	114
2.5	134
4.6	45
5.5	45
7.0	26
8.5	33
10.0	14

The many and varied processes used in isolation of the major tetracyclines will be made clearer by reference to the succeeding sections.

2.4---Isolation of chlortetracycline.

Generally, in high-yielding commercial CTC fermentations, at harvest the drug is present partly in solution and partly as precipitated metal chelates (especially with Ca^{++} ion) admixed with mycelia. The CTC is freed from the complexes and solubilized by addition of HCl to a pH less than 3 and the mash is filtered. The drug is recovered from the resulting beer filtrate in a number of ways in which combinations of solvent extractions, precipitations at neutral pH's, adsorptions, complexation with metal ions and crystallizations are used.

In the original processes, the cells were removed from the mash and CTC was adsorbed, for example, on charcoal or florisil, etc., at pH 4.5 and the column was washed with water and then acetone, to remove lipid contaminants, and methanolic HCl elutes the activity in a brilliant yellow band. This is concentrated to dryness _in vacuo_ and the activity is taken up in n-BuOH. After washing with some water, the solution is concentrated to a small volume and the CTC is precipitated with anhydrous ether.[36,37] The precipitate is dried and taken up in dilute HCl and the HCl salt is recovered by lyophilization. This process is surely only of historical interest. In a later process,[38] the beer solids are filtered after adjustment to pH 8.5 and then acidified to pH 1.4 with sulfuric acid and the precipitate is removed by filtration. Salt is added to the filtrate and the CTC-HCl is extracted into n-BuOH. The butanol layer is concentrated under vacuum at less than 20°C and the concentrate is adjusted to pH 1 with HCl and chilling produces crystalline CTC·HCl. Later this was refined[39] by showing that concentrated aqueous-acidic solutions of impure CTC will deposit pure CTC-HCl if the solution is saturated with NaCl and a small amount of cold n-BuOH is added. Another modification[40] involves suspending crude CTC-HCl in cold $EtOCH_2CH_2OH$, carefully making this alkaline to pH 7.8 and filtering insoluble impurities. Upon acidification with HCl to pH 1.5 and chilling good quality crystals are obtained. Colored impurities can be removed by charcoal treatment of the mildly alkaline solution. Instead of the crude HCl salt, the CTC can be precipitated from filtered beer with an alkyl sulfonic acid and then treated as indicated with $EtOCH_2CH_2OH$ and base, etc.

Another variation[41] involves taking the alkalinized fermentation mash and adding n-BuOH and adjusting the mixture to pH 1.4 with H_2SO_4. The filtrate is enriched by an acid-butanol wash of the fermentation mash solids and the pooled butanol layers are washed with a concentrated NaCl solution and then concentrated until CTC-HCl separates. This is completed by acidification with HCl and chilling.

Ca, Ba, Sr and Mg ions at a pH range of 6-10 and above form particularly insoluble CTC chelates. A process utilizing this[42] involves alkalinizing a fermentation broth to pH 8.5 with $Ca(OH)_2$, filtering and washing. The solids are suspended in dilute H_2SO_4, filtered and washed. The filtrate is reprecipitated by alkalinization with $Ca(OH)_2$ to pH 10 and filtration. The drug is solubilized by suspension in aqueous acidic acetone, concentrating and crystallizing. CTC must be handled rapidly at high pH's to avoid destruction.

Rather than acidify the mash in order to sharpen the separation, later it was found possible to extract the CTC directly without a filtration step.[43] The mash is acidified to pH 1.4 and ammonium oxalate is added to tie up Ca^{++} ion. Next, Arquad 16 (a liquid ion-exchanger) in 50% i-PrOH solution is added and the pH adjusted to 8.5 with NaOH. Methylisobutylketone is added along with filter-aid. After filtration and suitable washings, the MIBK layer has the activity. This is recovered as CTC-HCl by acidification. Recoveries of pure material are excellent.

Many refinements have been patented (for example, 44-46) but these are sufficient to illustrate the scope of the work.

2.5---Isolation of tetracycline.

Most of the CTC processes work reasonably well with TC itself. In fact, because TC is somewhat more stable, they work somewhat better. The original process[47] involved catalytic hydrogenolysis of CTC to TC, but this will be discussed later under chemical properties.

Use of a liquid ion exchange process,[48,53] extraction from filtered beer at pH 8.5 with n-BuOH or MIBK and precipitation with a non-polar solvent as the free base,[49] fractional precipitation of the less soluble TC-HCl from CTC-HCl (coproduced in the fermentation),[50] precipitation as the Ca^{++} complex,[51] or as the quaternary ammonium ion,[52,53] direct mash extraction,[43] and purification of crude TC preparations by pH solubilization-precipitations and charcoal treatments,[54] are sufficiently similar to those briefly described under CTC that they require no special comment. The tendency of TC fermentations to produce sufficient quantities of CTC also renders refining difficult on a commercial scale. This has resulted in careful attention to the conditions of the final crystallizations so as to avoid the necessity of using expensive chromatographic means.[55,56] TC oxalate is less soluble than CTC oxalate so that fractional crystallization is quite effective.[57]

Precipitation at about pH 4 in the presence of citrate,[58] urea,[59] and phosphate[60] have also been presented. These, presumably, tie up complexing ions preferentially so that salt-free product is formed. Precipitation of the cupric complex in the presence of detergents has been described[61] as has been the use of formamide complexes.[62] The dibutylnaphthalene sulfonate salt crystallizes in strongly acid solutions.[63] Just as with CTC, the precipitation with quaternary ammonium salts is advantageous.[64,65]

2.6---Isolation of 6-demethylchlortetracycline.

This antibiotic is more stable than either of those just described and it is produced by an artificial mutant descended from the original CTC producing culture. Orginally, isolation involved acidifying the beer and filtering. The filtrate was treated with salt and then extracted with butanol which was concentrated and the antibiotic was purified by column partition chromatography on acid-washed diatomaceous earth.[66] This process is hardly viable on a commercial scale and was quickly superceded by direct crystallization (at pH 0.65) as the HCl salt.[67] Another process destroys coproduced CTC by acid treatment so as to make chromatography unnecessary.[68] A liquid ion exchange process,[69] recrystallization using the urea sulfate complex to help purify,[70] butanol extraction of alkalinized beer filtrate followed by acid extraction, adjustment to pH 5.0 and crystallization of the free-base,[71] and so on, have also been described.

2.7---Isolation of oxytetracycline.

With the foregoing in mind, the isolation and refining processes for OTC are readily comprehended. OTC may be extracted from alkaline solutions with n-BuOH,[72] or using liquid ion exchangers,[73] or precipitated by Ba^{++} or Ca^{++} ions,[74] or quaternary ammonium salts with various chelating ions,[75] arylazosulfonic acids,[76] crystallized from butanol,[77] or from pH 4 solutions with, say, sodium citrate or sodium lauryl sulfate,[78] and so on.

REFERENCES

1. R. C. Evans, The Technology of the Tetracyclines, Quadrangle Press, New York, N. Y., 1968.
2. Anon., Tetracycline Manufacturing Processes, Noyes Development Corporation, Park Ridge, N. J., 1969. Vol. 1 and Vol. 2.
3. U. S. Patent 2,970,947 (1961).
4. U. S. Patent 2,987,449 (1961).
5. U. S. Patent 3,050,446 (1962).
6. U. S. Patent 3,145,154 (1964).
7. U. S. Patent 2,739,924 (1953).
8. U. S. Patent 2,734,018 (1956).
9. J. J. Goodman, M. Matrishin, R. W. Young and J. R. D. McCormick, J. Bacteriol., 78, 492 (1950).
10. U. S. Patent 2,923,667 (1960).
11. U. S. Patent 2,923,668 (1960).
12. U. S. Patent 2,940,905 (1960).

13. U. S. Patent 2,940,906 (1960).

14. U. S. Patent 2,940,907 (1960).

15. U. S. Patent 2,940,908 (1960).

16. U. S. Patent 2,940,909 (1960).

17. U. S. Patent 2,949,406 (1960).

18. U. S. Patent 2,949,407 (1960).

19. U. S. Patent 2,956,930 (1960).

20. U. S. Patent 2,970,946 (1961).

21. U. S. Patent 3,019,173 (1962).

22. U. S. Patent 3,037,916 (1962).

23. U. S. Patent 3,425,911 (1969).

24. U. S. Patent 3,429,780 (1969).

25. U. S. Patent 3,019,172 (1962).

26. U. S. Patent 2,923,688 (1960).

27. C. R. Stephens, K. Murai, K. J. Brunings and R. B. Woodward, J. Am. Chem. Soc., 78, 4155 (1956).

28. P. P. Regna and I. A. Solomons, Ann. N. Y. Acad. Sci., 53, 229 (1950).

29. W. H. Barr, J. Adir and L. Garrettson, Clin. Pharmacol. Ther., 12, 779 (1971).

30. S. Miyazaki, M. Nakano and T. Arita, Chem. Pharm. Bull., 23, 1197 (1975).

31. P. J. Weiss, M. L. Andrew and W. W. Wright, Antibiotics Chemother., 7, 376 (1957).

32. A. P. Doerschuk, J. R. D. McCormick, J. J. Goodman, S. A. Szumski, J. A. Growich, P. A. Miller, B. A. Bitler, E. R. Jensen, M. Matrishin, M. A. Petty and A. S. Phelps, J. Am. Chem. Soc., 81, 3069 (1959).

33. J. R. D. McCormick, N. O. Sjolander, U. Hirsch, E. R. Jensen and A. P. Doerschuk, J. Am. Chem. Soc., 79, 4561 (1957).

34. J. R. D. McCormick, S. M. Fox, L. L. Smith, B. A. Bitler, J. Reichenthal, V. E. Origoni, W. H. Muller, R. Winterbottom and A. P. Doerschuk, J. Am. Chem. Soc., 79, 2849 (1957).

35. P. P. Minieri, M. C. Firman, A. G. Mistretta, A. Abbey, C. E. Bricker, N. E. Rigler and H. Sokol, Antibiotics Annual, 81 (1953-4).

36. U. S. Patent 2,482,055 (1949).

37. U. S. Patent 2,586,766 (1952).

38. U. S. Patent 2,655,535 (1953).

39. U. S. Patent 2,658,077 (1953).

40. U. S. Patent 2,671,806 (1956).

41. U. S. Patent 2,740,816 (1956).

42. U. S. Patent 2,763,681 (1956).

43. U. S. Patent 2,875,247 (1959).

44. U. S. Patent 2,988,569 (1961).

45. U. S. Patent 2,992,274 (1961).

46. U. S. Patent 3,005,025 (1961).

47. U. S. Patent 2,699,054 (1955).

48. U. S. Patent 2,734,018 (1956).

49. U. S. Patent 2,739,924 (1956).

50. U. S. Patent 2,804,476 (1957).

51. U. S. Patent 2,847,471 (1958).

52. U. S. Patent 2,866,738 (1958).

53. U. S. Patent 2,871,264 (1959).

54. U. S. Patent 2,886,595 (1959).

55. U. S. Patent 2,905,714 (1959).

56. U. S. Patent 2,897,234 (1959).

57. U. S. Patent 2,929,837 (1960).

58. U. S. Patent 3,013,074 (1961).

59. U. S. Patent 3,037,973 (1962).

60. U. S. Patent 3,230,254 (1966).

61. U. S. Patent 3,272,862 (1966).

62. U. S. Patent 3,301,899 (1967).

63. U. S. Patent 3,349,127 (1967).

64. U. S. Patent 3,454,639 (1969).

65. U. S. Patent 3,458,572 (1969).

66. U. S. Patent 2,878,289 (1959).

67. U. S. Patent 3,023,239 (1962).

68. U. S. Patent 3,028,311 (1962).

69. U. S. Patent 3,050,558 (1962).

70. U. S. Patent 3,053,899 (1962).

71. U. S. Patent 3,070,514 (1962).

72. U. S. Patent 2,516,080 (1950).

73. U. S. Patent 2,658,078 (1953).

74. P. P. Regna, I. A. Solomons, K. Murai, A. E. Timreck, K. J. Brunings and W. A. Lazier, J. Am. Chem. Soc., 73, 4211 (1951).

75. U. S. Patent 2,873,276 (1959).

76. U. S. Patent 2,649,480 (1953).

77. U. S. Patent 2,867,661 (1959).

78. U. S. Patent 2,988,569 (1961).

CHAPTER 3

BIOSYNTHESIS

3.1---Introduction.

Intensive examination of the biosynthetic mode of the tetracyclines has been carried out. The initial studies had a very practical objective in mind -- the production of the highest feasible quantities of these agents with the minimum cost in time, labor and materials. Coupled with genetic manipulation of the cultures themselves, this work has been highly productive and the discovery of commercially useful 6-demethylchlortetracycline (DMCTC) resulted. The second and more laborious phase involved elucidation of the various intermediates lying between the crude culture constituents and the finished antibiotics and has been very productive from a scientific standpoint. The directed biosynthesis of 5-hydroxychlortetracycline is an example of the potential of this approach to achieve practical results. Given the relative ease with which the pretetramides can be synthesized, it is clearly possible that significant new tetracyclines could be produced in this somewhat artificial manner.

The evidence is now overwhelming that the tetracyclines are polyketides derived essentially from a shunt in fatty acid biosynthesis which occurs when the producing organisms go into secondary metabolism. Much of the evidence relating to the discrete order of intermediates through which acetate passes into tetracyclines is circumstantial but the data fit together to make a self-consistent story which must be essentially correct. A number of useful reviews have been published.[1-7]

3.2---The fundamental units.

Even before any significant biological evidence was in hand, several investigators posited on theoretical grounds that the tetracyclines arose from "acetate units or their biological equivalents."[8-10] Soon, however, it was shown using radioisotopes that acetate was indeed incorporated efficiently into the tetracyclines.[11-13] The N-methyls and the C_6-methyl group were subsequently shown to be methionine derived.[13,14] The origin of the nitrogen atoms is not entirely clear, but it has been shown that ammonium ion in a synthetic medium consisting primarily of glycerol and salts will suffice.[15] When a chlorine atom is present, it comes from inorganic chloride ion in the medium.[7,15,16]

3.3---The overall polyketide process to tetracycline.

According to basic polyketide theory[17,18] as modified in light of the details of fatty acid biosynthesis, McCormick[2] proposed a multienzyme complex which would utilize malonamyl CoA, nine malonyl CoA units, methionine and hydrogen to produce 6-methylpretetramide (5) as the first isolable intermediate (Figure 3-1). At least six further operations are required before oxytetracycline (6) results. The incorporation of radioactivity required by polyketide theory is indicated in the figure. The order in which the steps take place is assigned somewhat arbitrarily. Deletion of the C-methylating enzyme produces a parallel set of metabolites leading, if one includes subsequent chlorination

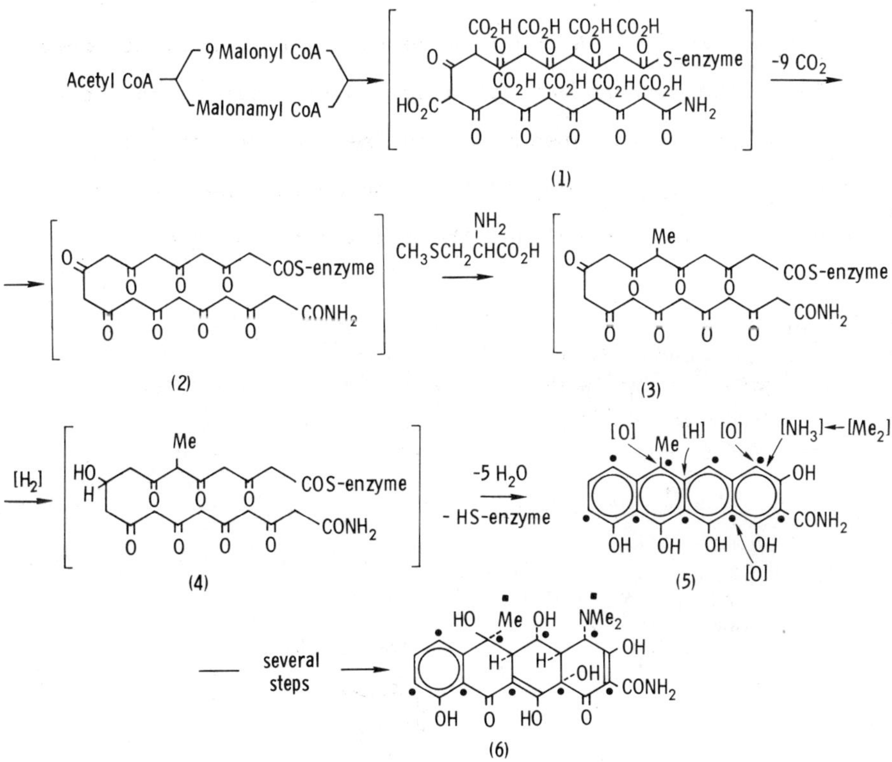

Figure 3-1. Overall biosynthetic scheme for oxytetracycline. Carbons derived from the methyl group of acetate (•) and methionine (■) are identified.

and omits a hydroxylation, to DMCTC. The CTC and TC series result by inclusion or deletion of key chlorinating enzymes as will be detailed subsequently. The import of this at this point is that a single basic pathway, suitably modified, is accepted as followed by all natural tetracyclines and that establishment of the details for one gives applicable results for all.

Birch et al. degraded oxytetracycline produced by fermentation with radiolabeled acetate (Figure 3-2) and the results were entirely consistent with the pattern indicated in Figure 3-1.[14,19] A complete degradation to show the fate of all of the carbons was not done. Nevertheless, the results are in quantitative agreement with the requirements of theory. Kuhn-Roth and Hoffman degradations on methionine-derived OTC showed that the C-methyl and the two N-methyls were

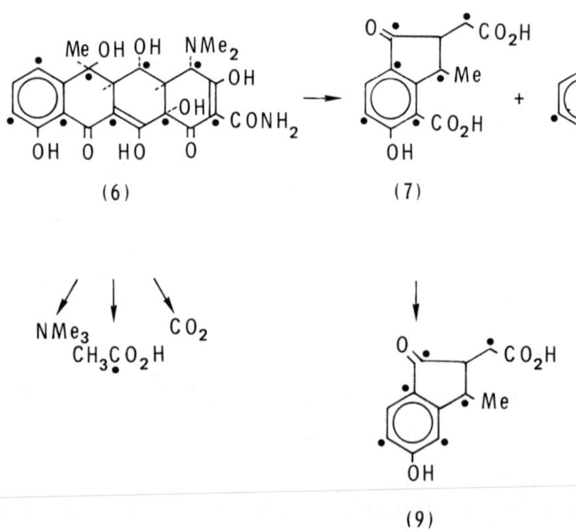

Figure 3-2. Degradation of radiolabeled oxytetracycline.

approximately equally labeled. Unfortunately, the A ring is not degradable to easily characterized products. In this scheme, only the carboxamide carbon and the N-methyl groups could be gotten out cleanly. This led to some initial confusion. There is no direct evidence for the involvement of malonamyl CoA as starter unit. Direct studies with malonic acid semiamide have failed perhaps due to lack of cellular penetration or the necessary activating enzymes.[20] It had been observed that the radioactivity incorporated into ring A was often lower than one would have expected when acetate was fed. When glutamic acid 2-^{14}C was fed, most of the radioactivity incorporated was present in the A ring. It was not yet generally appreciated that malonate rather than acetate units are involved in fatty acid and polyketide biosynthesis so it was ingeneously proposed that glutamine as primer unit made up most of ring A (10).[5] Later, Gatenbeck[21] showed that $NaHCO_3$ efficiently supplied the carboxamide carbon and suggested that the fluctuation in A-ring labeling with acetate resulted from metabolic degradation into CO_2 followed by fixation into malonate *via* the tricarboxylic acid cycle. The glutamate results are explained on the same basis. The only molecule of CO_2 which is retained on going from hypothetical polyketide 1 to oxytetracycline (6)

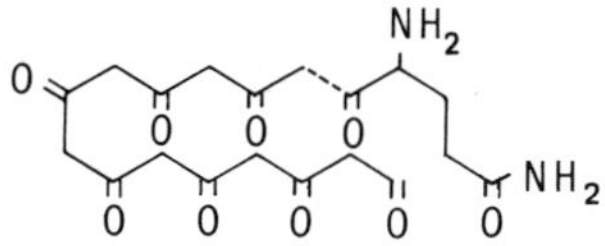

(10)

is that in the A-ring starter unit. A ^{13}C-biosynthetic experiment followed by Fourrier transform CMR would establish these inferences unambiguously, but has not been reported.

The production of 2-acetyl-2-decarboxamidotetracyclines (11, e.g.) is consistent with these ideas if one presumes that malonamyl CoA is not found in these strains but that acetyl CoA substitutes for it.[22,23,24]

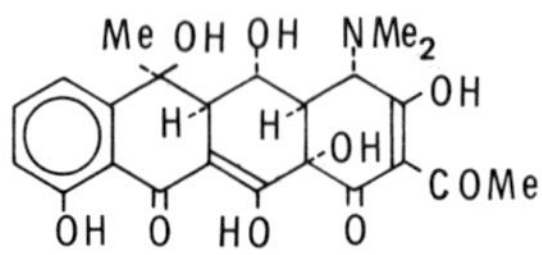

(11)

In later experiments, Hassall also prepared oxytetracyclin from methyl-^{14}C acetate and sodium fusion led to 3-acetylsalicylic acid (12) whose radioactivity was in accord with expectation.[25]

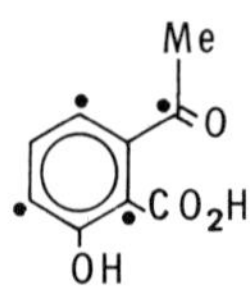

(12)

3.4---Pretetramides not capable of biotransformation to finished tetracyclines.

Use of a number of mutant organisms obtained by chemical mutagen exposure, irradiation or heat provide the next pieces of evidence. These mutants are not able to produce finished antibiotics but accumulate intermediates whose structural identity is most revealing in a biosynthetic sense. Several of these isolated intermediates can produce active antibiotics when fed to other blocked strains thus providing presumptive evidence for their intermediacy in non-blocked strains. This technique, called cosynthesis, has been particularly valuable and is illustrated in Figure 3-3. A wide variety of blocked mutants were available and it was inherently unlikely that they could all be blocked at the same point in the sequence. If a stable intermediate were elaborated by strain A, this could be partially purified and fed to strain B. If strain B were capable of taking up the intermediate and were blocked at an earlier point in the sequence, the necessary enzymes would be present to complete the biosynthesis. This could be

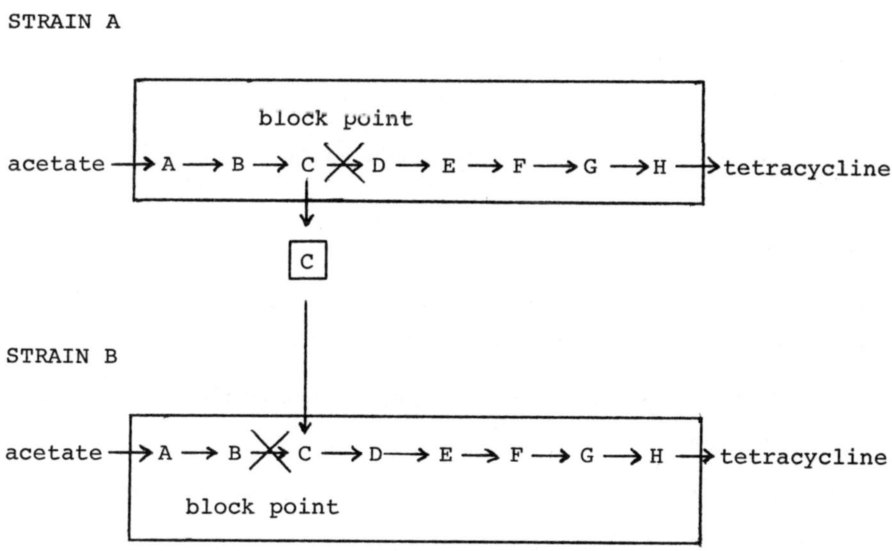

Figure 3-3. A schematic representation of the cosynthesis technique as it applies to tetracycline biosynthetic studies.

detected by the production of antimicrobial activity. Neither strain A nor strain B is capable of producing TC by itself. This technique provides a ready assay so that the intermediate can be isolated and identified.

Reference to Figure 3-1 shows that 6-methylpretetramide (5) is the earliest intermediate capable of independent existence. Intermediates produced by cultures blocked previous to this point would either be disassembled and the acetate used for some other purpose, or, in some cases, could be set free and be isolable. Protetrone (13) appears to be such a substance.[26] When fed back to apparently suitable strains, it cannot be transformed further to a bioactive tetracycline. Note that the carboxamide function is already present while no methyl group is present at pro C_6. The hydroxyl group at pro C_8 is also missing. This is, incidentally, the great missing link in that no tetracycline substituted at C_8 has ever been made either biosynthetically or by chemical manipulation. The cell line from which protetrone was derived has chlorinating capacity so the absence of Cl in 13 suggests this to be a later step while the absence of CH_3 is known from other evidence to be an earlier step. In any case, the protetrone producing strain does not produce C_6 methylated tetracyclines. It is of some interest also that 13 is capable of undergoing non-enzymatic cyclization to 14 when treated with strong acid.[26]

Another shunt metabolite with a suggestive structure is 15.[27] In this substance, produced by a different strain, the pro C_6 methyl group is in place. As will be seen,

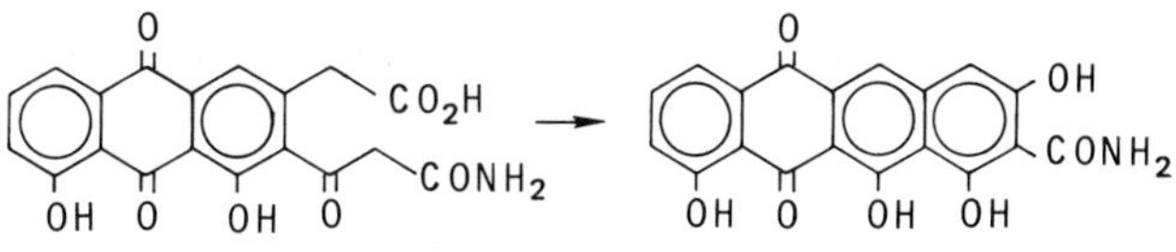

(13) (14)

hydroxylation at C_6 is surely a later step and it is meaningful in this regard that 15 is not optically active despite having an asymmetric center. This implies a non-enzymatic origin for the OH group. Cyclization *in vitro* to 16 can be accomplished by acid treatment.

The naphthacenic pretetramides of biosynthetic intermediacy have been prepared by total synthesis, partial degradation of tetracyclines, transformation of other pretetramides and isolation from blocked mutants.

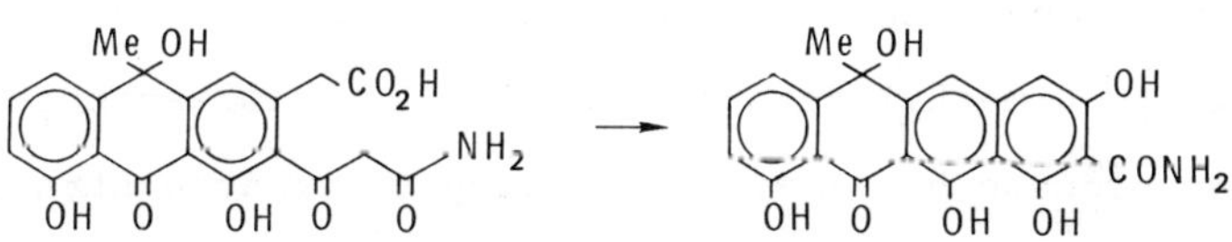

(15) (16)

3.5---Pretetramides prepared by total synthesis.

The structurally simplest of the pretetramides for which intermediacy has been established is pretetramide itself (20).[28] Obviously, the Friedel-Crafts condensation of 17 with 18 could have proceeded in two fashions although 19 is the only product reported. The synthesis of 20 was completed by strenuous reduction with KI and KH_2PO_2. When 20 was fed to *S. aureofaciens* strain V828, 6-DMCTC was formed in 8%

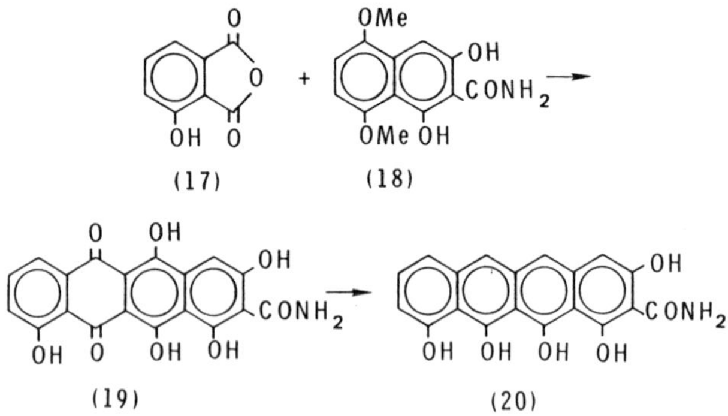

yield. The fact that chlorination, but not methylation, could be accomplished by this culture is quite revealing.

3.6---Pretetramides prepared by partial degradation of tetracyclines.

Acid catalyzed dehydration of dedimethylamino-12a-deoxyoxytetracycline (21), preparable from OTC, leads directly to 6-methylpretetramide (5).[29] This essentially circular process has limited capacity to produce structurally novel tetracyclines but has been very useful in elucidating the normal sequence. 6-Methylpretetramide is extremely useful in that it has been converted to a variety of tetracyclines depending on the cell-line used. *S aureofaciens* strain V828 gives a 75% conversion to CTC when fed 5 while strain ED1369 gives a 50% conversion. Strain F-198-1, which lacks chlorinating enzyme, gives

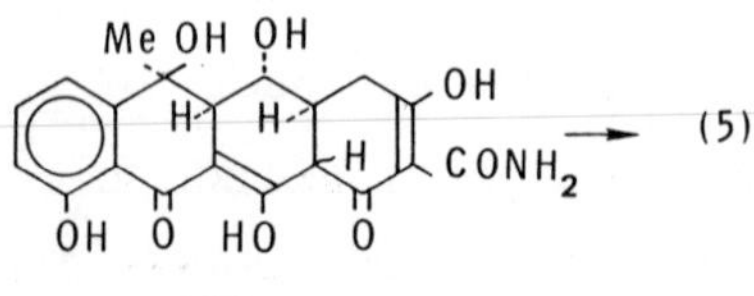

(21)

28% of TC. The intermediate status of 5 seems well substantiated by these studies even though it has not been isolated as yet from a blocked mutant.

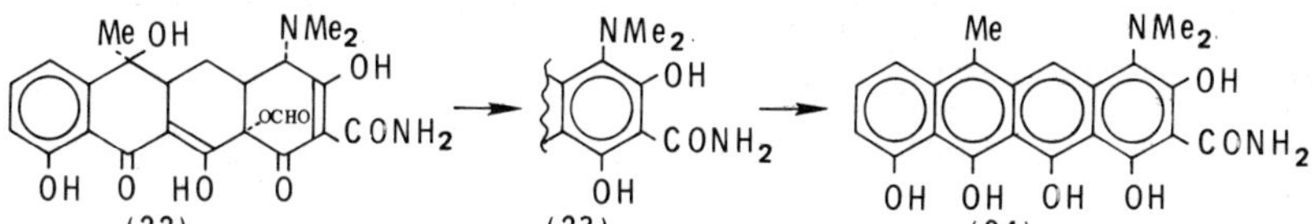

(22) (23) (24)

Tetracycline forms a 12a-formyl ester (22) when heated with acetic formic anhydride. Pyrolysis of the latter aromatizes the A ring to give 23. Acid treatment dehydrates the tertiary alcohol group at C_6 to produce 4-dimethylamino-6-methylpretetramide (24). When fed to various strains, a 6-15% yield of TC or CTC was achieved. Careful examination of this reaction showed this result to be fortuitous as, when the transformation is carried out in the presence of labeled methionine, the N-methyl groups become radioactive. Thus, partial biological degradation followed by resynthesis is taking place and 24 is not a true intermediate.

Similar work with 4-dimethylamino-7-chloropretetramide (25), prepared from DMCTC, led to a 7-10% bioconversion back to DMCTC.

These findings engendered an interest in preparing novel pretetramides and exploring their biological properties.

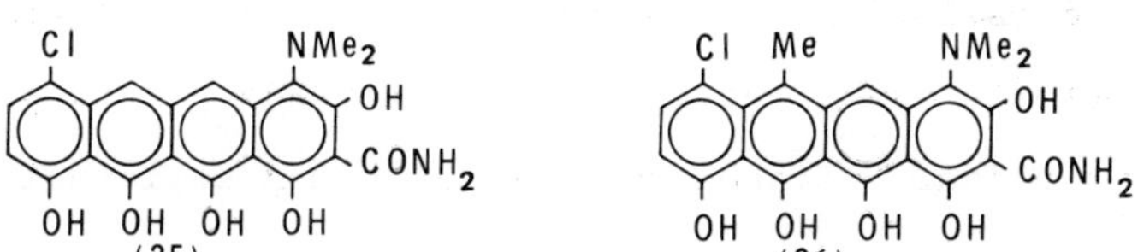

(25) (26)

Subsequently, in addition to a number of alternate paths to 6, 20, 24 and 25, analog 26 was also made.[30] The principle chemical lesson from this work is that pretetramides can be formed from a variety of partially alicyclic substances under fairly strenuous acidic dehydrating conditions and that OH and NMe_2 groups para to a phenolic OH group can be selectively removed.

The biosynthetic results obtained with these pretetramides all speak to the early inclusion of the pro C_6 methyl and that this step is optional - the biosynthesis proceeding apparently as well without it as with it, although use of methylation inhibitors such as aminopterin, sulfonamides or ethionine to divert the biosynthesis to production of DMCTC may result in lower overall yields.[31-35] Amusingly, such efforts with ethionine occasionally lead to substitution as well as inhibition. The N-ethyl-N-methyl analog of OTC has been isolated following fermentation under these conditions.[36] These studies represent successful attempts to apply fundamental biosynthetic knowledge to practical purposes although the final products have not seen clinical use.

3.7---Pretetramides isolated from blocked mutants-4-hydroxypretetramides.

The power of cosynthesis as a technique[37] for genetic mapping and isolation of biosynthetic intermediates from blocked mutants where the block is in secondary metabolism and not in primary metabolism where it would be lethal and obvious, was shown by the discovery of the next substance in the sequence, 4-hydroxy-6-methyl pretetramide (27).[38,39] When isolated from mutant V655 and fed to mutant ED1369, a 75% bioconversion to CTC was achieved. This provided convincing experimental support for the polyketide-pretetramide theory and suggested that the next biosynthetic step from 5 is para-hydroxylation, a step with ample biological precedent. Chlorination is obviously still to come.

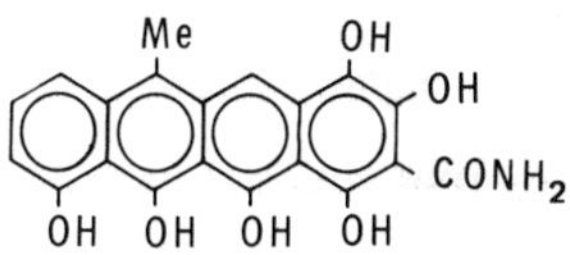

(27)

Fortunately, a convenient partial synthesis of 27 has been developed so these materials are fairly easily available.[40-42] Anhydro TC or CTC can be quaternized with methyl iodide and converted to their betaines (28) by careful pH adjustment. Refluxing this in acetonitrile led to 27. It is postulated that this proceeds via a Hoffman/Cope elimination to 29 followed by scission of ring B to form ketene 30 which then acylates highly reactive ring A, after rotation about the C_{4a} bond, to give 27. The same compound was obtained by heating TC betaine followed by acid elimination.

Some unusual pretetramides were made in the same fashion by using the betaine (31) derived from DMCTC or its deschloro analog. Heating eliminated trimethylamine and

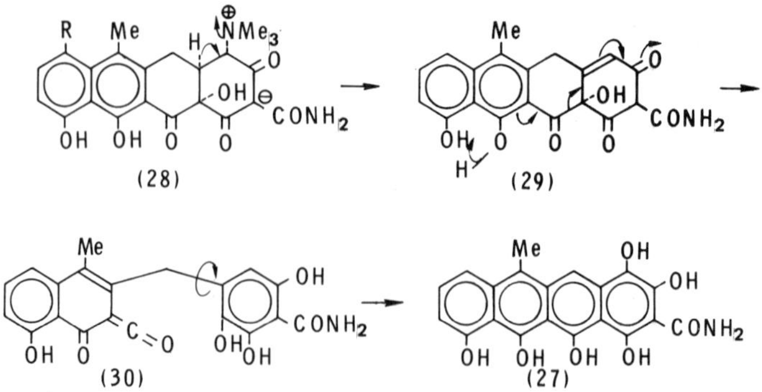

rearranged the molecule to 32. Next, chlorination at the highly reactive C_{11a} position was accomplished with N-chlorosuccinimide and dehydrohalogenation with tetraethylammonium bromide led to 4,6-dihydroxypretetramide (34) with or without a Cl at C_7. Unfortunately, attempts to convert these hydroquinones to new tetracyclines using blocked cultures were unsuccessful.

Some oxidative studies have been made on these compounds but the results are not of biosynthetic interest.[43,4] This work did, however, show that compounds of this type which have a methyl group at C_6, add oxygen readily at that

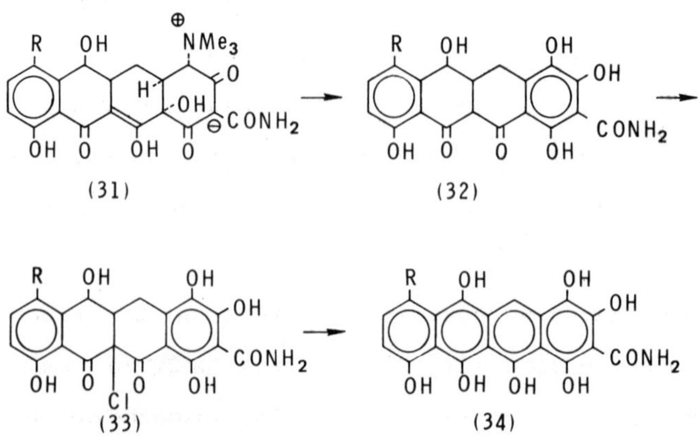

position. This is suggestive in light of the structures of the protetrones described earlier.

3.8---4-Ketoanhydrotetracyclines.

Those intermediates which logically appear to belong next in the sequence and for which precursor activity has been demonstrated in vivo are the 4-ketoanhydrotetracyclines. These have been prepared synthetically from anhydrotetracyclines (35) by use of mercuric acetate oxidation[45] and by dehydration of the tetracycloxides (38),[46] which are themselves formed under enamine generating conditions from DMCTC (37).[47-50] When fed to whole cell or cell-free preparations, successful bioconversion to tetracycline and chlortetracycline has been achieved.[4,51] These experiments are rather difficult to perform because 36 and its analogs are extremely unstable. Warming in solution, or even performing an nmr leads to lactone formation (40), probably via ketene 39.[52] Perhaps this explains failure to synthesize the 4-ketoanhydrotetracyclines by oxidation of the corresponding 4-hydroxy-6-methylpretetramide.[53]

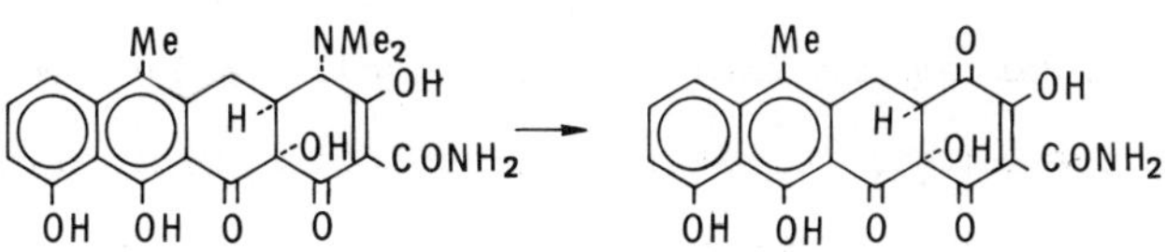

(35) (36)

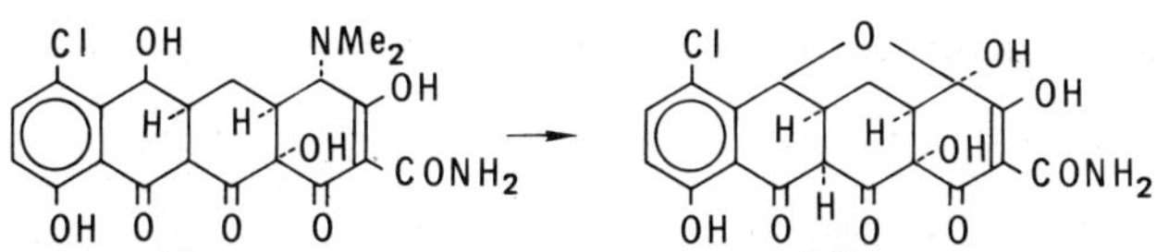

(37) (38)

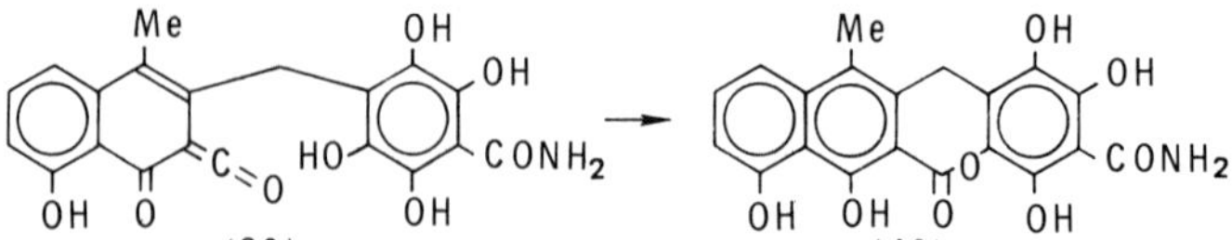

(39) (40)

3.9---The 4-aminoanhydrotetracyclines.

The next piece of evidence bearing on the proposed sequence was provided by experiments using genetically competent strains. Addition of ethionine at a suitable point in the fermentation antagonizes methionine utilization and tetracycline biosynthesis is shut off at an intermediate stage.[54] Precursors accumulated and could be detected conveniently and quantitatively by assaying cellular extracts in the presence of radiolabeled methionine in a cell-free enzyme preparation made by sonication of suitable tetracycline producing streptomyces.[4] The competence of these cell-free systems was a powerful tool as diffusion and permiability barriers were no longer factors of concern. A variety of these intermediates were isolated and characterized and 41 is typical. They are apparently reductive transamination products of 36. These materials could be converted to finished tetracyclines but neither the cell-free system nor blocked mutants could chlorinate them so this step must lie between 36 and 41. Various degrees of methylation are present in these substances showing that the three methionine derived carbons of the tetracyclines are sensitive to differing extents to the inhibitory effect of ethionine. In the cell-free system, it could be shown that N-methylation occurs stepwise via 42 to 43, but no C-methylation of the C_6 demethyl analogs of 41 (for example, 44) could be demonstrated.

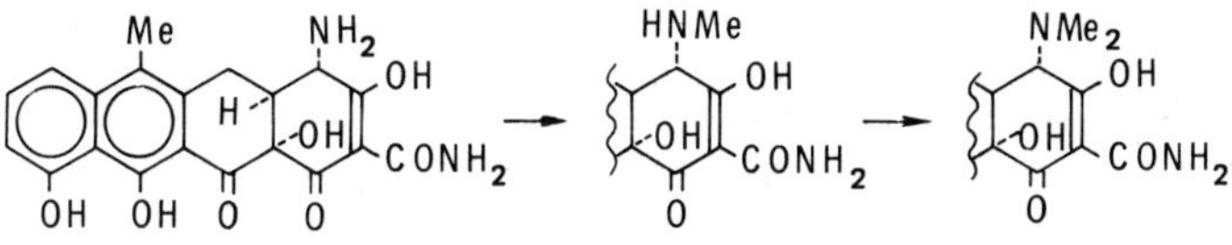

(41) (42) (43)

This data received strong additional support when blocked S. aureofaciens mutant 1E 1407 was shown to accumulate 44 and that 44 could be converted by S. aureofaciens mutant V828 to DMCTC in 34% yield.[55]

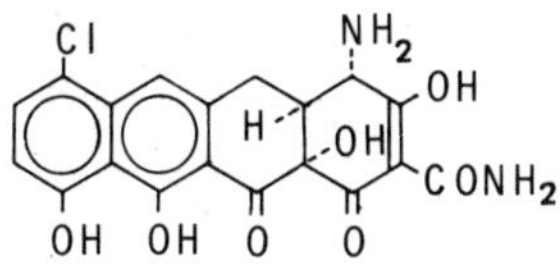

(44)

The biologically unnatural 4-epi series (45) could be prepared by epimerization of the 4-aminoanhydrotetracyclines and were inert as precursors.[56] Subsequent work showed that the analogs 4-dedimethylaminoanhydrotetracycline (46) and 4-hydroxy-4-dedimethylaminoanhydrotetracycline (47) were also inert.

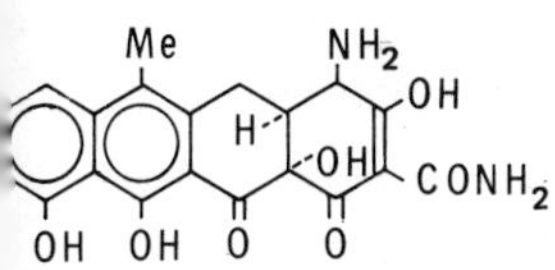

(45)

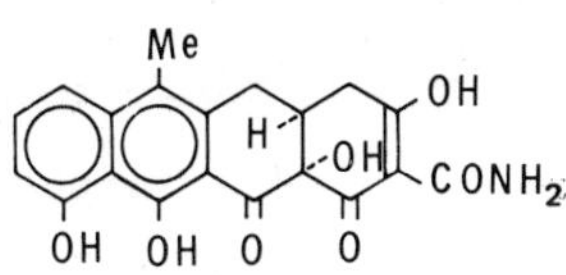

(46)

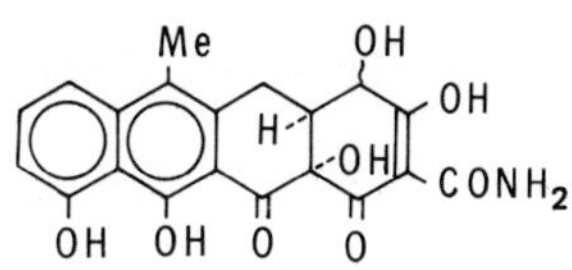

(47)

3.10--The anhydrotetracyclines.

The products of stepwise biological methylation of the 4-amino precursors, the anhydrotetracyclines (43), are readily prepared from the tetracyclines themselves and had been shown quite early to be converted back to the parent antibiotics by the appropriate cell lines.[57] The results obtained are collected in Table 3-1. Note especially that while anhydrotetracycline was a suitable precursor for either TC or OTC depending upon whether S. aureofaciens or S. rimosus strains are employed, S. aureofaciens will convert anhydrochlortetracycline to CTC, S. rimosus will not accept it as a substrate. This was taken as explaining why oxychlortetracycline (50) had never been encountered as a natural product.

Subsequently, 6-demethylanhydrochlortetracycline was isolated from blocked mutant S. aureofaciens strain 1E-6113 to provide welcome additional support for the biological intermediacy of the anhydrotetracyclines.[58]

3.11--The dehydrotetracyclines.

Of the two steps remaining in the sequence, hydroxylation at C_6 preceeds 5a,lla-reduction. It will be recalled from Table 3-1 that S. aureofaciens strain S-1308 did not convert anhydrochlortetracycline to CTC, but stopped at 5a,lla-dehydrochlortetracycline (48). This substance was one of the first biosynthetically incomplete tetracyclines to be isolated and characterized.[59] Its further bioconversion to CTC was soon demonstrated.[60] Apparently, the biochemical lesion which leads to accumulation of 48 can either be lack of the appropriate reductase, or its coenzyme, known as cofactor 1.[61]

Table 3-1. Bioconversion of some anhydrotetracyclines to tetracyclines using blocked mutant cultures.[51]

Substrate	Product	Culture
Anhydrotetracycline	TC	_S._ _aureofaciens_ BC-41
Anhydrotetracycline	OTC	_S._ _rimosus_ T1686B
Anhydro-7-chloro-tetracycline	None	_S._ _rimosus_ T1686B
Anhydro-7-chloro-tetracycline	CTC	_S._ _aureofaciens_ BC-41
Anhydro-7-chloro-tetracycline	5a,11a-dehydroCTC	_S._ _aureofaciens_ S-1308
Anhydrodemethyl-tetracycline	DMTC	_S._ _aureofaciens_ S-2242
Anhydrodemethyl-tetracycline	None	_S._ _rimosus_ T1686B
Anhydrodemethyl-chlortetracycline	DMCTC	_S._ _aureofaciens_ S-2311
Anhydrooxytetracycline	OTC	_S._ _aureofaciens_ V-828
4-Epianhydrotetracycline	None	_S._ _aureofaciens_ T-219

The dehydrotetracyclines are often difficult to work with because of their instability, but dehydrotetracycline has been isolated in microgram quantities and precursor activity was demonstrated.[62] Dehydrooxytetracycline has likewise been characterized. Dehydrotetracycline has been reported to rearrange to 5β-hydroxyanhydrotetracycline in acid solution.[63] This interesting reaction appears to be without biosynthetic significance.

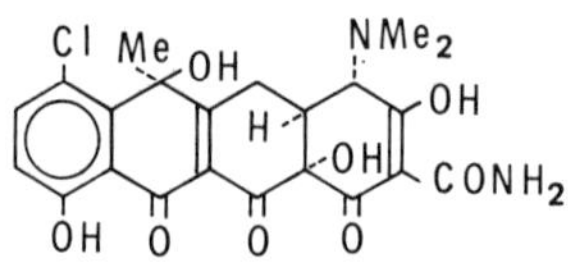

(48)

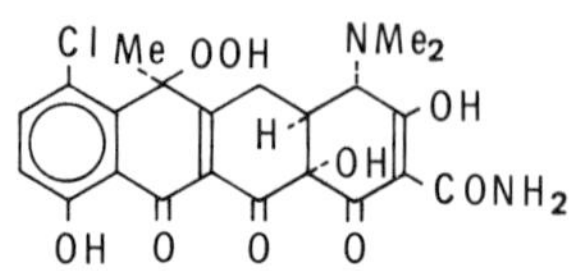

(49)

In a biogenetic-like synthesis, anhydrochlortetracycline has been photooxygenated to its 6-hydroperoxy analog (49) and conditions could be found by which reduction to TC could be accomplished.[64] No conversion of 49 could, however, be achieved in cell-free biosynthetic experiments.[4]

3.12--Biosynthetic preparation of oxychlortetracycline.

A practical application of these methods which promise to be an important research technique for the future led to the development of oxychlortetracycline (50) a long sought but previously elusive antibiotic.[65] It will be recalled that cultures frequently produce mixtures of CTC and TC, or CTC and DMCTC or TC and OTC, but no *S. rimosus* culture ever produced a chlorinated tetracycline. As it was also known that anhydrochlortetracycline was not a suitable substrate for *S. rimosus*, there remained only the hope that 5a,11a-dehydrochlortetracycline (48) would be accepted by the S. rimosus reductase. Ultimately, conditions were found whereby 50 could be so produced and tested. It is quite active as an antibiotic, but its pronounced instability precludes any practical application of this substance in the clinic.[66,67]

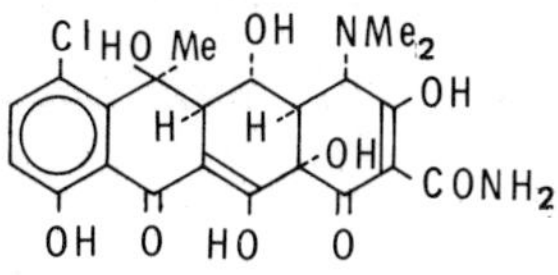

(50)

Hopefully, other semiartificial studies will be reported in the future -- perhaps involving artificial pretetramides.

3.13--Summary.

The overall sequence and its branch points can be summarized as in the scheme. The branches occur when a step is missing. The branch products then go on in parallel. Thus, the biosynthesis of the tetracyclines is a network of biochemical reactions rather than a single discreet pathway.

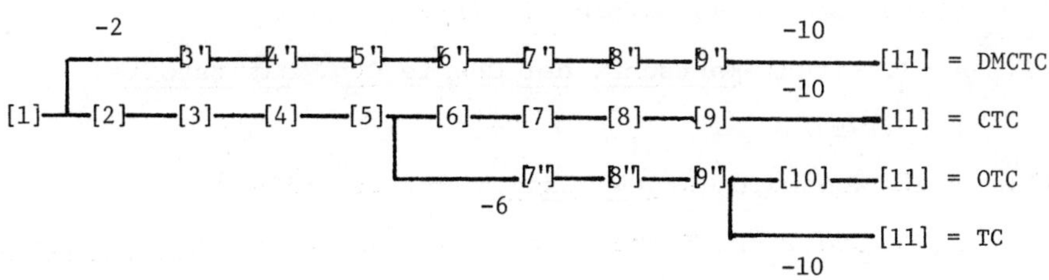

1 = Raw culture materials (acetate, etc.)
2 = Polyketide processing - especially methylation
3 = Pretetramide
4 = Hydroxylation at C_4
5 = C_{12a}-Hydroxylation
6 = C_7-Chlorination
7 = Reductive amination at C_4
8 = N-Methylation
9 = C_6-Hydroxylation
10 = C_5-Hydroxylation
11 = 5a,11a-Reduction

REFERENCES

1. J. R. D. McCormick *in* "Antibiotics, Advances in Research, Production, and Clinical Use," M. Herold and Z. Gabriel, Eds., Butterworths, London, 556 (1966).
2. J. R. D. McCormick *in* "Biogenesis of Antibiotic Substances, Z. Vanek and Z. Hostalek, Eds., Academic Press, N. Y., Ch. 8 (1965).
3. J. R. D. McCormick *in* "Antibiotics II. Biosynthesis," D. Gottlieb and P. D. Shaw, Eds., Springer Verlag, N. Y. 111 (1967).
4. P. A. Miller, *Developments in Industrial Microbiology*, *8*, 96 (1967).
5. R. H. Turley and J. F. Snell *in* "Biosynthesis of Antibiotics. I," J. F. Snell, Ed., Academic Press, N. Y., 95 (1966).
6. L. A. Mitscher, *J. Pharm. Sci.*, *57*, 1633 (1968).
7. M. A. Petty, *Bacteriol. Revs.*, *25*, 111 (1961).
8. R. Robinson, "Structural Relations of Natural Products," Clarendon Press, Oxford, 58 (1955).
9. A. J. Birch, *Fortschr. der Chemie Org. Naturstoffe*, *14*, 186 (1957).
10. R. B. Woodward, *Angew. Chem.*, *68*, 13 (1956).
11. J. F. Snell, R. Wagner and F. A. Hochstein, *Proc. Internat. Conf. Peaceful Uses of Atomic Energy*, *12*, 431 (1955).
12. J. F. Snell, *Atompraxis*, *7*, 460 (1961).
13. P. A. Miller, J. R. D. McCormick and A. P. Doerschuk, *Science*, *123*, 1030 (1956).

14. A. J. Birch, J. F. Snell and P. J. Thompson, J. Chem. Soc., 425 (1962).

15. J. R. D. McCormick, N. O. Sjolander, S. Johnson and A. P. Doerschuk, J. Bacteriol., 77, 475 (1959).

16. A. P. Doerschuk, J. R. D. McCormick, J. J. Goodman, S. A. Szumski, J. A. Growich, P. A. Miller, B. A. Bitler, E. R. Jensen, M. Matrishin, M. A. Petty and A. S. Phelps, J. Am. Chem. Soc., 81, 3069 (1959).

17. A. J. Birch, Proc. Chem. Soc., 3 (1962).

18. A. J. Birch, Science, 156, 202 (1967).

19. J. F. Snell, A. J. Birch and P. J. Thompson, J. Am. Chem. Soc., 82, 2402 (1960).

20. N. Behal, M. Podojil, Z. Hostalek, Z. Namek and F. Lynen, Folia Microbiol., 19, 146 (1974).

21. S. Gatenbeck, Biochem. Biophys. Res. Commun., 6, 422 (1962).

22. F. A. Hochstein, M. Schach von Wittenau, F. W. Tanner and K. Murai, J. Am. Chem. Soc., 82, 5934 (1960).

23. M. W. Miller and F. A. Hochstein, J. Org. Chem., 27, 2525 (1962).

24. G. C. Lancini and P. Sensi, Experientia, 20, 83 (1964).

25. E. R. Catlin, C. H. Hassall and D. R. Parry, J. Chem. Soc., Ser. C., 1363 (1969).

26. J. R. D. McCormick and E. R. Jensen, J. Am. Chem. Soc., 90, 7126 (1968).

27. J. R. D. McCormick, E. R. Jensen, N. H. Arnold, H. S. Corey, U. H. Joachim, S. Johnson, P. A. Miller and N. O. Sjolander, J. Am. Chem. Soc., 90, 7127 (1968).

28. J. R. D. McCormick, J. Reichenthal, S. Johnson and N. O. Sjolander, J. Am. Chem. Soc., 85, 1694 (1963).

29. J. R. D. McCormick, S. Johnson and N. O. Sjolander, J. Am. Chem. Soc., 85, 1692 (1963).

30. U. S. Patent 3,345,409 (1968).

31. S. J. Neidleman, E. Albu and E. Bienstock, Biotechnol. Bioengineering, 5, 87 (1963).

32. S. L. Neidleman, E. Bienstock and R. E. Bennett, Biochem. Biophys. Acta, 71, 199 (1963).

33. D. Hendlin, E. L. Dulaney, D. Dreschler, T. Cook and L. Chaiet, Biochem. Biophys. Acta, 58, 635 (1962).

34. W. A. Zygmunt, J. Bacteriol., 84, 1126 (1962).

35. J. J. Goodman and P. A. Miller, Biotechnol. Bioengineering 4, 391 (1962).

36. E. L. Dulaney, I. Putter, D. Dreschler, L. Chaiet, W. J. Miller, F. J. Wolf and D. Hendlin, Biochem. Biophys. Acta, 60, 447 (1962).

37. J. R. D. McCormick, U. Hirsch, N. O. Sjolander and A. P. D. Doerschuk, J. Am. Chem. Soc., 82, 5006 (1960).

38. J. R. D. McCormick, U. H. Joachim, E. R. Jensen, S. Johnson and N. O. Sjolander, J. Am. Chem. Soc., 87, 1793 (1965).

39. J. R. D. McCormick and E. R. Jensen, J. Am. Chem. Soc., 87, 1794 (1965).

40. J. J. Hlavka, P. Bitha and J. H. Boothe, J. Am. Chem. Soc., 90, 1034 (1968).

41. J. J. Hlavka, P. Bitha and J. H. Boothe, J. Am. Chem. Soc., 87, 1796 (1965).

42. J. J. Hlavka, P. Bitha and J. H. Boothe, Tet. Letts., 1139 (1967).

43. J. E. Baldwin, D. H. R. Barton, L. Bould and P. D. Magnus, Chem. Commun., 319 (1967).

44. C. H. Hassall and T. E. Winters, J. Chem. Soc., Ser. C., 1558 (1968).

45. L. A. Mitscher and J. H. E. J. Martin, Unpublished experiments.

46. R. K. Blackwood and C. R. Stephens, J. Am. Chem. Soc., 86, 2736 (1964).

47. R. C. Esse, J. A. Lowery, C. R. Tamorria and G. M. Sieger, J. Am. Chem. Soc., 86, 3875 (1964).

48. R. C. Esse, J. A. Lowery, C. R. Tamorria and G. M. Sieger, J. Am. Chem. Soc., 86, 3874 (1964).

49. R. K. Blackwood and C. R. Stephens, Can. J. Chem., 43, 1382 (1965).

50. J. S. P. Schwarz, H. E. Applegate, J. L. Bouchard and F. L. Weisenborn, J. Org. Chem., 32, 1238 (1967).

51. Reference 3, p. 117.

52. A. I. Scott, E. Yamaguchi and S. -K. Chung, Tet. Letts., 1369 (1975).

53. D. H. R. Barton, L. Bould, D. L. J. Clive, P. D. Magnus and T. Hase, J. Chem. Soc., Ser. C., 2206 (1971).

54. P. A. Miller, A. Saturnelli, J. H. Martin, L. A. Mitscher and N. Bohonos, Biochem. Biophys. Res. Commun., 16, 285 (1964).

55. J. R. D. McCormick, E. R. Jensen, S. Johnson and N. O. Sjolander, J. Am. Chem. Soc., 90, 2201 (1968).

56. F. Barbatschi, M. Dann, J. H. Martin, P. A. Miller, L. A. Mitscher and N. Bohonos, Experientia, 21, 162 (1965).

57. J. R. D. McCormick, P. A. Miller, S. Johnson, N. Arnold and N. O. Sjolander, J. Am. Chem. Soc., 84, 3023 (1962).

58. J. R. D. McCormick and E. R. Jensen, J. Am. Chem. Soc., 91, 206 (1969).

59. J. R. D. McCormick, P. A. Miller, J. A. Growich, N. O. Sjolander and A. P. Doerschuk, J. Am. Chem. Soc., 80, 5572 (1958).

60. J. R. D. McCormick, N. O. Sjolander, P. A. Miller, U. Hirsch, N. H. Arnold and A. P. Doerschuk, J. Am. Chem. Soc., 80, 6460 (1958).

61. P. A. Miller, N. O. Sjolander, S. Nalesnyk, N. Arnold, S. Johnson, A. P. Doerschuk and J. R. D. McCormick, J. Am. Chem. Soc., 82, 5002 (1960).

62. P. A. Miller, J. H. Hash, M. Lincks and N. Bohonos, Biochem. Biophys. Res. Commun., 18, 325 (1965).

63. Reference 2, page 82.

64. A. I. Scott and C. T. Bedford, J. Am. Chem. Soc., 84, 2271 (1962).

65. L. A. Mitscher, J. H. Martin, P. A. Miller, P. Shu and N. Bohonos, J. Am. Chem. Soc., 88, 3647 (1966).

66. J. H. Martin, L. A. Mitscher, P. A. Miller, P. Shu and N. Bohonos, Antimicrob. Agts. Chemother., 563 (1966).

67. L. A. Mitscher, J. H. Martin, A. Dornbush, L. Leeson and G. Redin, Antimicrob. Agts. Chemother., 568 (1966).

CHAPTER 4

SPECTROSCOPY AND ANALYSIS

4.1---Introduction.

Spectroscopy plays a strong role in the structural analysis of tetracyclines as it does, indeed, with most classes of complex natural products. Initially, the spectra were utilized for identification of individual agents and then for analysis. More recently, more subtle questions of conformation and binding sites are being addressed. As each new technique is developed, it quickly becomes applied to the tetracyclines so that structural characterization is now a relatively simple task.

4.2---Infrared spectra.

The tetracyclines are not sufficiently soluble in convenient solvents such as chloroform, so their IR spectra are usually determined in KBr wafers or mineral oil mulls. The spectra are primarily used for identification purposes, relatively little structural information being directly discernable in the spectra themselves. The carbonyl region

(5.5 to 6.0 microns) is of greatest value to chemists, but the several carbonyl groups of the tetracyclines are amide in character, or conjugated to double bond systems, or strongly hydrogen bonded. Thus, the amide band, at about 6 microns, and the large carbonyl envelope near 6.2 microns are virtually identical for almost all the tetracyclines whose spectra, then, differ mostly in the fingerprint regions below 6 microns. This relatively unfortunate circumstance has resulted in there being no papers in the literature in which detailed discussion of their IR is set forth. On the other hand, in specific molecules, carbonyl or other singular absorptions appear and because of their unusual nature are important structural clues.

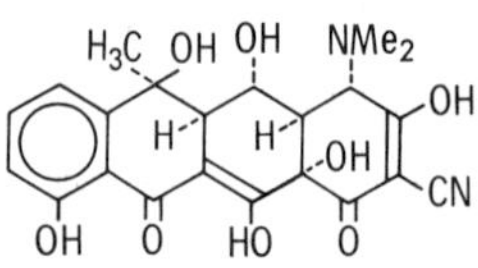

(1)

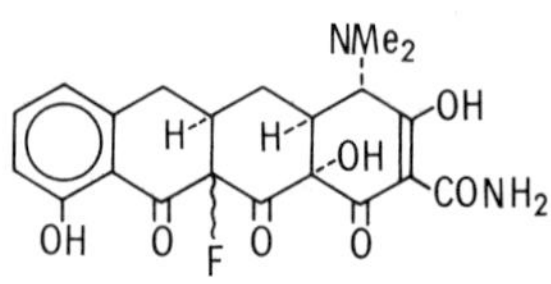

(2)

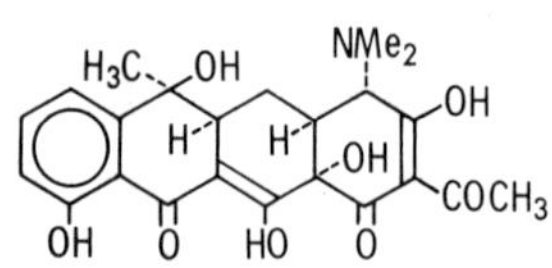

(3)

For example, the tetracycline nitriles (1) have a typical C≡N band at 4.5 microns.[1] The C_{12} carbonyl group of 11a-fluoro-6-demethyl-6-deoxytetracycline (2) cannot enolize toward C_{11a} and so it appears at 5.7 microns, well away from the other carbonyl frequencies.[2] The C_{12a} formyl ester of OTC has the formate ester band at about 5.8 microns.[3] The C-acetyl function of the naturally occurring 2-acetyl tetracyclines, such as 3, occurs at 5.95 microns.[4]

In each of these cases, the band has diagnostic value because it lies in a region which is otherwise transparent amongst tetracyclines.

4.3---Ultraviolet spectra.

The quaternary carbon at C_{12a} separates the chromophores of the tetracyclines into two relatively distinct regions. The β-tricarbonyl system of ring A contributes a strong absorption band at about 260 nm while the aromatic ring D conjugates with the β-diketone moiety in rings B and C to produce a visible band at about 360 nm (accounting for the pale to bright yellow color of the tetracyclines), a series of shoulders and inflections at about 310 nm and two strong bands at about 260 and 230 nm. The 260 nm band overlaps with the 260 nm band of the A ring chromophore.

Selected spectra are recorded in Table 4-1.

When base is added to such solutions, ionization results in a characteristic bathochromic shift of the visible peak. Chelating metals also produce a bathochromic shift, but, as would be expected from their greater

Table 4-1. Ultraviolet visible spectra of representative tetracyclines in alcoholic 0.01 N HCl.[5]

Tetracycline	UV-Vis Maxima
TC	363 nm (log ε 4.14), 268 (4.27)
CTC	355 (4.0), 270 (4.0)
OTC	357 (4.10), 267 (4.32)
MOTC	345 (4.19), 253 (4.37)
DOOTC	351 (4.12), 267 (4.24)
4-Epitetracycline	365 (4.2), 255 (4.2)
Anhydrotetracycline	425 (3.9), 275 (4.6)

efficiency at displacing protons, the shifts occur at lower pH's than with base alone.[6] From the bands involved, most investigators have come to believe that the BCD chromophore is actively involved as a chelating site,[7-11] while some investigators infer a supplimentary or alternate A ring binding site on various grounds.

The point is of theoretical import, but also of practical interest on a variety of grounds. It has long been known that some metal ions can neutralize the anti-bacterial effect of tetracyclines on bacterial cultures.[12,13] The dramatic effect of chelation on bioavailability and solubility of the tetracyclines has been alluded to in Chapters 1 and 2 and is reinforced in pharmaceutical terms,[14-16] in studies of the effect of Ca ion on absorption from the small intestine,[17,18] and in back-epimerizing the 4-epi-tetracyclines,[19] for example.

The pronounced lengthening of the visible band position upon dehydration at 5a, 6 is quite understandable and the ratio of the peaks at 425 and 363 nm provides an assay for the presence of these two drugs in mixtures.

The essential correctness of the uv band assignments is supported on very many grounds including the coincidence of the uv spectrum of synthetic 2-acetyl-8-hydroxyindanone (4) in acidic and alkaline methanolic solutions and in the

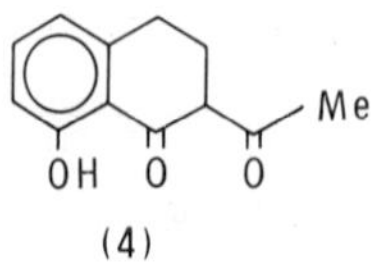

(4)

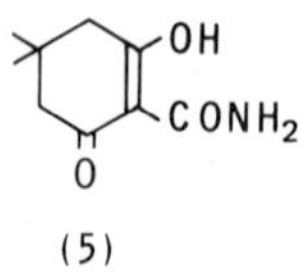

(5)

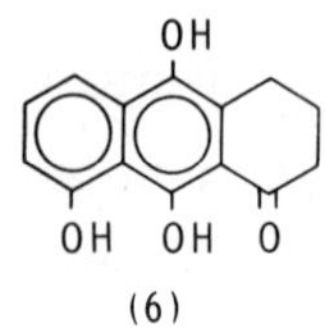

(6)

presence of chelating ions with the BCD bands of the tetracyclines.[6] Likewise, the uv of 2-carboxamidodimedone (5) lies in the expected 260 nm region.[1*] Hydroquinone 6 is virtually the same in the visible region as that of anhydrotetracycline.[20]

As might be expected, for example, the uv spectrum of 7 is dramatically different from that of MOTC showing instead bands at 374 (3.60), 274 (4.27), and 237 (4.34) nm.[6] The uv spectrum provided, in this case, prima facia evidence that the BCD moiety had been dramatically altered.

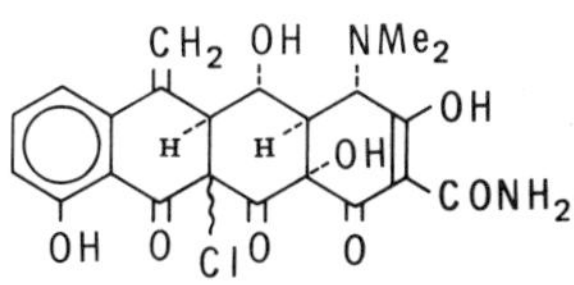

(7)

4.4---Nuclear magnetic resonance spectra.

Limitations of solubility and the relatively few strategically placed hydrogen atoms somewhat hindered the most effective use of proton magnetic resonance measurements in the days before the general availability of Fourier-transform and computer-of-average-transients techniques. Nevertheless, use of dimethyl sulfoxide, trifluoroacetic acid and pyridine solutions has been extremely useful. Table 4-2 lists some of the more significant findings.

Particularly notable is the substantial downfield shift in the resonance due to the C_4 proton when the tetracyclines epimerize at C_4. This is especially

---

* See G. O. Dudek and G. P. Volpp, J. Org. Chem., 30, 50 (1965).

Table 4-2. PMR spectra of selected tetracyclines and degradation products.[21]

Substance	Solvent	Chemical Shift						
		$C_4\underline{H}$	$C_{4a}\underline{H}$	$C_5\underline{H}$	$C_{5a}\underline{H}$	$C_6\underline{H}$	$N\underline{Me}_2$	$C_6\underline{Me}$
TC	Pyridine	3.6	2.2-3.2	2.2-3.2	2.2-3.2	-	2.6	1.8
4-EpiTC	Pyridine	4.6	2.2-3.2	2.2-3.2	2.2-3.2	-	2.7	1.8
OTC	Pyridine	4.1	3.1	5.3	3.4	-	2.7	2.2
OTC•HCl	DMSO	3.8	2.9	4.8	2.9	-	2.9	1.7
α•DOOTC	Pyridine	3.9	2.8-3.1	4.5	2.8-3.1	2.8-3.1	2.7	1.7
β•DOOTC•HCl	Pyridine	3.9-4.3	3.0-4.3	5.3	3.0-4.3	3.0-4.3	3.3	1.0
AnhydroTC	TFA	4.2	3.1-3.7	3.1-3.7	-	-	3.3	2.4
4-EpianhydroTC	TFA	5.2	3.0-3.9	3.0-3.9	-	-	3.5	2.3

convenient as both isomers are usually available and can be distinguished easily in this way. Of course, they can also be distinguished readily microbiologically and, as will be seen shortly, by circular dichroism spectroscopy. The nmr shift appears to be general regardless of solvent being seen in pyridine,[21] trifluoroacetic acid,[21] and dimethyl sulfoxide.[22]

The contiguous hydrogen series on the upper periphery, especially of oxytetracycline, at C_4, C_{4a}, C_5, C_{5a} and, sometimes, C_6 are potentially suitable for settling conformational questions through use of the well-known Karplus relationship between coupling constant and dihedral angle. Unfortunately, the cis-AB ring juncture gives the tetracyclines considerable flexibility and the necessity of using concentrated non-aqueous solvents leaves prudent doubt about the general applicability of the findings to dilute physiological fluids and the question of tetracycline conformations have been attacked by a wide variety of experimental methods with variable results and the question of the most meaningful tetracycline conformation, unfortunately, must still be regarded as open. Under the conditions used in Table 4-2,[21] oxytetracycline clearly has conformation 8 as shown by the appropriate coupling constants (J_{4-4a}=9Hz; J_{4a-5}=0-2Hz; J_{5-5a}=4Hz).[21] The conformation of tetracycline, however, was different, being in accord with X-ray studies to be discussed later in this chapter. Conformation 9 is in accord with J_{4-4a}=4.5Hz.

More recently, carbon magnetic resonance measurements have been performed using the natural ^{13}C abundance.[23]

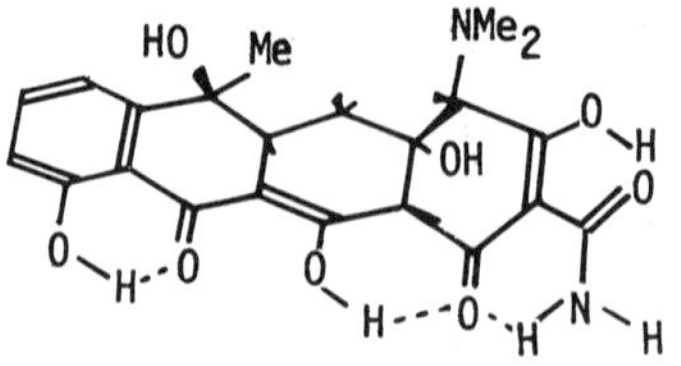

(8)

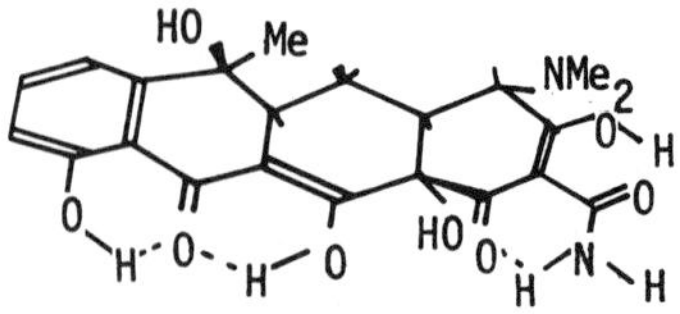

(9)

Many more resonances are present in these spectra compared with the pmr. The data for TC-HCl are set out in Table 4-3.

The β-shifts are useful in determining the order of deprotonation when the pH profile is measured.[23] These measurements have also been used to determine binding sites with complexing ions.[24] This subject is also one of vexing complexity and remains unclear. By this technique, clear evidence for a binding site in the A ring is clear from the selective broadening and shifting of signals when DMSO-d_6 is used as solvent. These findings confirm earlier work with the more limited pmr spectroscopy[25,26] but are of uncertain generality in aqueous solvents, especially as the conclusions are different from those seen in a number of other laboratories using other techniques.

In an attempt to overcome the inherent limitations of solubility, resort has been made to formation of the trimethylsilyl derivatives of the tetracyclines.[27] These derivatives are easily formed and are sufficiently soluble in CCl_4 for useful spectra to be obtained and the groups are removed easily using 50% aqueous methanol and a trace of acid. There is, however, the complicating feature of multiple reacting sites coming into play at different rates. This is illustrated with anhydrotetracycline (<u>10</u>) which reacts

Table 4-3. CMR spectrum of TC•HCl, 0.2 M in D_2O solvent. The signals are slightly different in DMSO.[22]

Carbon	Resonance	Gated Decoupling Complexity
1	193.9	
2	97.1	
$\underline{C}ONH_2$	173.0	
3	187.3	
4	70.7	
$H\overset{+}{N}\underline{Me}_2$	43.1	quartet
4a	35.0	doublet
5	27.3	triplet
5a	42.3	doublet
6	70.4	
$C-\underline{C}H_3$	22.1	
6a	146.7	
7	118.6	
8	138.4	
9	116.8	
10	161.9	
10a	115.1	
11	194.3	
11a	107.3	
12	172.3	
12a	74.4	

rapidly to form 11 and more sluggishly to form 12. Meaningful measurements cannot be carried out until equilibrium has been established.

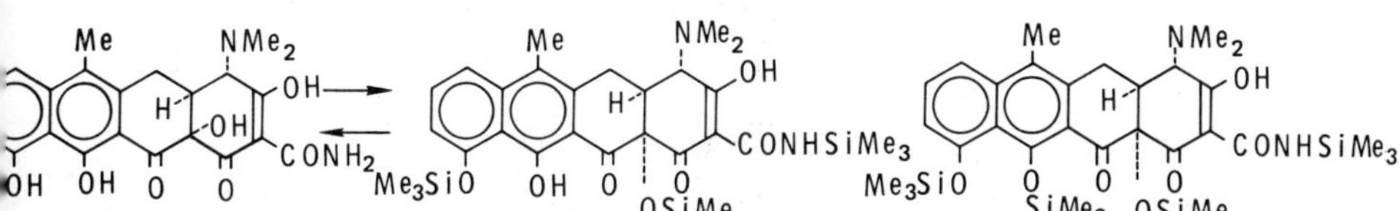

(10) (11) (12)

4.5---Mass spectrometry.

The tetracyclines are relatively non-volatile and are thermally unstable so that their electron-impact mass spectra are rich in fragment ions and weak in molecular ion intensity.[28] The identity of the various peaks in the fragmentation scheme is supported by high resolution mass measurements, substituent labeling and metastable ions. In common with most tertiary amines, this function dominates the fragmentation. Thermal dehydration at $C_{5a,6}$ is prominent and the majority of the spectrum of TC is identical with that of anhydroTC. In the highest mass region, then, one sees m/e 426 for dehydration followed by ions 409 and 391 resulting from loss of NH_3 and water from the carboxamide function as well as 381 for loss of the whole group as $CONH_3$. In addition, one sees m/e 366 for the loss of $MeNCH_2$ from 409 and 364 for the loss of Me_2NH also from 409. Ion 366 loses CO to produce 364. The only other peak still containing all four rings is m/e 320 which represents loss of CH_3NCH_2 and CO from 391.

The linear annelation of the rings inhibits fragmentations involving more than a single ring. Most of the fragments seen involve rings A and B because rings C and D so quickly become naphthalenoid. Fragments 13-18 clearly come from the A ring and are very intense. Ion 19

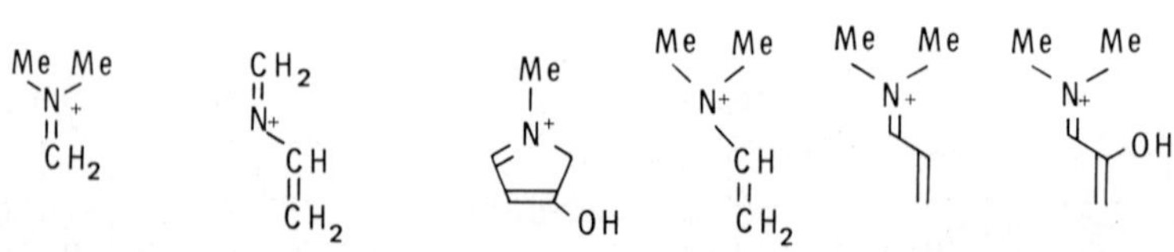

(13) (14) (15) (16) (17) (18)

and its McLafferty rearrangement product 20 are also significant. Ions 256 (21) and 170 (22) result from a retro Diels-Alder reaction and are structurally very revealing.

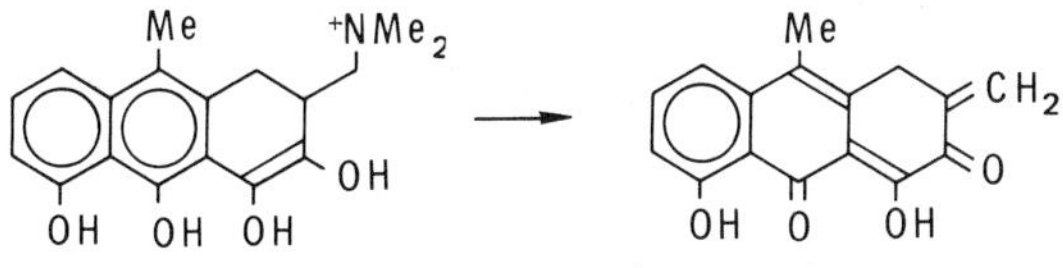

(19) (20)

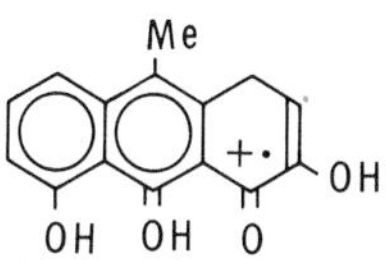

(21)

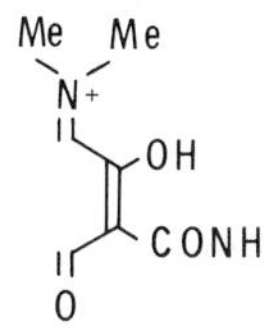

(22)

The chemical ionization (isobutane) mass spectra of the tetracyclines under ideal conditions produce intense molecule ions and, when fragmentation occurs, the retro Diels-Alder products 21 and 22 are often the dominant ions.[29] Unfortunately, the underivatized antibiotics do not give truly reproduceable spectra under standard conditions, diminishing the value of the method. The silyl ethers of Hassall promise one solution to this dilemma.[27]

4.6---Circular dichroism spectra.

Given the chiral nature of the tetracyclines and their complex chromophores, the tetracyclines provide excellent ORD-CD spectra. It was quickly concluded that the major bioactive tetracyclines all possess the same absolute configuration and solution conformation in acid solutions.[30,31] The composite nature of the 265 nm uv band was easily demonstrated as the BCD and A ring bands in this region are of opposite sign.

The intensity of the A ring band and its relative absence in 4-epitetracycline ultimately provided a sensitive assay for epimeric mixtures[32] and was rationalized in terms of the somewhat twisted A-ring chromophore of conformation 9.[30,31] Progressive disappearance of the 262 nmr band on raising the pH was consistent with a less twisted conformation wherein the C_{12a} OH and C_4NMe_2 groups are colinear in the physiological range. The ability of this technique to reflect subtle conformational shifts in dilute hydroxylic solvents under a wide variety of conditions is a particular strong point. Interaction with complexing ions gave dramatic changes in the spectral bands from both chromophoric regions providing evidence for chelation in both areas. Quantitative studies of ion binding led to the conclusion that little if any binding takes place below pH 3, that BCD binding takes place at pH 5 and that the A ring binds at physiological pH's.[33] It was also apparent that Mg ions induced a different conformation than Ca ions and that this phenomenon was particularly apparent with OTC.[33,34]

Other investigators have come to roughly the same conclusions with respect to the effect of ion binding on CD spectra of tetracyclines.[10,35]

More recently, the large differences in the CD spectra of the anhydrotetracyclines have been used to study the kinetics of epimerization of these materials.[36]

4.7---Potentiometric titrations and pKa determinations.

The macroscopic pKa values of the tetracycline antibiotics in aqueous solution are agreed to be approximately 3.3, 7.5 and 9.3 (Table 4-4).[9,37,38,39] After an initial misassignment,[40] the assignments were remade[41] and are now generally accepted.

The most acidic value is attributable to the unusual β-tricarbonyl system in ring A which is vinylogously like a carboxylic acid moiety in three directions in that loss of a proton produces a carbanion in which the negative charge can be distributed over C_1-C_3 and their pendant groups as illustrated in formula 23. The middle pKa is associated with the vinylogous acidic β-dicarbonyl system of rings B and C (24). The highest pKa is then assigned to the protonated dimethylamino function at C_4. Subsequent work has defined the microscopic dissociation constants[41] by use of pmr measurements of the chemical shifts of various non-labile protons as a function of pH.[42] The latter work[42] also reports a fourth pKa at 10.7 attributed to the phenolic OH groups at C_{10}.

Table 4-4. pKa values of selected tetracyclines in water at 25°.[39,40]

Antibiotic	pKa Values		
TC	3.30	7.68	9.69
CTC	3.30	7.44	9.27
OTC	3.27	7.32	9.11

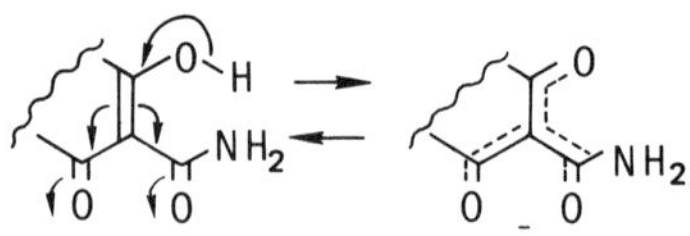

(23)

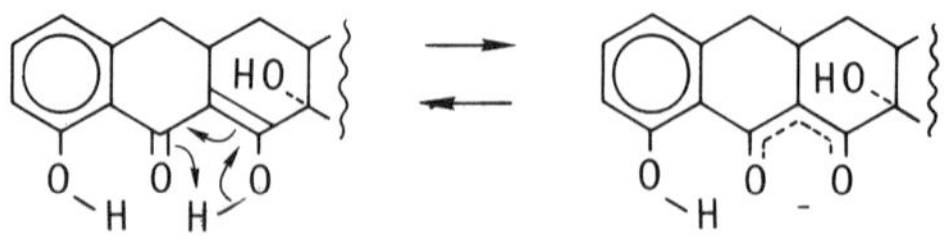

(24)

Having established these, the influence of chelating ions could be measured, as the ions displace protons in the act of binding.[9,37,38,43] Although the measurements become imprecise at higher pH's, clear evidence for BCD involvement was adduced.

4.8---X-ray crystal analysis.

The structures and solid state conformations of the tetracyclines have been carefully studied. CTC-HCl was determined first[44,45,46,47] and resulted in assignment of a conformation identical to 9. Subsequently, OTC-HCl was determined[47-50] but the configuration of the C_5OH was ambiguous. This was subsequently established beyond question by pmr measurements of 12a-epi OTC in which the conformational flexibility which complicates spectral interpretation is no longer a problem.[51] More recently, an X-ray study of 5,12a-diacetyloxytetracycline has settled this question beyond any reasonable doubt.[52] It is unlikely, however, if the unusual conformation adopted by this derivative has any biological relevance.

A brief report of the crystal structure of DMCTC-HCl has indicated the same solid state conformation as was reported for CTC and OTC.[53] TC-HCl also has the same solid state conformation as the rest and use of anomalous dispersion measurements confirmed the absolute configuration to be as generally depicted.[54]

An X-ray study has been published on 7-chloro-4-hydroxytetracycloxide, an interesting tetracycline synthon,[55] and one on anhydrotetracycline.[56]

One of the limitations of X-ray crystal studies is the static nature of the measurements. One normally cannot get much information regarding solution dynamics except by inference. A recent ambitious attempt to make a study of this type has given much useful information about the tetracyclines.[57,58] TC and OTC free bases were determined. The hydrated Zwitterions held conformations rather similar to that of the protonated antibiotics whereas the anhydrous form was rather like the 5,12a-diacetylOTC conformation.[57] It was felt that this form would be biologically relevant in cell compartments having a high lipid content. A crystal study of the mercuric chloride complex of OTC showed chelation only to A ring sites, however, the uv data presented was sufficiently atypical of other complexes to indicate that this data should not be generalized to include the Ca, Mg and Al ion complexes. At the same time, a crystal study of the dipotassium salt indicated binding to both the ring A and BCD sites -- one through O_1, O_{12} and O_{11}; and the other through O_1, O_{12a} and O_{12}. There was, unfortunately, high thermal motion in the crystal, however, hydrogen binding between the C_{12a}-OH and the C_4-NMe_2 groups was established making these groups colinear as in the flattened, non-twist form of 6 inferred from circular dichroism studies. There were, however, differences in the degree of puckering of the B ring and the 5,12a-diacetylOTC type conformation was clearly not seen.[58]

Work is needed in which X-ray data can be found for the Ca, Mg or Al ion complexes of the tetracyclines, but this work is difficult because of the enormous difficulty of growing suitable crystals.

4.9---Miscellaneous spectroscopic methods.

Because of their insolubility in almost all reasonable solvents, the cobalt and nickel ion complexes of the tetracyclines have been studied by reflectance methods leading to the conclusion that binding occurs in the A ring.[59] Magnetic moments have also been published.[59] In addition to uv wavelength shifts, the tetracycline Ca and Mg ion complexes give discrete fluorescence spectra which are quite characteristic.[10]

Solutions of tetracyclines in aqueous NaOH contain a surprisingly large concentration of free radicals which have been characterized by electron spin resonance methods.[60] As the tetracyclines may cleave under these conditions, it is dangerous to speculate as to the structure of the products with the data in hand.

4.10--Analytical methods - introduction.

In the United States, the law relegates responsibility for analytical standards of antibiotics to the Food and Drug Administration. The legal compendium, The United States Pharmacopea, simply is required to follow the F.D.A. in this. The regulations dealing with antibiotics are revised from time to time and are published in the Code of Federal Regulations, Title 21, which is available for purchase from the Superintendent of Documents, U. S. Government Printing Office, Washington, DC, 20402.

While the law places its primary reliance on microbiological methods, quite a number of other assays have been developed for special purposes and these have been critically reviewed.[61,62]

4.11--Microbiological methods.

The microbiological methods are generally the first applied to an antibiotic substance because of their sensitivity and because they can be applied long before any secure knowledge is obtained about the chemistry of the substance. They are corresondingly non-specific but are convenient and reflect the end use of the agents so remain the legal and practical basis of analysis of the tetracyclines, i. a. As an example, CTC-HCl is assayed by the cylinder plate method in the official compendium. A working standard is established compared to a primary standard antibiotic sample (1000 mcg/mg by definition). Suitable dilutions are prepared in 0.01N HCl and then working solutions are prepared from this stock by dilution to various concentrations in 1% phosphate buffer at pH 4.5 just before use. These are pipetted into stainless steel cylinders standing on an agar bed in a sterile petri dish. The surface layer of the agar has been diluted with a spore suspension of *Bacillus cereus var. mycoides* (ATCC 11778). After incubation, clear zones of inhibition are seen and the diameters of these zones are related to the log of the concentration of the antibiotic. Thus, it is possible to determine the potency of unknown samples.

An alternate assay procedure which has legal status is the turbidimetric method. In this case, various concentrations of antibiotic are incubated in liquid medium using the test organism, *Staphylococcus aureus* (ATCC 6538-P). After about four hours time, the cell density is read photoelectrically at 530 nm.

Both of these methods are standard and well known to microbiologists.

4.12--UV assays.

A simple procedure for CTC was developed by Levine in which the antibiotic is dehydrated by heating in acid and the resulting solution examined spectrophotometrically at 440 nm.[63] This is preferred to direct spectrophotometric examination at 360 nm because there are fewer interferences at longer wavelengths. The same method works for TC. Later advantage was taken of the wavelength shift which occurs with chelating metals and OTC, TC and CTC were assayed using the orange to brown color at 490 nm developed with ferric chloride.[64] When CTC is present in solutions of TC, it can be made non-interfering by heating at pH 7.5 whereupon it degrades to isoCTC (see Chapter 5). TC survives and is subsequently degraded with acid to anhydro TC and absorbance is read at 440 nm.[65] OTC degrades to non-interfering apoOTC in acid (see Chapter 5) so does not interfere when it is mixed with TC. The simplest method of all is simply to measure absorbance directly at 355 nm in dilute acid solutions when relatively "clean" pharmaceutical formulations are involved.[66]

A rather more drastic use of the dehydration technique has been developed for measuring the amount of 6-demethyl-tetracycline in DMCTC in which the sample is heated with 4<u>N</u> HNO_3. The DMCTC is destroyed while its deschloro analog gives a product absorbing at 425 nm which is believed to be 7-nitroanhydrodemethyltetracycline.[67]

Use of thorium complexes as auxochromes[68] and a cerium complex of OTC have been recommended,[69] as has even uranium salts.[70]

It should be obvious that direct measurement of anhydrotetracyclines as degradation products is possible,[71,72] but this is better done by methods involving separations (v.i.). McCormick developed a spectrophotometric method for determining the amount of 4-epitetracycline in TC samples, however, the differences in spectrum are slight.[73] Another application of absorbancy ratios determines the amount of tetracyclines in the presence of the anhydrotetracyclines, but the amounts found are large compared to those in other studies.[74]

TC forms a rose color with diazobenzene sulfonic acid in acid solutions which can be measured spectrophotometrically, especially as CTC and OTC form yellow solutions which do not interfere.[75] Another dye reaction used for analysis is the butanol soluble blue color developed by TC in neutral solutions with p-aminodimethylaniline and sodium hypochlorite.[7] Boric acid in concentrated sulfuric acid produces an orange-red color, but the conditions needed limit the use of this method.[77]

4.13--Fluorimetric assays.

CTC produces an intensely fluorescent solution when heated at pH 7.5 in aqueous buffers.[63] This method has been used to measure the antibiotic in feeds. The method was then improved by adding Ca ion and barbiturates whereupon the fluorescence could be extracted into ethyl acetate.[78,79] The method does not seem to pick up some of the major degradation products, however.[80]

For OTC, a procedure with better recovery involves extraction from acidic solutions with amyl alcohol followed by back extraction with base and the addition of Mg ion before reading the fluorescence. EDTA is then added as a quenching agent to establish a background.[81]

Taking advantage of the greater lipophilicity of anhydrotetracycline, one method dehydrates TC by heating in acid, extracting at about pH 4-5 with chloroform and then measuring the fluorescence of the Al chelate.[82]

4.14--Non-aqueous titrations.

Of limited value are the titration of tetracyclines in non-aqueous solvent mixtures with methylene blue-quinaldine red indicator using perchloric acid as titrant.[83]

4.15--Polarography.

A number of papers describe the polarographic determination of tetracyclines claiming excellent sensitivity and reproducability.[84-90] Under ideal conditions, mixtures can be analyzed rapidly and the method is adaptable to automated analysis.

4.16--Circular dichroism.

The use of this chiroptical method for convenient analysis of epimers in the TC and anhydrotetracycline groups has been alluded to.[32,36] Use of the method will be limited to those who have the expensive equipment required.

4.17--Paper chromatography.

The methods heretofore described are potentially limited in that no real separation of mixtures is performed so the assays lack generality and specificity. Paper partition chromatographic methods have been very widely applied to qualitative analysis of tetracyclines although elution of the separated antibiotics and spectroscopic analysis has also been performed. This subject has been thoroughly reviewed in an authoritative fashion.[61,91] In this author's experience, impregnation with EDTA to tie up chelating ions in the paper and the use of ammonia vapor to enhance the fluorescence is particularly valuable.[92] Pressing the developed plate to a seeded agar sheet to develop a bioautogram is also useful for location of the bioactive components.

4.18--Thin layer chromatography.

Despite its relative lower reproducibility, tlc has gained popularity because of its speed and flexibility. Amongst the many publications in this area, those using wetting agents and sequestering agents, although requiring fanatic adherence to conditions, are among the best.[93] This area has also been reviewed.[61,91]

4.19--Column chromatography.

Washed diatomaceous earth impregnated with buffered stationary phases containing EDTA have been used to separate and quantify tetracycline mixtures in the presence of degradation products.[94-96] Adaption of tlc systems to column use have also been proposed.[97] A further elaboration allowed automation to increase the number of samples which could be processed.[98] Some have found it advantageous to use a preseparation by solvent extraction to lessen the demand on capacity and resolution.[99]

Sephadex G-25 buffered at alkaline pH's has excellent resolving power for some purposes.[100-102]

4.20--High performance liquid chromatography.

This technique is the only one to my knowledge which can rapidly, repeatedly and sensitively resolve and quantitate not only mixtures of tetracyclines, but also TC from its most significant degradation products, 4-epiTC, anhydroTC and 4-epianhydroTC. Thus, it has rapidly found application and a large literature has developed. Butterfield separated fifteen tetracyclines using ion exchange systems.[103] Later workers included EDTA in the system to prevent binding with the metal columns.[104] Other modifications are available.[105-107] One of these involves an application to serum level determination where as little as 0.3 mcg/ml could be determined.[106] Another demonstrates some advantages of reverse phase HPLC over ion exchange techniques.[107]

This versatile method cannot fail to grow in importance and use and may eventually reach compendial status despite conservative ennui.

REFERENCES

1. F. A. Hochstein, C. R. Stephens, L. H. Conover, P. P. Regna, R. Pasternack, P. N. Gordon, F. J. Pilgrim, K. J. Brunings and R. B. Woodward, J. Am. Chem. Soc., 75, 5455 (1953).

2. C. R. Stephens, J. J. Beereboom, H. H. Rennhard, P. N. Gordon, K. Murai, R. K. Blackwood and M. Schach von Wittenau, J. Am. Chem. Soc., 85, 2643 (1963).
3. R. K. Blackwood, H. H. Rennhard and C. R. Stephens, J. Am. Chem. Soc., 82, 5194 (1960).
4. F. A. Hochstein, M. Schach von Wittenau, F. W. Tanner and K. Murai, J. Am. Chem. Soc., 82, 5934 (1960).
5. R. K. Blackwood, "Tetracyclines" in Kirk-Othmer Encyclopedia of Chemical Technology, 2nd Ed., Vol. 20, p. 3.
6. L. H. Conover, Symp. Antibiotics and Mould Metabolites, Spec. Publ. No. 5, The Chemical Society, London, 48 (1956).
7. J. L. Colaizzi, A. M. Knevel and A. N. Martin, J. Pharm. Sci., 54, 1425 (1965).
8. K. H. Ibsen and M. R. Urist, Proc. Soc. Exp. Biol. Med., 109, 797 (1962).
9. J. T. Doluisio and A. N. Martin, J. Med. Chem., 6, 16 (1963).
10. A. H. Caswell and J. D. Hutchison, Biochem. Biophys. Res. Commun., 43, 625 (1971).
11. M. Ishidate and T. Sakaguchi, Pharm. Bull. Jap., 3, 147 (1955).
12. F. Jacob and J. Monod, J. Mol. Biol., 3, 318 (1961).
13. E. F. Gale and J. P. Folkes, Biochem. J., 53, 493 (1953).
14. E. G. Remmers, W. C. Barringer, G. M. Sieger and A. P. Doerschuk, J. Pharm. Sci., 53, 1452 (1964).

15. E. G. Remmers, W. C. Barringer, G. M. Sieger and A. P. Doerschuk, J. Pharm. Sci., 53, 1534 (1964).

16. E. G. Remmers, W. C. Barringer, G. M. Sieger, N. Anagnostakos, J. J. Corbett and A. P. Doerschuk, J. Pharm. Sci., 54, 49 (1965).

17. K. Kakemi, H. Sezaki, H. Ogata and T. Nadai, Chem. Pharm. Bull., 16, 2200 (1968).

18. K. Kakemi, H. Sezaki, M. Hayashi and T. Nadai, Chem. Pharm. Bull., 16, 2206 (1968).

19. M. M. Noseworthy, U. S. Patent, 3,009,956 (1962) via Chem. Abs., 56, 6101 (1962).

20. C. R. Stephens, L. H. Conover, R. Pasternack, F. A. Hochstein, W. T. Moreland, P. P. Regna, F. J. Pilgrim, K. J. Brunings and R. B. Woodward, J. Am. Chem. Soc., 76, 3568 (1954).

21. M. Schach von Wittenau and R. K. Blackwood, J. Org. Chem. 31, 613 (1966).

22. F. Barbatschi, M. Dann, J. H. Martin, P. A. Miller, L. A. Mitscher and N. Bohonos, Experientia, 21, 162 (1965).

23. G. L. Asleson and C. W. Frank, J. Am. Chem. Soc., 97, 6247 (1975).

24. J. Gulbis and G. W. Everett, Jr., J. Am. Chem. Soc., 97, 6248 (1975).

25. J. Gulbis and G. W. Everett, Jr., Tetrahedron, 32, 913 (1976).

26. D. E. Williamson, G. W. Everett, Jr., J. Am. Chem. Soc., 97, 2397 (1975).

27. C. H. Hassall and G. J. Thomas, J. Chem. Soc., Ser. C., 636 (1970).

28. D. R. Hoffman, J. Org. Chem., 31, 792 (1966).

29. L. A. Mitscher and R. Foltz, Unpublished experiments.

30. L. A. Mitscher, A. C. Bonacci and T. D. Sokoloski, Tet. Letts., 5361 (1968).

31. L. A. Mitscher, A. C. Bonacci and T. D. Sokoloski, Antimicrob. Agts. Chemother., 78 (1968).

32. R. F. Miller, T. D. Sokoloski, L. A. Mitscher, A. C. Bonacci and B. A. Hoener, J. Pharm. Sci., 62, 1143 (1973).

33. L. A. Mitscher, A. C. Bonacci, B. Slater-Eng, A. K. Hacker and T. D. Sokoloski, Antimicrob. Agts. Chemother., 111 (1970).

34. L. A. Mitscher, B. Slater-Eng and T. D. Sokoloski, Antimicrob. Agts. Chemother., 2, 66 (1972).

35. D. Sompolinsky and Z. Samga, J. Bacteriol., 110, 468 (1972).

36. T. D. Sokoloski, L. A. Mitscher, P. H. Yuen and B. Hoener, J. Pharm. Sci., in press (1977).

37. A. Albert and C. W. Reese, Nature, 172, 201 (1973).

38. A. Albert and C. W. Reese, Nature, 177, 433 (1956).

39. T. V. Parke and W. W. Davis, Anal. Chem., 26, 642 (1954).

40. C. R. Stephens, K. Murai, K. J. Brunings and R. B. Woodward, J. Am. Chem. Soc., 78, 4155 (1956).

41. L. J. Leeson, J. E. Krueger and R. A. Nash, Tet. Letts., 1155 (1963).

42. N. E. Rigler, S. P. Bag, D. E. Leyden, J. L. Sudmeier and C. N. Reilley, Anal. Chem., 37, 872 (1965).

43. L. Z. Benet and J. E. Goyan, J. Pharm. Sci., 54, 983 (1965).

44. S. Hirokawa, Y. Okaya, F. M. Lovell and R. Pepinsky, Acta Cryst., 12, 811 (1959).

45. S. Hirokawa, Y. Okaya, F. M. Lovell and R. Pepinsky, Z. Krist., 112, 439 (1959).

46. J. Donohue, J. D. Dunitz, K. N. Trueblood and M. S. Webster, J. Am. Chem. Soc., 85, 851 (1963).

47. Y. Takauchi and M. T. Buerger, Proc. Natl. Acad. Sci. U. S. A., 46, 1366 (1960).

48. J. Robertson, I. Robertson, P. F. Eiland and R. Pepinsky, J. Am. Chem. Soc., 74, 841 (1952).

49. J. D. Dunitz and J. H. Robertson, J. Am. Chem. Soc., 74, 1108 (1952).

50. H. Cid-Dresdner, Z. Kristallogr., Kristallgeometrie, Krystallphys., Krystallchem., 121, 170 (1968).

51. M. Schach von Wittenau, R. K. Blackwood, L. H. Conover, R. H. Glanert and R. B. Woodward, J. Am. Chem. Soc., 87, 134 (1965).

52. R. E. Hughes, H. Muxfeldt and R. B. Von Dreele, J. Am. Chem. Soc., 93, 1037 (1971).

53. C. J. Palenick and M. Mathew, Acta Crystallogr. Sect. A, 28, 547 (1972).

54. K. Kamiya, M. Asai, Y. Wada and M. Nishikawa, Experientia, 27, 363 (1971).

55. J. H. Van den Hende, J. Am. Chem. Soc., 87, 929 (1965).

56. R. Restivo and G. J. Palenik, Biochem. Biophys. Res. Commun., 36, 621 (1969).

57. J. J. Stezowski, J. Am. Chem. Soc., 98, 6012 (1976).

58. K. H. Jogun and J. J. Stezowski, J. Am. Chem. Soc., 98, 6018 (1976).

59. W. A. Baker, Jr. and P. M. Brown, J. Am. Chem. Soc., 88, 1314 (1966).

60. C. Lagercrantz and M. Yhland, Acta Chem. Scand., 17, 2568 (1963).

61. D. W. Hughes and W. L. Wilson, Can. J. Pharm. Sci., 8, 67 (1973).

62. I. C. Dijkhuis, Pharm. Weekbl., 102, 907 (1967).

63. J. Levine, E. A. Garlock, Jr. and H. J. Fischbach, J. Am. Pharm. Ass., Sci. Ed., 38, 473 (1949).

64. F. Monastero, J. A. Means, T. C. Greenfell and H. F. Hedger, J. Am. Pharm. Ass., Sci. Ed., 40, 241 (1951).

65. F. S. Chiccarelli, M. H. Woolford, Jr. and M. E. J. Avery, J. Am. Pharm. Ass., Sci. Ed., 48, 263 (1959).

66. I. Cruceanu, M. Medianu, E. Aiteanu and A. Moldovan, Pharmazie, 24, 733 (1969).

67. F. S. Chiccarelli, J. Pharm. Sci., 57, 1046 (1968).

68. L. G. Chatten and S. I. Krause, J. Pharm. Sci., 60, 107 (1971).

69. B. Janik and D. Holiat, Acta Polon. Pharm., 29, 168 (1972).

70. A. E. -S. Mahgoub, E. M. Khairy and A. Kasem. J. Pharm. Sci., 63, 1451 (1974).

71. I. C. Dijkhuis, Pharm. Weekblad., 102, 1308 (1967).

72. V. C. Walton, M. R. Howlett and G. V. Selzer, J. Pharm. Sci., 59, 1160 (1970).

73. J. R. D. McCormick, S. M. Fox, L. L. Smith, B. A. Bitler, J. Reichenthal, V. E. Origoni, W. H. Muller, R. Winterbottom and A. P. Doerschuk, J. Am. Chem. Soc., 79, 2849 (1957).

74. M. Pernarowski, R. O. Searl and J. Naylor, J. Pharm. Sci., 58, 470 (1969).

75. H. Vogth, Arch. Pharm., 289, 502 (1956).

76. K. Murai, Yakugakku Zasshi, 80, 544 (1960).

77. K. Sakaguchi, Yakugakku Zasshi, 78, 970 (1958).

78. K. W. Kohn, Anal. Chem., 33, 862 (1961).

79. D. M. Wilson, M. Lever, E. A. Brosnan and A. Stillwell, Clin. Chem. Acta, 36, 260 (1972).

80. A. Regosz, Acta Pol. Pharm., 31, 259 (1974).

81. K. H. Ibsen, R. L. Saunders and M. R. Urist, Anal. Biochem., 5, 505 (1963).

82. R. G. Kelly, L. M. Peets and K. D. Hoyt, Anal. Biochem., 28, 222 (1969).

83. F. Yokoyama and L. G. Chatten, J. Am. Pharm. Ass., Sci. Ed., 47, 548 (1958).

84. J. Doskocil and M. Vondracek, Chem. Listy, 46, 564 (1952).

85. J. Doskocil, Die Pharmazie, 9, 394 (1954).

86. O. Krestynova-Telupilova, V. Macak and F. Santavy, Chem. Listy, 47, 636 (1953).

87. D. Doskocilova, Die Pharmazie, 13, 548 (1958).

88. J. S. Hetman, Lab. Pract., 12, 740 (1963).

89. M. E. Caplis, H. S. Raghels and E. D. Schall, J. Pharm. Sci., 54, 694 (1965).

90. S. Silvestri, Pharm. Acta Helv., 47, 209 (1972).

91. Tetracyclines, in "Chromatography of Antibiotics," by G. H. Wagman and M. J. Weinstein, Elsevier, New York (1973).

92. R. G. Kelly and D. A. Buyske, Antib. and Chemother., 10, 604 (1960).

93. P. P. Ascione, J. B. Zagar and G. P. Chrekian, J. Pharm. Sci., 56, 1393 (1967).

94. W. W. Fike and N. W. Brake, J. Pharm. Sci., 61, 615 (1972).

95. R. G. Kelly, J. Pharm. Sci., 53, 1551 (1964).

96. F. Bailey, J. Pharm. Pharmacol., 121, 40s (1969).

97. P. P. Ascione, J. B. Zagar and G. P. Chrekian, J. Pharm. Sci., 56, 1396 (1967).

98. P. P. Ascione, J. B. Zagar and G. P. Chrekian, J. Chromatog., 65, 377 (1972).

99. L. J. Leeson and J. F. Weidenheimer, J. Pharm. Sci., 58, 355 (1969).

100. B. W. Griffiths, R. Brunet and L. Greenberg, Can. J. Pharm. Sci., 5, 101 (1970).

101. B. W. Griffiths, J. Pharm. Sci., 55, 353 (1966).

102. B. W. Griffiths, J. Chromatog., 38, 41 (1968).

103. A. G. Butterfield, D. W. Hughes, N. J. Pound and W. L. Wilson, Antimicrob. Agts. Chromatog., 4, 11 (1973).

104. K. Tsuji, J. H. Robertson and W. F. Beyer, Anal. Chem., 46, 539 (1974).

105. A. G. Butterfield, D. W. Hughes, W. L. Wilson and N. H. Pound, J. Pharm. Sci., 64, 316 (1975).

106. I. Nilsson-Ehle, T. T. Yolshikawa, M. C. Schotz and L. B. Guze, Antimicrob. Agts. Chemother., 9, 754 (1976).

107. E. R. White, M. A. Carroll, J. E. Zarembo and A. D. Bender, J. Antibiot., 28, 205 (1975).

CHAPTER 5

DEGRADATION AND STRUCTURE PROOFS

5.1---Introduction.

Considering the complexity and relative instability of the tetracyclines and the fact that there were no compounds quite like them in the literature upon which to draw chemical experience, it is remarkable that their structures were elucidated so quickly. Only two years elapsed between the announcement of the discovery of OTC and publication of its structure (1950-1952). This work represents a fine example of the combined power of spectral analysis and deductive logic. The structural chemistry of the tetracyclines has been the subject of several good reviews which may be consulted for additional perspective.[1-9]

Aside from those reactions of practical significance because they take place in dilute aqueous solutions and therefore are of pharmaceutical and clinical significance (Sections 5.2 to 5.4), most of the more deep-seated degradations of the tetracyclines are now of historical and chemical interest only. The wealth of spectroscopic methodology available in the field makes it uncommon for anyone to undertake a classical degradation today unless the structure be truly unusual or one be pursuing the labeling pattern in a biosynthetic scheme. Even in the latter case, the impact of ^{13}CMR has lessened the utility of deep-seated degradation for most biosynthetic studies. Still, classically trained chemists are reluctant, often rightly so, to place complete reliance on spectroscopy alone. Further, the synthetic chemist will find the data of some interest in that it reveals some of the conditions that a tetracycline cannot withstand.

It is clear from Chapter 3 that tetracyclines are polyketides. Classically, such compounds, being essentially aldol products, are stable within reason to acids but quite sensitive to alkali. If this is kept in mind, much tetracycline chemistry falls into place.

5.2---Reversible epimerization at C_4.

The dimethylamino function at C_4 of all bioactive tetracyclines (1) stands 1,3-diaxially eclipsed with respect to the C_{12a}OH group in acidic solutions. Epimerization relieves this interaction and takes place *via* enol 2.[10-14] The product, 4-epitetracycline (3) has no significant antibacterial activity. The reaction takes place most rapidly

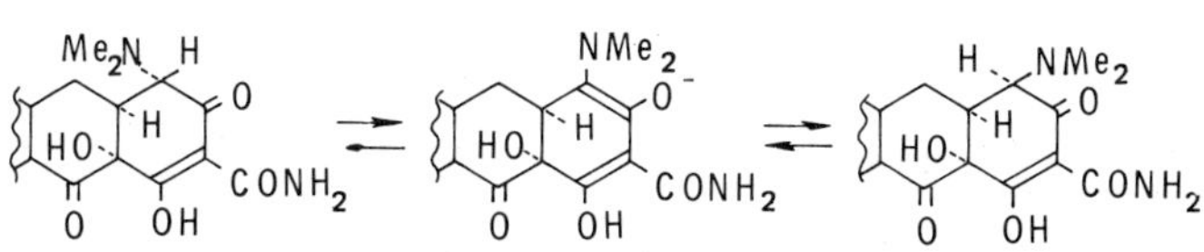

(1) (2) (3)

at pH 3-5 in aqueous solutions and is a reversible first-order reaction.[15,16]

The most convincing proof of the site of the epimerization was provided by the conversion of 1 and 3 to their respective quaternary methiodides followed by conversion to the identical 4-dedimethylaminotetracycline (4) by reaction with zinc in aqueous acetic acid.[12] It was shown that the two methiodides did not equilibrate in the aqueous acetic acid used for the reaction. This was particularly important as acetic acid alone, *i. a.*, is an excellent medium for the epimerization of nonquaternary tetracyclines.[11]

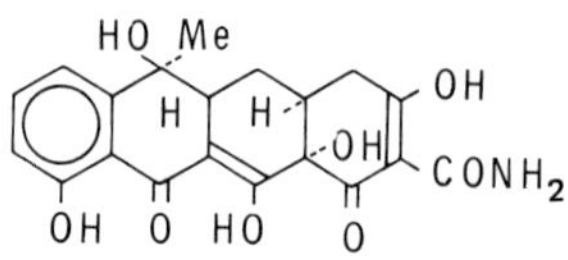

(4)

In alkaline solutions using precise conditions, epitetracyclines are converted almost completely back to the bioactive isomer (1) in the presence of chelating metals.[17] This has been rationalized as being due to the complexing metal tying together the C4-dimethylamino and C_{12a}-hydroxy functions thus overcoming their steric repulsion.[18] Other groups which influence the epimerization include phosphate,[15] citrate,[15] urea,[19] and some pharmaceutical ingredients.[20]

5.3---Dehydration at $C_{5a,6}$.

The C_6OH group is axial and antiperiplanar trans to the H at C_{5a} so that it is sterically ideal for an E_2

reaction. In tetracycline, the group not only is tertiary, but the double bond character imparted to C_{10}-C_{10a} by the enolic β-dicarbonyl function facilitates the reaction also by making the C ring aromatic as the reaction proceeds. The anhydrotetracyclines (5) produced possess in vitro bioactivity, but have not found clinical application. They are formed progressively at pH's lower than 2, especially upon heating.[21-27]

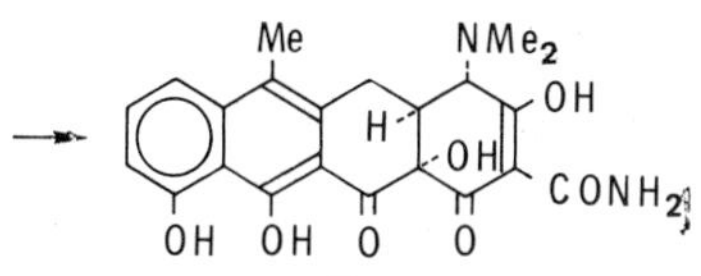

(5)

DMCTC has a secondary OH group at C_6 and so it is more stable to acid dehydration.[28] Minocycline totally lacks the OH group and so cannot degrade in this fashion.

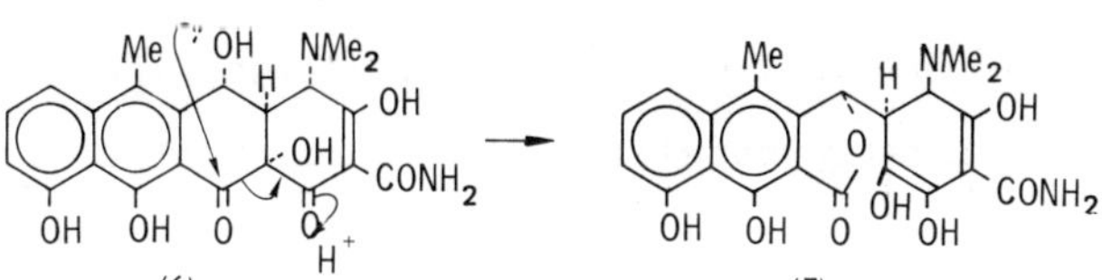

(6) (7)

OTC dehydrates in the same manner as TC, but anhydrooxytetracycline (6) is quite unstable under the reaction conditions, undergoing scission of ring B mediated through the C_5OH group to produce the isomeric phthalides, α- and β-apoterramycins (7) (IR band at 5.75μ). Given the manifold opportunities for isomerism inherent in formula 7, the precise nature of the difference between α- and β-apoterramycin remains unclear. In hydroxyl-free media, anhydrooxytetracycline (6) can be isolated. When subsequently placed in dilute aqueous or alcoholic acid 6 goes rapidly to 7.[20,27]

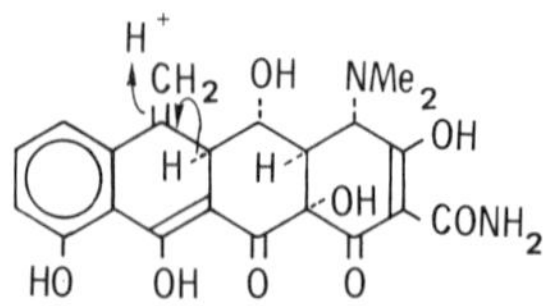

(8)

MOTC (8) undergoes a prototropic shift in acid solution which leads to α- and β-apoterramycin (7) via anhydrooxytetracycline (6). This, apparently, requires more vigorous conditions than simple dehydration of OTC.[29] α-DOOTC, obviously, cannot undergo $C_{5a,6}$ dehydration.

The C_{12a}-hydroxyl in the tetracyclines is cis to the C_{4a} hydrogen and very vigorous conditions are required for its dehydration. The proximity of the protonated C_4-dimethylamino function may also play a significant role by electrostatically repelling the approach of a proton to C_{12a}.

5.4---Phthalide formation in base.

In alkaline solutions, tetracyclines having a C_6 hydroxyl group cleave readily to the isotetracyclines. CTC (9) is specially prone to this.[30,31] A transanular attack implicit in formula 9 is presumed to be the mechanism.

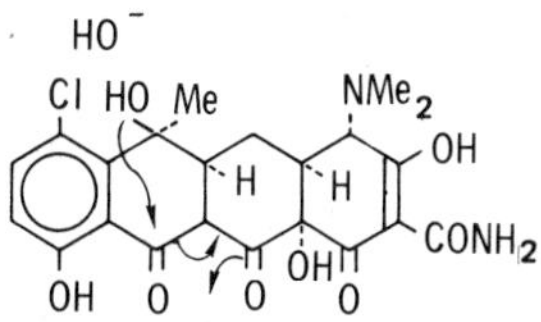

(9)

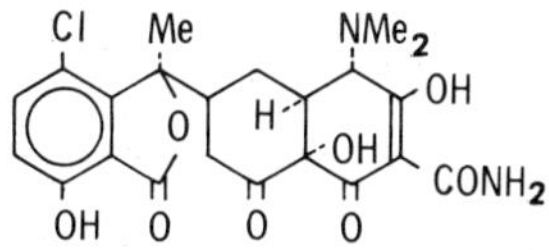

(10)

5.5---Deep-seated degradations of OTC.

Alkali treatment of OTC caused progressively more and more damage to the aliphatic rings A and B. The isolated products retained ring D and fragments of rings B and C.[32]

The molecular formula of OTC was established to be $C_{22}H_{24}O_9N_2$. Customarily, one attempts to account for the hetero atoms first in such a formula and preliminary examination was directed to this end. One of the nitrogen atoms was basic, for the antibiotic formed a well-defined monohydrochloride salt. Strong base treatment of OTC liberated one mole of dimethylamine and one of ammonia. The latter function was considered to be part of a primary amide group as treatment with benzenesulfonyl chloride gave a nitrile (infra red band at 4.5 microns), apparently by dehydration of the carboxamide function. By inference, then, the dimethylamino group was responsible for the basic properties of the antibiotic.

The ultraviolet absorption spectrum of OTC indicated a complex, highly conjugated chromophore of a type not previously encountered in the literature. The infra red spectrum was characteristically ill-defined but did reveal the lack of non-conjugated carbonyl groupings (such as aldehyde, acid, ester, ketone, lactone, etc.). Two of the oxygen atoms were alcoholic hydroxyls for a diester formed which could be shown, by titration, to have retained the mildly acidic functions. The nature of the latter was partly revealed by the formation of a dimethyl ether. Active hydrogen determination revealed eight such groupings, of which four were involved in the etherification and acetylation reactions. Only two of the active hydrogens could be titrated. Taken along with the ultraviolet spectrum, it was apparent that a complex, readily-enolizable, assembly must be present in the molecule. Kuhn-Roth oxidation revealed one methyl group attached to carbon. These preliminary findings can be summarized in partial formula 11. All attempts to find the carbon skeleton to which these groups were appended were unsuccessful at this stage. This considerable handicap was not successfully overcome until the structural analysis was far along.

	$-CH_3$	
	$-OH$	—acidic
	$-OH$	
$C_{18}H_9O_4$	$-OH$	—alcoholic
	$-OH$	
	$-N(CH_3)_2$	
	$-CONH_2$	

(11)

Deep-seated structural changes accompanied treatment with alkali and, when these reactions were finally understood, they revealed a great deal about the ring system. Low temperature alkaline fusion[36] gave 3-hydroxyphthalic acid (12) while more drastic conditions gave additional fragments 13-16.[32]

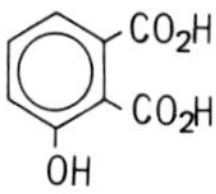
(12)

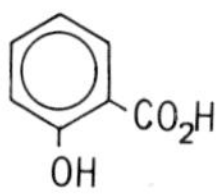
(13)

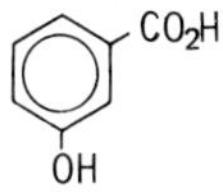
(14)

$MeCO_2H$
(15)

$HO_2CCH_2CH_2CO_2H$
(16)

Less drastic alkaline treatment (with 4% aqueous sodium hydroxide solution) gave terracinoic acid (17) which is the main nitrogen-free product that can be obtained by base treatment of OTC. This material was formed under quite mild conditions and yet its formation was mystifying at first for the infrared spectrum of OTC and 17 clearly showed that terracinoic acid could not be present as such in the molecule. Its formation must clearly be the result of a rearrangement.[32] More significantly, despite the presence of two potentially asymmetric centers, 17 was isolated in racemic form. There is no easily visualized means by which both optical centers could racemize, so either these atoms were racemic in OTC itself, or, more likely, the rearrangement which led to formation of terracinoic acid involved loss of optical activity. The rationalization of its formation and the care with which its structure were determined were central to further progress in the structural chemistry of OTC.

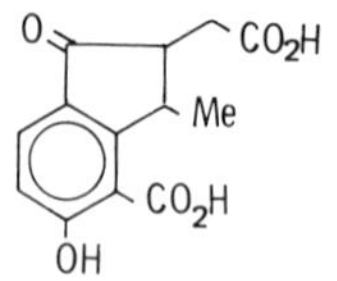

(17)

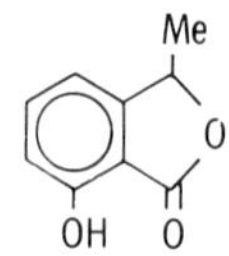

(18)

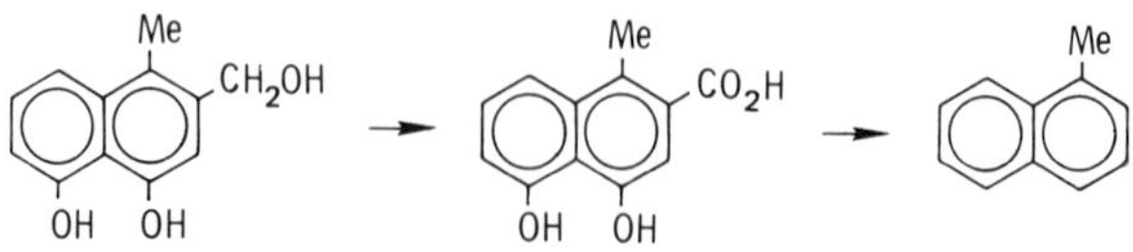

(19) (20) (21)

Strenuous alkaline hydrolysis under reducing conditions (zinc dust present) gave two additional fragments, 3-methyl-7-hydroxyphthalide (18)[32,38] and terranaphthol (19).[35] The structure of 18 was readily confirmed by synthesis.[37] Terranaphthol's structure (19) was more revealing of the structure of OTC. It was clearly a naphthol from its ultraviolet absorption spectrum. It contained one C-methyl group (as does OTC) and formed a triacetate. Two of the hydroxyls were phenolic and their *peri*-relationship to one another was easily demonstrated for it caused a dramatic increase in the acidity of borate solutions. It could be oxidized to an acid whose ultraviolet and infrared spectra were clearly different from those of 2-carboxy-1,8-dihydroxynaphthalene, and zinc dust distillation led to 1-methylnaphthalene (21). These relationships are best rationalized by structure 19.

It was inherently probable that significant portions of the structure of terracinoic acid overlapped with those of 18 and 19. Terracinoic acid contained three carbonyl infrared bands, two in regions where OTC was blank, and thus could not exist as such in the molecule. It contained two carboxyl groups and one phenolic hydroxyl for stepwise methylation of 17 with increasing amounts of diazomethane produced a mono- (22), di- (23) and trimethyl derivative (24). The first two compounds could be hydrolyzed back to terracinoic acid, while the third had one methyl group which was not easily removed and was therefore part of an aromatic methoxyl group.

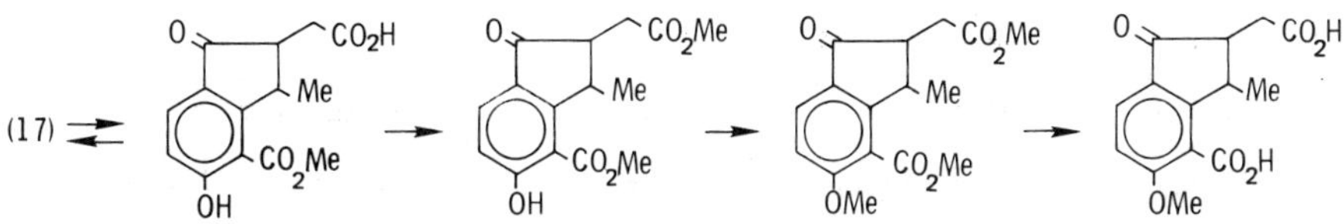

(22) (23) (24) (25)

These findings agreed with titration data which revealed a strong, medium, and weakly acidic group (pKa=2.6, 4.7 and 9.5). The strongest acidic group was lost as carbon dioxide upon heating in acid. The resulting monocarboxylic acid (25) could only be decarboxylated with some difficulty. The decarboxylated product (26) still possessed carbonyl absorption in the infrared at a suitable frequency for an indanone. The presence of a ketonic oxygen in terracinoic acid was confirmed by the formation of a monooxime. Monodecarboxyterracinoic acid (26) formed a pyrazolone (28)

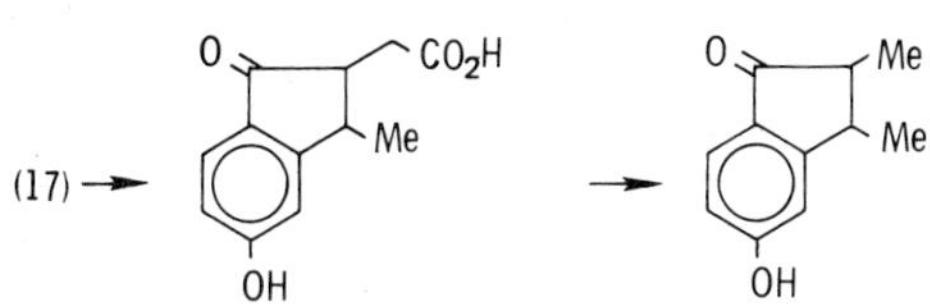

(26) (27)

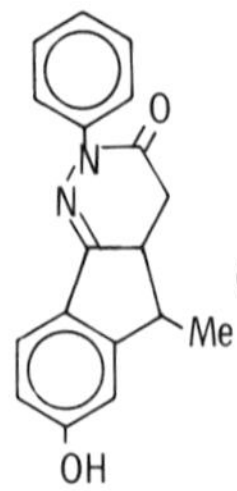

(28)

upon reaction with phenylhydrazine indicating that the remaining carboxyl group was near the ketone function. This inference was confirmed by studying the bromination of 17 whereupon a monobromo derivative (29) was formed, demonstrating that the ketone had only one enolizable hydrogen on an α-carbon. Treatment of the bromoketone (29) with aqueous base led to loss of HBr with simultaneous decarboxylation. The facile loss of CO_2 involved the formerly recalcitrant carboxyl group as shown by titration data on the product (30) for the strongest and weakest acidic groups were still present (pKa=3.1, 10). This indicated that the newly introduced double bond took up a β,δ-position relative to the weaker carboxyl group for this is known to facilitate decarboxylation of acids through a cyclic mechanism.

Treatment of the bromoketone with milder base (aqueous sodium acetate) resulted in replacement of Br by OH rather

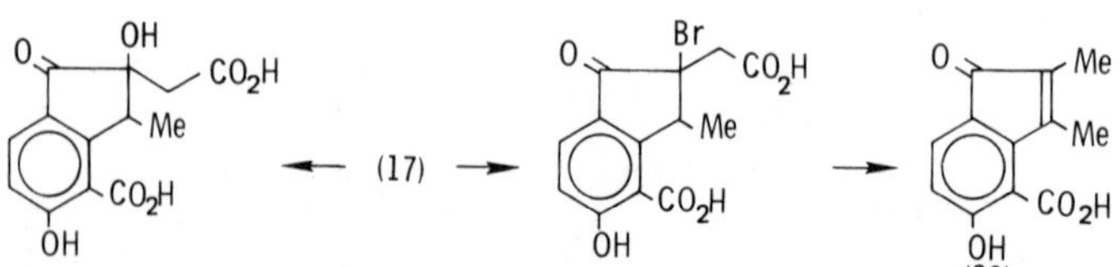

(31) (29) (30)

than elimination. The same product (31) could be formed directly from terracinoic acid by alkaline permanganate oxidation. This material liberated a molecule of acetic acid upon pyrolysis, suggesting a position β to the carbonyl group for the newly introduced hydroxyl (and therefore the bromine atom as well) and showed that the α-carbon was not occupied. Terracinoic acid does not liberate acetic acid upon pyrolysis.

Drastic hydrogenation of 16 led to the uptake of about six moles of hydrogen and the formation of a dicarboxylic acid, $C_{13}H_{20}O_4$, whose hydrogen content was only consistent with a bicyclic formulation. Under milder conditions, the ketone function was reduced to a methylene group (32). This ready hydrogenolysis is consistent only with the carbonyl group being adjacent to the aromatic ring so that the intermediate benzylic alcohol would undergo facile hydrogenolysis.

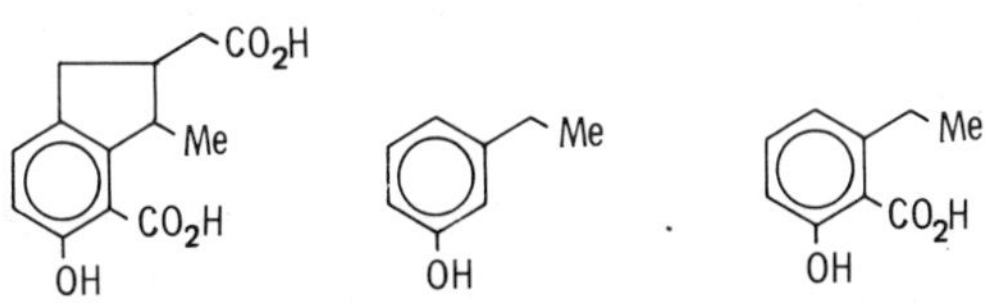

(32) (33) (34)

Kuhn-Roth oxidation of terracinoic acid (17) liberated one mole of acetic acid showing one methyl group attached to carbon. This was, presumably, the same C-methyl group that was present in OTC and terranaphthol. The attachment of the two rings was discernible from the products of KOH fusion of terracinoic acid. In addition to m-ethyl-

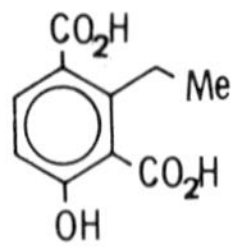

(35)

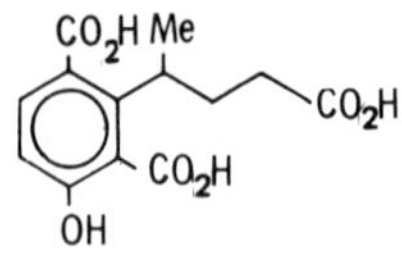

(36)

phenol (33) and 6-ethylsalicylic acid (34) two new dicarboxylic acids (35 and 36) were formed whose carboxyl groups were not *ortho* disposed to one another as they did not form phthalic anhydrides upon heating. These products demonstrated that the carbocyclic ring had to be fused to the aromatic ring in a *ortho* fashion for there is not enough carbon in 16 to construct a ring large enough to reach to a *meta* or *para* position. The strongest acid dissociation constant of terracinoic acid was attributable to a salicylic acid function and this explains its ready decarboxylation by heating in acid (27). This requires closing the aliphatic ring *meta* and *para* to the phenolic hydroxyl. The aliphatic character of the side chains *meta* to the hydroxyl in the fusion products required the ketone function to be placed *para* to the phenolic hydroxyl as did the placement of the carboxyl groups of 35 and 36.

The only formulation which satisfies all of these varied requirements is 17.

The correctness of this structure was confirmed by synthesis.[39]

With the structure of these fragments in hand, partial structure 37 could be put forth at this stage to represent the OTC molecule. The formation of the fragments was rationalized by breaking the various bonds labeled a-d.

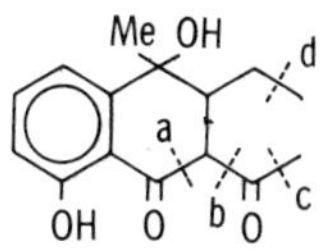

(37)

The observations that a) terracinoic acid was racemic, b) was not present in OTC as such, and c) that 3-methyl-7-hydroxyphthalide (18) was formed under reductive conditions (and carried an oxygen atom in a position where it is lacking in terracinoic acid (17)) were highly significant and had to be rationalized. That all of these fragments came from the same part of the OTC molecule was strongly suggested by the finding that they all possessed a C-methyl group and only one C-methyl group is present in OTC.

Formation of terranaphthol was postulated to have occurred by splitting bonds b, c, and d as shown in the following formulae. A 1,5-fragmentation reaction split ring B and eliminated dimethylamine to give 39. Retroaldolation would give a β-ketoacid from which loss of CO_2 would give 40. Aldoldehydration would give aldehyde 41 which would be reduced by zinc to give terranaphthol (19). Formation of 3-methyl-7-hydroxyphthalide (18) requires splitting of bonds a, c and d. After alkaline cleavage of 39, further base cleavage rather than decarboxylation would give dicarboxylic acid 43. Retroaldolation would give 44 which, in its phthalide or pseudoacid form, would form the phthalide (18) on reductive loss of the benzylic OH.

Formation of terracinoic acid (17) requires splitting bonds a, c and d with subsequent formation of a

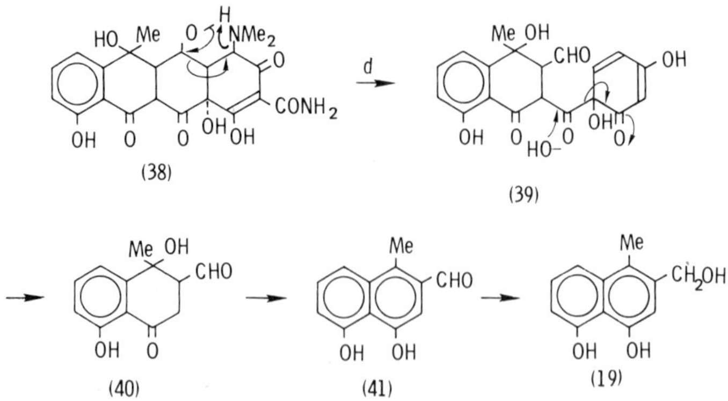

new ring between the activated <u>para</u> position of the phenolic ring and the newly generated aldehyde function. Aldoldenydration rather than retroaldolation would convert <u>43</u> to <u>45</u> with an accompanying loss of both asymmetric centers. Base catalyzed cyclization of the activated <u>para</u>-position with the aldehyde function would give <u>46</u>. The rearrangement of the double bond in <u>46</u> to give rise to <u>17</u> has ample precedent and is due to the ease with which hydrindene double bonds migrate. The origin of the various atoms from the OTC molecule is indicated by the maintenance of the corresponding numbers in formulae <u>45</u> and <u>17</u>.

In seeking additional experimental support for this ingenious proposal, it was predicted on mechanistic grounds that another indanone should be present in the mother-liquors. This was proposed to have arisen by <u>ortho</u> ring formation from <u>45</u> as opposed to the <u>para</u> closure which leads to <u>17</u>. The intermediate β-ketoacid (<u>47</u>) would decarboxylate to <u>48</u>. Indenol-indanol rearrangement would give <u>49</u>. Careful investigation was rewarded by discovery of the missing indanone. The new indanone (<u>49</u>) lacked the salicylic acid function of <u>17</u> for its

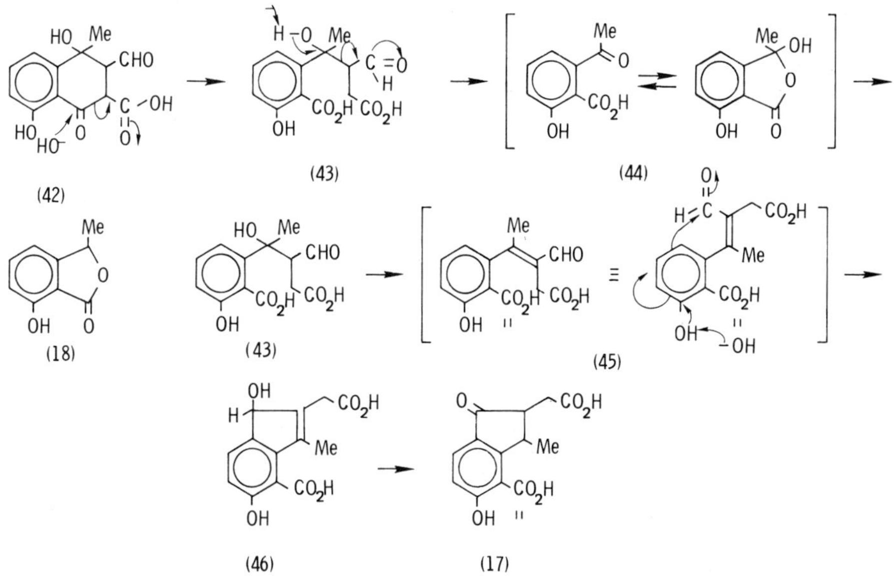

pKa values lay at 5.5 and 9.6. Alkaline fusion led to 3-ethylphenol and bromination-dehydrobromination, in a similar fashion to terracinoic acid, led to facile decarboxylation to give indenone <u>50</u>.

Additional support for the presence of partial structure <u>37</u> in OTC came upon comparison of the ultraviolet absorption spectrum of synthetic model <u>51</u> with that of OTC itself. The close correspondence of the curves provided convincing evidence for the presence of this chromophore in OTC. There is additional absorption in the 250-300 nm region of the spectrum of OTC which was attributed to the presence in the molecule of an additional chromophoric group insulated from the acetyltetralone chromophore. The nature of this chromophore will be discussed later. It obviously lay in the region not yet revealed by the degradations.

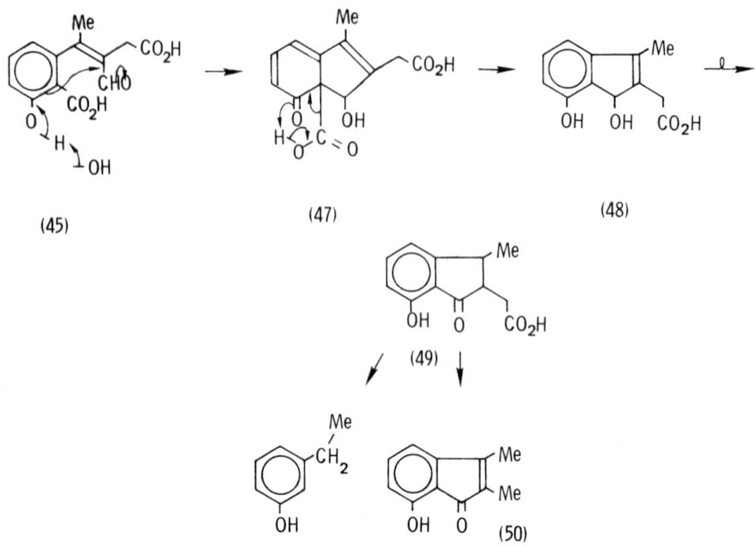

(45) (47) (48) (49) (50)

Combining all of these structural features and the other information obtained to this point leads to partial expression 52.

Acid degradations unlocked most of the rest of the structure.[40,41,34] Under mildly acidic conditions in non-hydroxylic solvents, a molecule of water is readily eliminated from OTC to form anhydrooxytetracycline (53), ($C_{22}H_{22}N_2O_8$), as discussed in Section 5.3. This result is explicable readily from formulation 52. Comparison of the ultraviolet spectrum of 53 with that of model substance 54 showed close correspondence and indicated that the two materials possessed essentially the same chromophore.

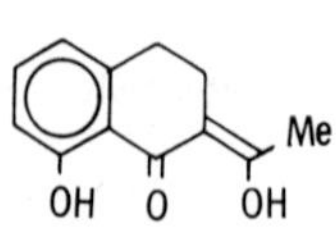

(51)

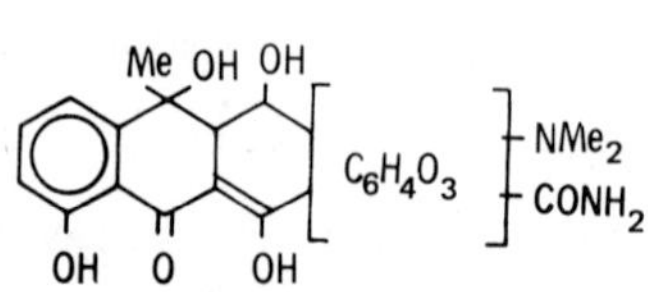

(52)

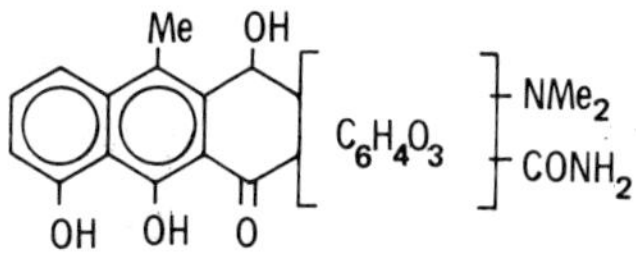

(53)

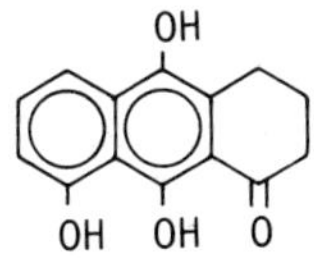

(54)

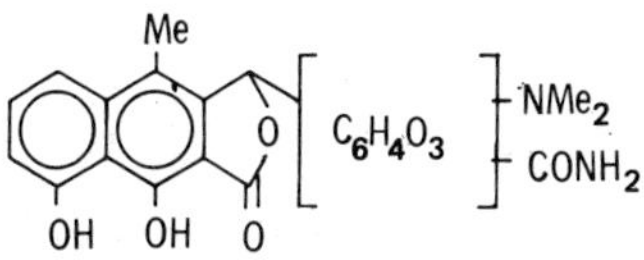

(55)

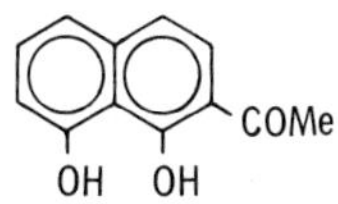

(56)

It will also be recalled from Section 5.3 that anhydro-oxytetracycline rearranges in acidic hydroxylic media to two isomers, α- and β-apoterramycin (55). These materials possess the same empirical formula as anhydrooxytetracycline and can be formed directly from OTC itself by treatment with acid in hydroxylic solvents. Interestingly, alkaline treatment of anhydrooxytetracycline also leads to the apoterramycins. It is readily apparent from their spectral properties that the apo-derivatives are phthalides. Comparison of their ultra-violet spectra with model substance 56 showed the same chromophore was present. The *peri*-situation of the phenolic hydroxyls of 55 were demonstrated by an increase in the acidity of borate solutions by 3.2 pH units. Alkaline fusion of either isomer led to terranaphthoic acid (20). Therefore, the source of the isomerism of the two compounds must lie in the portion of the molecule which is not yet accounted for by the degradations discussed to this point.

When more strongly acidic conditions were used to degrade OTC, terrinolide (57) ($C_{20}H_{15}NO_8$), decarboxyamidoterrinolide (58) ($C_{19}H_{14}O_7$), ammonia, carbon dioxide and dimethylamine were produced. The infrared spectra of 57 and 58 indicated that both compounds are phthalides. They both have a pKa at about 4.5 and they form pentaacetates, pentamethoxyethers and pentatosylates. Nitric acid oxidation of the pentamethoxy ether produced a bisanhydride (59) whose infrared spectrum (four bands at 5.35-5.60 microns) and ultraviolet spectrum closely resembled that of 2,5-dimethoxypyromellitic anhydride (60).

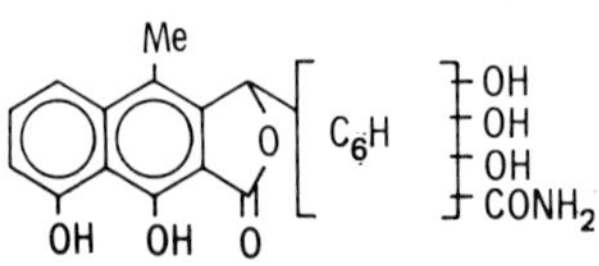

(57)

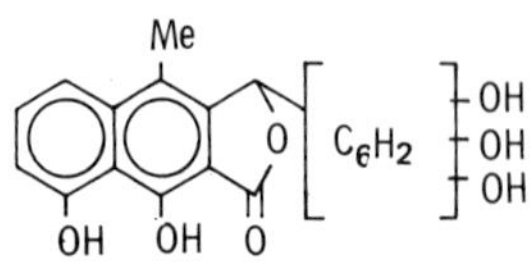

(58)

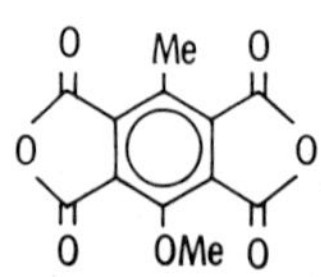

(59)

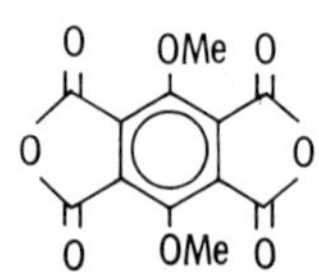

(60)

The pentamethyl ether of descarboxamidoterrinolide gave a diol (61) upon reduction which then formed a cyclic ether (62) on acid treatment. The ultraviolet spectrum of the ether contained two insulated chromophores. Summation of the ultraviolet spectra of the dimethylether of terranaphthol (63) and 1,2,4-trimethoxybenzene produced a very close match to that of 62. Summation with the alternate possibilities (1,2,3- and 1,3,5-trimethoxybenzene) produced curves which differed significantly. This allowed one to formulate descarboxamidoterrinolide as 64.

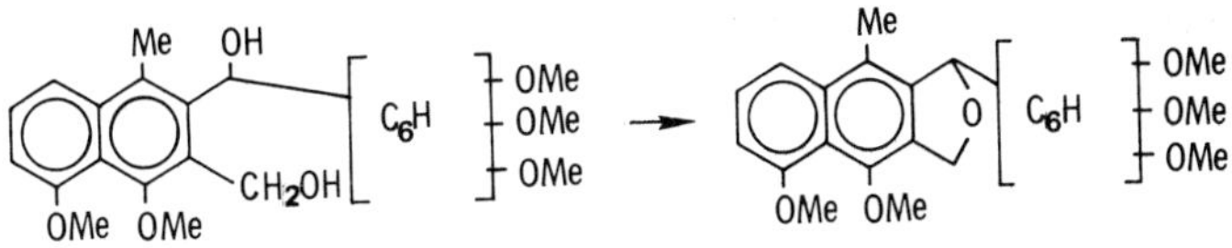

(61) (62)

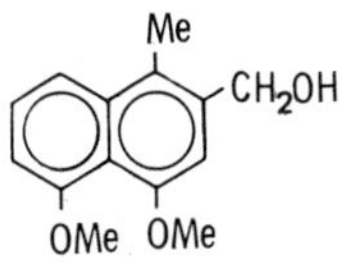 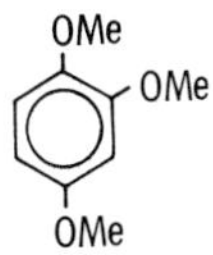 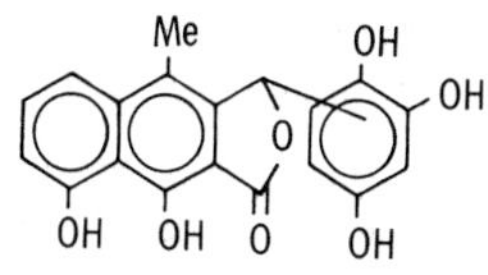

(63) (64)

The exact placement of the carboxamido function on the phenolic ring of terrinolide was greatly assisted by comparison of acidity data. The *peri*-naphtholphthalide function of 57 gave rise to pKa = 4.7. This compared well with model substance 65 which has pKa = 4.5. The phenolic ring, then, is responsible for the other acid function, pKa = 10.2. Descarboxamidoterrinolide (58), by contrast, had pKa values of 4.7 and 7.5. The greater acidity of the phenolic system of terrinolide (57) (2.7 pKa units) had to be a consequence of the presence of the carboxamide function in the aromatic ring. Model studies showed that placing a carboxamide function *ortho* or *para* to a single phenolic hydroxyl group only increases the acidity of the phenolic group by 1 pKa unit. On the other hand, placing the carboxamide group between two *ortho*-hydroxyl groups, as in model substance 66, leads to

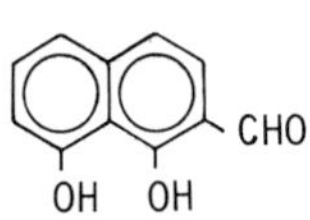 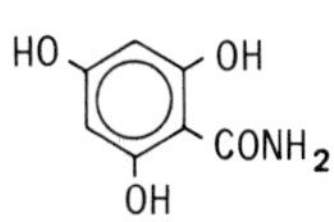 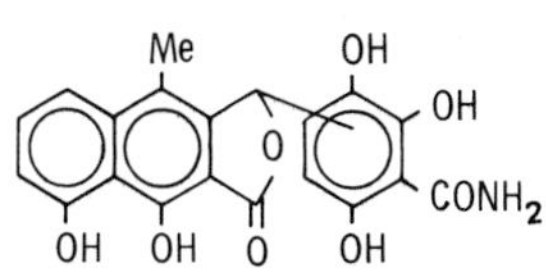

(65) (66) (67)

considerable enhancement of acid strength (pKa = 8.2). This amplifies the formulation of terrinolide to 67. The point of attachment of the phthalide to the remanent of ring A was still ambiguous at this point.

The spectra of the terrinolides clearly showed that the third ring could not be aromatic. Indeed, the facile loss of dimethylamine from the apoterramycins in their transformation to the terrinolides was only consistent with its presence on an aliphatic ring system. Titration data were only consistent with an enolized α- or β-diketo system (α = pKa 4.0, 5.1 and 8.4 β = 3.6, 5.2 and 7.8). KOH fusion of the apoterramycins led to the formation of terranaphthoic acid (20) and 2,5-dihydroxybenzoquinone (68). It was highly unlikely that either isomer had a hydroxyl or dimethylamino group β-situated to a carbonyl group for the apoterramycins survived unchanged in 0.5*N* hydrochloric acid solution for *six weeks* at 60° in the absence of oxygen! These facts could only be rationalized in terms of formula 69 for the apoterramycins. This formulation could only be realistically related to OTC by requiring formula 70 for the antibiotic itself. The remaining point of uncertainty was the relative placement of the last OH and the dimethylamino groups.

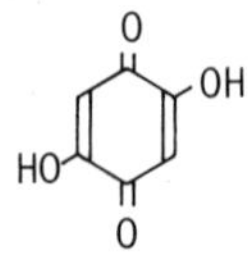

(68)

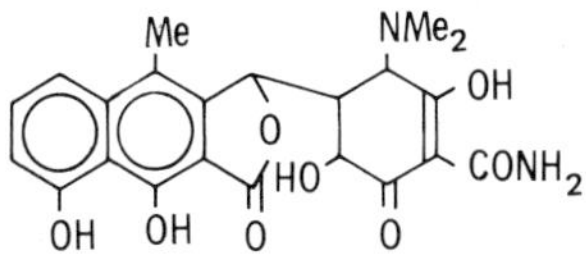

(69)

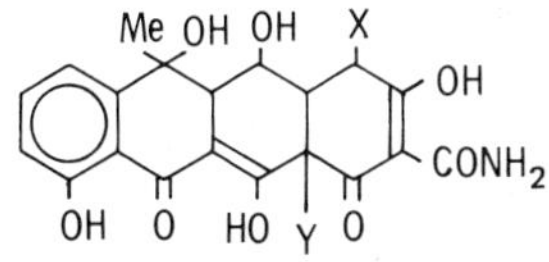

(70)

To decide the identities of X and Y, one additional mode of degradation was needed, reduction. Treatment of OTC with zinc dust under progressively more severe conditions led first to loss of the dimethylamino function and then loss of the hydroxyl group as well. Loss of the dimethylamino function hardly affected the ultraviolet spectrum while loss of the hydroxyl group made a substantial difference. Inspection of formula 70 shows that moiety Y insulates the two chromophoric regions from one another while X is not directly attached to either chromophore. The only reasonable explanation for the spectral consequences of the reduction study is that X was the dimethylamino function and Y represented the hydroxyl. On this basis, the formula for OTC must be 71. The stereochemistry implied in this formula is not justified by the data presented so far and, in fact, was not established with certainty until considerably later.

The hydroxyl group which was removed reductively to give 72 was not that at C-6, for phthalide formation (76) still occurred on treatment with base, and, in any case, this hydroxyl is not on the chromophore. The phthalide was still a β-diketone based upon pKa measurements.

Treatment of 72 with mineral acid now took a different course than that followed by OTC, for loss of two molecules of

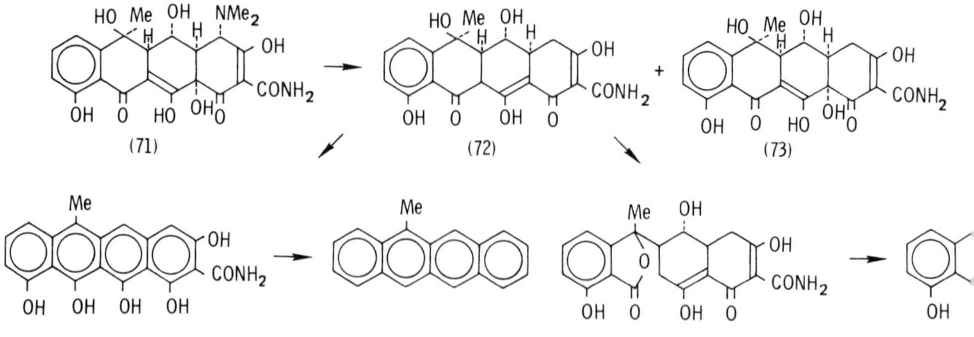

(71) (72) (73) (74) (75) (76) (18)

water occurred and a highly colored, fully aromatic derivative, initially called terrarubein (74), was generated. This deeply colored polyphenol gave a naphthacene (75) upon zinc dust distillation. Here, at last, after all of these studies, was direct evidence for the carbon skeleton of the molecule! The name tetracycline is a consequence of the antibiotics possessing this linear four-ring aromatic system.

The general features of the structure were subsequently amply confirmed by X-ray crystallography as detailed in Chapter 4. During the period when there was some uncertainty regarding the relative stereochemistry of the C-5 hydroxyl group, this point was settled independently by a combination of chemical means and spectral analysis.[42] Treatment of 72 with peracids leads to chemical reintroduction of the C-12a-hydroxyl group, but, in this case, in the unnatural β-orientation. This is

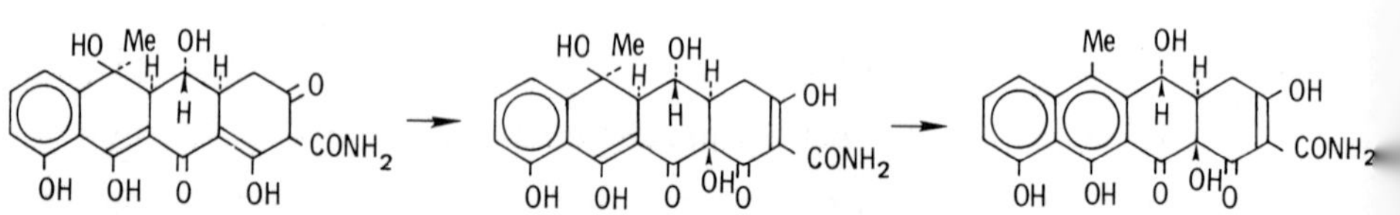

(72) (77) (78)

unfortunate from the standpoint of resynthesis of the molecule itself, but has a fortunate consequence for the study of the stereochemistry at C-5. Whereas cis-fused six-membered ring systems are flexible and can occupy a number of possible conformations by simple ring inversion, trans-fused derivatives are much more rigid for it is not possible for trans-fused decalins to isomerize in the same way without breaking at least one of the rings open.

The product (77) was converted to its 5a,6-anhydro derivative (78) in the usual way. In its pmr spectrum, a coupling constant of 8 Hz was determined between H_{4a} and H_5. A coupling constant of this magnitude is only consistent with a trans-diaxial relationship between the two hydrogens as illustrated in formula 78. Neither of these two centers in question have been affected directly by the reaction sequence, so their relative stereochemistry must be the same in OTC itself.

5.6---Degradative structure determination of CTC.

Very soon after the structure of OTC was reported, the structure of CTC was reported by the Harvard-Pfizer group.[43-45] Concurrently, a series of communications supporting and amplifying the structural assignment appeared eminating from the Lederle Laboratories.[46-51]

It was immediately apparent from a comparison of the biological properties and physicochemical properties of OTC and CTC that they were closely related. The molecular formula of CTC, $C_{22}H_{23}O_8N_2Cl$, contained a covalently bound chlorine atom that was not present in OTC and the latter possessed an additional oxygen atom over CTC. The position of the chlorine atom was quickly established by KOH fusion which produced 5-chlorosalicylic acid (79).[35] This finding was consistent with the ultraviolet absorption spectrum of CTC which is shifted to somewhat longer wavelengths than that of OTC. This would be expected if the halo group were on the BCD chromophore.

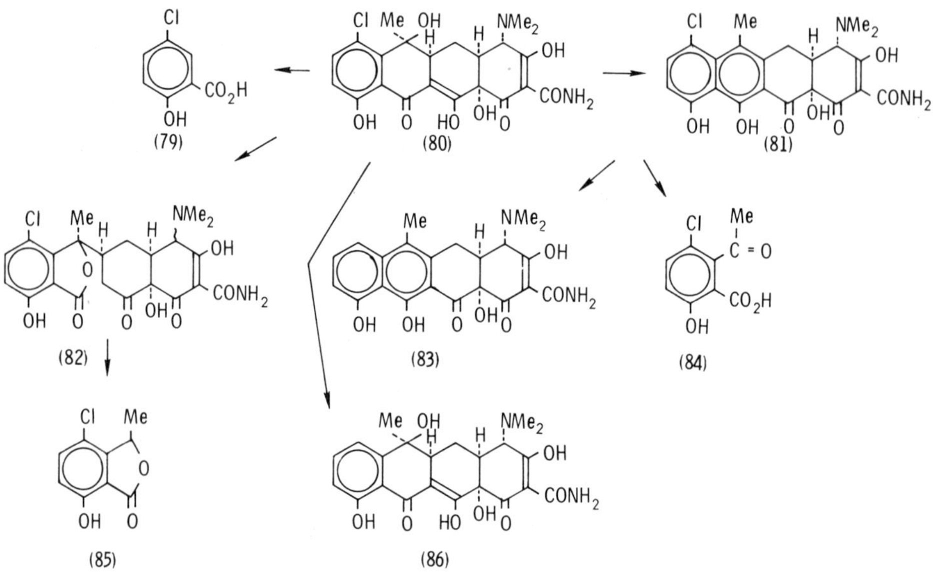

It was now necessary to decide which of the oxygen atoms of OTC was missing in the CTC molecule in order to complete the structure. Examination of the ultraviolet absorption spectrum of CTC and numerous of its degradation products clearly showed that the two chromophoric regions are essentiall the same as those of OTC. In support of this, the pKa values of CTC hydrochloride (3.4, 7.4, 9.2) and OTC hydrochloride

(3.4, 7.6, 9.2) were so similar that the only possible explanation encompassing these two lines of evidence is that the oxygen atoms at C-1, C-3, $CONH_2$ and at C-10, C-11, C-12 and C-12a must be the same in the two antibiotics. Only one oxygen atom of CTC remains to be accounted for. By analogy to OTC, it could only be at either C-5 or C-6.

The presence of the hydroxyl group at C-6 was easily demonstrated. Treatment with aqueous base, toward which CTC is much more sensitive than OTC, led to the formation of isoaureomycin (82) which was clearly a phthalide from its spectral and titration properties. In addition, treatment of CTC with acids led to dehydration and the formation of an anhydro derivative (81) whose properties were very similar to those of anhydro OTC except in one striking particular. Anhydro CTC showed no tendency to undergo subsequent scission of ring B with phthalide formation. This factor was strong evidence for the lack of a C-5 hydroxyl group. Another useful experimental observation followed dehydration of CTC with HI instead of HCl. This led to reductive loss of the chlorine atom and the ultraviolet absorption spectrum of the resulting anhydro derivative (83) was virtually superimposable on that of anhydroOTC.

This data in itself constitutes sufficient evidence from which to formulate aureomycin as 80.[43,44] Numerous other degradation reactions could be readily rationalized on this basis.

The dimethylamino and C-12a hydroxyl functions were present in CTC, as expected from the titration data, for reduction with zinc dust led to the anticipated changes in spectral and titration properties in direct parallel with the OTC reactions. Dedimethylamino-12a-deoxyCTC formed a phthalide on standing in dilute base. This derivative cleaved upon heating to give 3-methyl-4-chloro-7-hydroxyphthalide (85) whose structure was proven by synthesis.[52] The same phthalide could be obtained by pyrolysis of isoaureomycin (82).

Subtraction of the ultraviolet absorption curve of the chlorophthalide (85) from that of the parent phthalide (82) gave a curve which could be superimposed upon the curve obtained by similar subtraction of the corresponding OTC derivatives. This operation canceled the effect of differing ring D substitution and provided strong evidence that the A ring chromophore was the same in the two antibiotics.

An additional spectral finding of interest resulted from the observation that the chlorine atom in CTC could be replaced by a hydrogen by catalytic reduction in the presence of alkali and a noble metal catalyst. The resulting derivative, deschloroaureomycin (TC), had an ultraviolet spectrum which was virtually identical with that of OTC.

Treatment of isoaureomycin (82) with base in the presence of a reducing agent led to ketone cleavage and formation of the isomeric α- and β-aureomycininc acids (87).[47] Treatment of 87 with diazomethane followed by oxidation led to loss of the A ring and formation of the

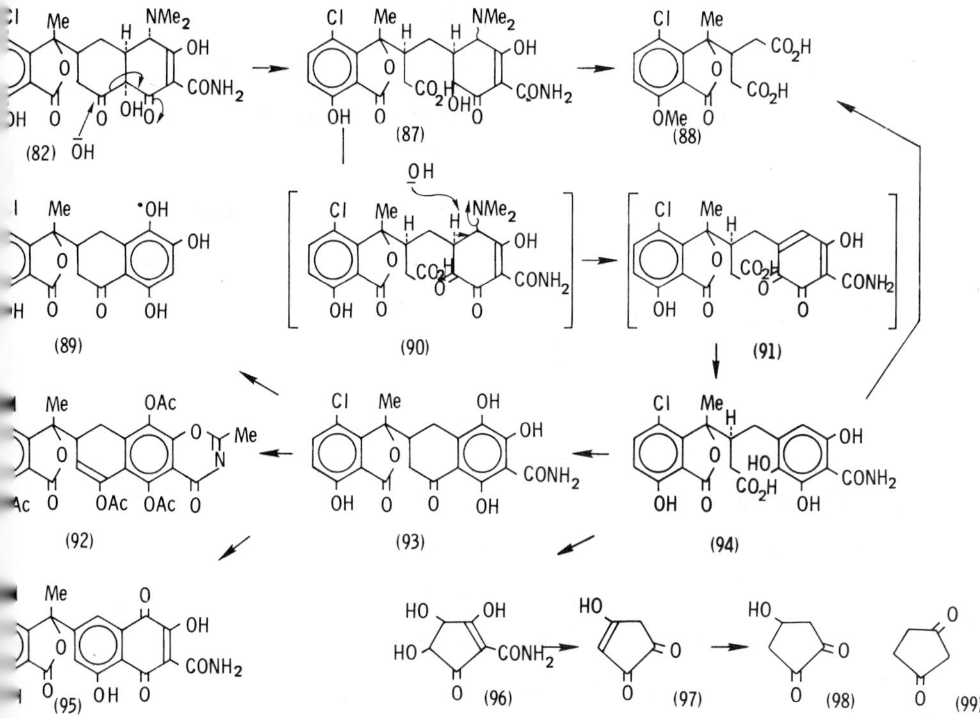

substituted glutaric acid derivative 88 which was subsequently synthesized. If air were present, treatment of isoaureomycin or the aureomycininc acids with base resulted in the liberation of dimethylamine and the formation of desdimethylaminoaureomycinic acid (94). This process is thought of as being autocatalytic once a small amount of the ortho-quinone (91) was formed. This situation, of course, is closely analogous to experience with OTC in similar reactions. The product isolated was desdimethylaminoaureomycinic acid (94) in which the phthalide function, the carboxylic acid, and the carboxamidated phenolic ring were easily recognizable from their spectral properties and the titration curve.[46] Further treatment with oxygen in base led to cleavage to the glutaric acid phthalide (88) and to a fragment of ring A in which ring contraction had occurred (96).[45] Acid treatment of 96 led to loss of the carboxamide function and a molecule of water with the formation of a cyclopentanetrione (97). The latter could be directly or indirectly (via 98) reduced to cyclopentane-1,3-dione (99) which was unknown at the time.

If desdimethylaminoaureomycinic acid (94) was treated with strong acid, a Friedel-Crafts like reaction ensued, and the cyclized product, aureonamide (93), was isolable.[46] This compound had a six-membered ketone function clearly visible in its infrared spectrum.

Acetylation of 93 led to the formation of a pentaacetylated derivative (92) in which not only had enol acetylation occurred, but the carboxamide function had participated in ring formation. The carboxamido function could be removed by alkaline treatment of 93 with base, giving rise to aureone (89). If the reaction were allowed to proceed in the presence of air or oxygen, aureonquinone amide (95) was isolated instead. The ultraviolet spectrum of 95 clearly contained a 2-hydroxy-1,4-naphthoquinone component. Reduction of the C_{12}-carbonyl of aureone (89) gave a product whose ultraviolet spectrum was the sum of the glutaric acid derivative (88) and 1,2,4-trihydroxybenzene, and, finally, the same operations on 94 provided evidence for a 2,6-dihydroxybenzoic acid moiety.

It is not possible to propose an alternate structure for CTC which will encompass all these findings. The structure is amply confirmed by single crystal X-ray analysis (Chapter 4).

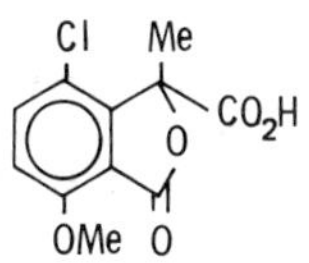

(100)

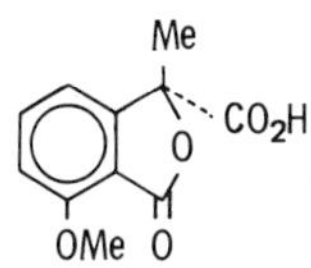

(101)

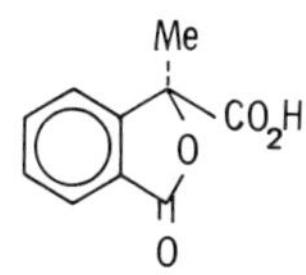

(102)

This, however, left open the question of the absolute configuration, as opposed to the relative configuration. This question was attacked by a Russian group.[54] It was known from the early degradation work that CTC gave rise to a number of acids when treated with methylating agents followed by oxidation. These reactions presumably left the configuration at C-6 unchanged and were suitable for investigation of the stereochemistry at that center. Since the X-ray study had revealed the relative configuration of all the centers in the molecule, it was only necessary to establish one of these in an absolute sense to establish them all. Treatment of CTC with dimethylsulfate and KOH followed by permanganate oxidation produced chlorophthalide 100, *i.a.* On catalytic hydrogenation 100 was converted to phthalide 101 whose optical rotatory dispersion curve was compared to that of 102 which had been synthesized for this purpose and had been related to L(+)-atrolactinic acid whose absolute configuration was known. The two curves were enantiomeric suggesting to the investigators that the configurations of the two compounds were opposite. Fortunately, this result is in agreement with the arbitrarily depicted stereochemistry in the literature. This work has been confirmed by subsequent X-ray analysis.[55] Coupled with circular dichroism measurements which show that all the major bioactive tetracyclines have the same absolute configuration,[18] this settles the stereochemical questions in the field.

5.7---Structure proof for TC.

Tetracycline was apparently encountered first, as detailed above, during the structural studies leading to the elucidation of the chemistry of CTC and OTC.[20,21,55] Subsequent to its preparation by catalytic hydrogenation of CTC, it was discovered in fermentation residues as a fermentation product.[56,57]

With the structure of CTC firmly known, conversion to TC by hydrogenolysis, a process which does not involve any optically active centers, is a sufficient proof of the latter's structure and stereochemistry.

5.8---Structure of 5a,11a-dehydrochlortetracycline.

Considerable genetic manipulation of the original *S. aureofaciens* strain was undertaken in order to improve yields of CTC or TC. Some of the descendant strains produced new tetracyclines. The first substance to be isolated from one of the progeny of the original Duggar strain was ultimately shown to be 5a,11a-dehydrochlortetracycline (103).[58] This material has relatively little bioactivity in its own right but has been of interest as an intermediate for chemical and microbiological conversions. The molecular formula contains two hydrogens less than CTC and the ultraviolet spectrum clearly was incompatible with the presence of the classical tetracycline BCD chromophore, for the spectrum was strongly altered in the 300-400 nm region.[59] Addition of $MgCl_2$ to the solution taken for the ultraviolet spectrum produced a bathochromic shift consistent with the view that the 11,12-diketo function was at least potentially present. The pKa values of the substance (3.3, 5.0, 9.6) were also consistent with this view. Catalytic hydrogenation produced a mixture of two dihydro dehalo products. One of these was TC itself (104, 5aH=α), while the other was clearly an isomer (104, 5aH=β). Isolation of tetracycline as a product of the reaction located all of the major structural features of the new metabolite. The isomeric product could be converted to anhydrotetracycline (5) by acid treatment, although the conditions were more vigorous than normally employed for this reaction. These findings meant that the double bond had C5a as one of its termini and the new isomer produced by reduction was 5a-epitetracycline.

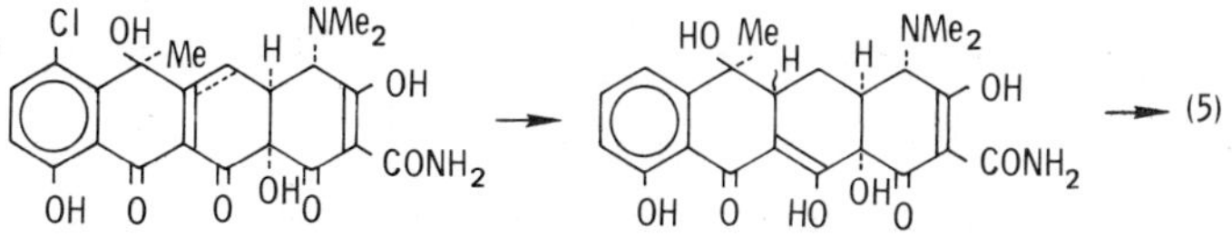

(103) (104)

Interestingly, two isomeric forms of dehydrochlortetracycline have actually been isolated.[60] When crystallized from chloroform, the C5a-11a isomer (infrared band at 1716 cm^{-1}) is formed, whereas crystallization from water leads to the isolation of the C5-5a isomer (no infrared band above 1660 cm^{-1}).

5.9---Degradation of 6-DMCTC.

Further work on mutant strains of *S. aureofaciens* resulted in strain Lederle-S-604 which produced a substance with substantial antibiotic activity. Ultimately, two products lacking the C_6-methyl group were isolated and characterized, DMCTC (105) and its deschloroanalog (106).[61] The two antibiotics were simply related to one another by catalytic halogenolysis.[62]

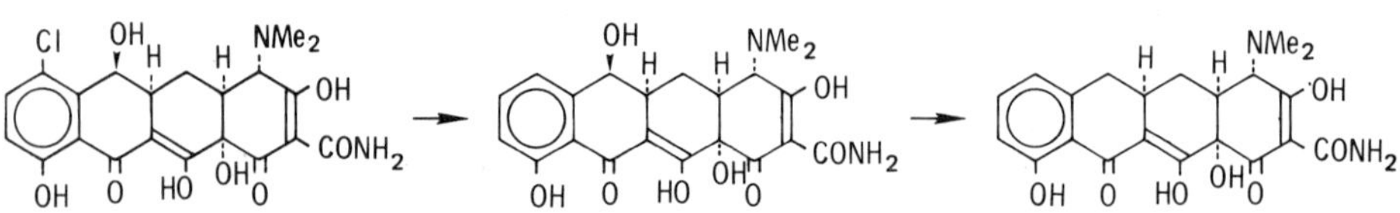

(105) (106) (107)

The classical tetracycline chromophore was present in these products. Significantly, Kuhn-Roth oxidation produced no acetic acid, indicating that there was no methyl group attached to carbon. The standard tetracycline degradation reactions were employed with the result that it was clear that the only novel feature about these new products was the absence of the methyl group at C-6. An important experimental finding was the observation that these antibiotics possessed enhanced acid and base stability over that of the previously encountered tetracyclines (see 5.3 and 5.4). When this increased stability was coupled with certain advantages in in vivo performance, DMCTC (105) was rapidly introduced into clinical use.

Reduction of either derivative under forcing conditions leads to hydrogenolysis of the C-6 hydroxyl group (which is benzilic) giving 6-demethyl-6-deoxytetracycline (107). This substance is the simplest member of the tetracycline family which possesses essentially all of the characteristic biological activities of the family. Because of its remarkable stability towards acid (it can be recovered unchanged from concentrated sulfuric acid), it has been extensively studied in attempts to produce new tetracyclines chemically.

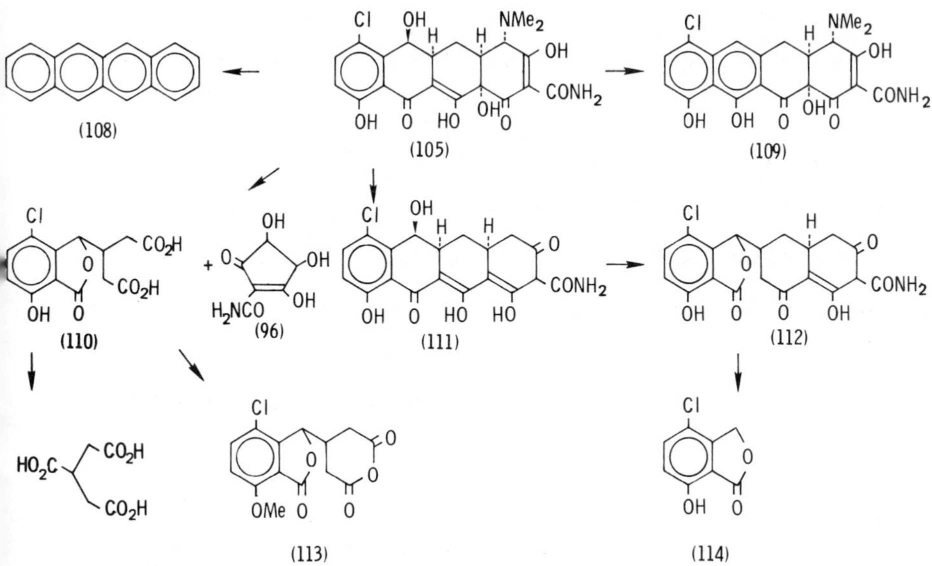

On distillation with zinc dust, DMCTC (105) produced naphthacene (108). Formation of the anhydroanalog (109) required heating in concentrated HCl. When degraded with NaOH in the presence of air, 110 and 96 were produced. These are quite analogous to the CTC degradation products. Product 110 could be further degraded to the glutaranhydride (113) showing the relationship of the two carboxyl groups and also to β-carboxyglutaric acid. On treatment with zinc and acetic acid, the dimethylamino and C_{12a}-OH groups were both lost and 111 resulted. Treatment with base led to phthalide 112. Pyrolysis of the latter produced 114 which was subsequently synthesized.[63] The identity of degradation product 114 was decisive when compared with 85.

As is found with all of the normal tetracyclines, epimers involving the dimethylamino function at C-4 form at intermediate pH's in solution. These products accompanied the parent antibiotics as originally isolated.

5.10--2-Acetyl-2-decarboxamidotetracycline.

An interesting group of naturally occurring tetracycline analogs which have been isolated from normal cultures and characterized are the C-2 acetyl derivatives. It is thought that to a certain extent acetate can serve as a "starter unit" in place of the postulated normal malonic acid semiamide with the result that a methyl ketone function appears at C-2 in the finished tetracyclines. Apparently, this occurs to a certain extent in virtually all strains for it has been reported that all commercial samples available to one group of investigators contained measurable amounts of the C-2 acetyl analogs.[64]

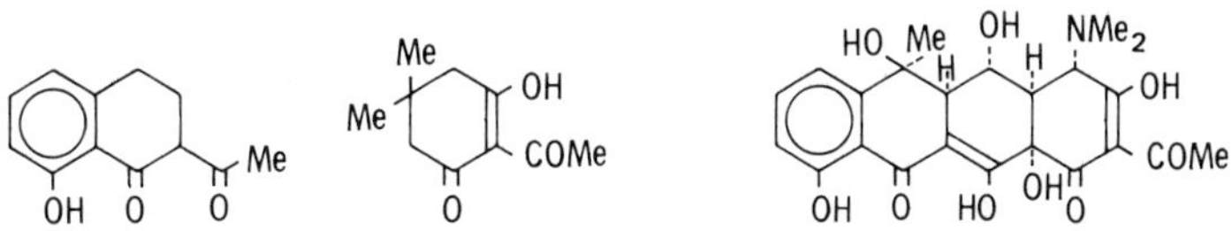

(115) (116) (117)

The C-2 acetyl analogs of CTC, OTC and TC have been isolated and characterized.[64-67] The ultraviolet chromophore associated with the BCD rings of these agents was normal, but there were small but definite aberrations in the A ring absorption maximum. Thus, the difference between these materials and the classical tetracyclines likely resided in the A ring. Kuhn-Roth oxidation demonstrated that there were now <u>two</u> methyl groups attached to carbon. Microanalyses revealed a single nitrogen to be present and titration data confirmed that it was basic. An infrared absorption band was present at 5.92μ (C=O) which is not present in the infrared spectrum of any of the major tetracyclines. These considerations suggested strongly that the carboxamide function was replaced by a methyl ketone moiety. This inference received strong support from the finding that addition of the ultraviolet spectrum of 2-acetyl-7-hydroxy tetralone (115) to that of 2-acetyl dimedon (116) produced a spectrum which was very nearly identical with that of the new antibiotics.

Confirmation that major portions of the BCD chromophore were indeed intact came from degradative reactions. Careful

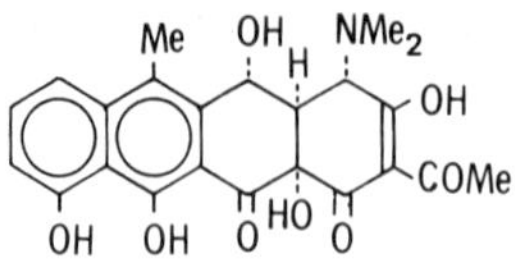

(118)

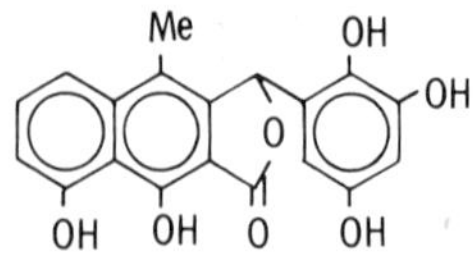

(64)

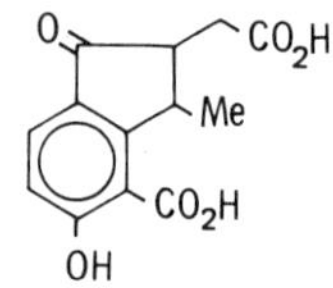

(17)

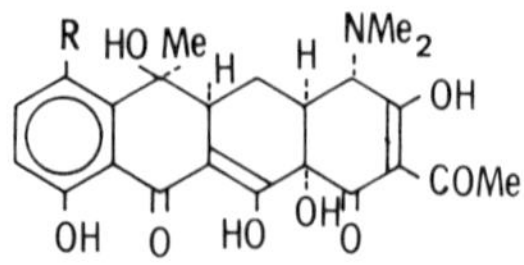

(119)

acid treatment led to an anhydro derivative (118) with its attendent spectroscopic changes and vigorous acid treatment led to the known OTC degradation product, decarboxamido-terrinolide (64). Thus, the presence of the majority of the structural features of the new substance was clearly demonstrated. Treatment with alkali led to formation of terracinoic acid (17). These findings are most consistent with the structures 117 and 119 for these interesting molecules.

REFERENCES

1. H. Muxfeldt and R. Bangert, Prog. Chem. Org. Nat. Prod., 21, 80 (1963).
2. G. C. Garrett, J. Pharm. Sci., 52, 309 (1963).
3. T. Money and A. I. Scott in "Progress in Organic Chemistry J. Cook and W. Carruthers, Eds., Butterworths, Washington, 1 (1968).

4. P. P. Regna *in* "Antibiotics. Their Chemistry and Non-Medical Uses," H. Goldberg, Ed., Van Nostrand, Princeton, 77 (1959).

5. J. H. Boothe, *Antimicrob. Agts. Chemother.*, 213 (1962).

6. D. L. J. Clive, *Quarterly Reviews*, *22*, 435 (1968).

7. J. J. Hlavka and J. H. Boothe, *Prog. Drug Res.*, *17*, 210 (1973).

8. W. Durckheimer, *Angew. Chem., Intnl. Ed., English*, *14*, 721 (1975).

9. R. K. Blackwood, "Tetracyclines," *in* Kirk-Othmer Encyclopedia of Chemical Technology, Second Ed.

10. A. P. Doerschuk, B. A. Bitler and J. R. D. McCormick, *J. Am. Chem. Soc.*, *77*, 4687 (1955).

11. C. R. Stephens, L. H. Conover, P. N. Gordon, F. C. Pennington, R. L. Wagner, K. J. Brunings and F. J. Pilgrim, *J. Am. Chem. Soc.*, *78*, 1515 (1956).

12. J. R. D. McCormick, S. M. Fox, L. L. Smith, B. A. Bitler, J. Reichenthal, V. E. Origoni, W. H. Muller, R. Winterbottom and A. P. Doerschuk, *J. Am. Chem. Soc.*, *78*, 3547 (1956).

13. M. A. Kaplan, A. P. Granatek and F. H. Buckwalter, *Antibiot. Chemother.*, *7*, 569 (1957).

14. J. R. D. McCormick, S. M. Fox, L. L. Smith, B. A. Bitler, J. Reichenthal, V. E. Origoni, W. H. Muller, R. Winterbottom and A. P. Doerschuk, *J. Am. Chem. Soc.*, *79*, 2849 (1957).

15. E. G. Remmers, G. M. Sieger and A. P. Doerschuk, *J. Pharm. Sci.*, *52*, 752 (1963).

16. D. A. Hussar, P. J. Niebergall, E. T. Sugita and J. T. Doluisio, J. Pharm. Pharmacol., 20, 539 (1968).

17. J. J. Korst, J. D. Johnson, K. Butler, E. J. Bianco, L. H. Conover and R. B. Woodward, J. Am. Chem. Soc., 90, 439 (1968).

18. L. A. Mitscher, A. C. Bonacci and T. D. Sokoloski, Antimicrob. Agts. Chemother., 78 (1968).

19. C. T. Agostini and C. R. Kowarski, Pharm. Acta Helv., 47, 560 (1972).

20. V. Naggar, N. A. Daabis and M. M. Motawi, Die Pharmazie, 29, 129 (1976).

21. L. H. Conover, W. T. Moreland, A. R. English, C. R. Stephens and F. J. Pilgrim, J. Am. Chem. Soc., 75, 4622 (1953).

22. J. H. Boothe, J. Morton, J. P. Petisi, R. G. Wilkinson and J. H. Williams, J. Am. Chem. Soc., 75, 4621 (1953).

23. M. W. Miller and F. A. Hochstein, J. Org. Chem., 27, 2525 (1962).

24. C. W. Waller, B. L. Hutchings, R. W. Broschard, A. A. Goldman, W. J. Stein, C. F. Wolf and J. H. Williams, J. Am. Chem. Soc., 74, 4981 (1952).

25. R. K. Blackwood and C. R. Stephens, Can. J. Chem., 43, 1382 (1965).

26. J. J. Hlavka and H. M. Krazinski, J. Org. Chem., 28, 1422 (1963).

27. A. Green, R. G. Wilkinson and J. H. Boothe, J. Am. Chem. Soc., 82, 3946 (1960).

28. J. R. D. McCormick, N. O. Sjolander, U. Hirsch, E. R. Jensen and A. P. Doerschuk, J. Am. Chem. Soc., 79, 4561 (1957).

29. R. K. Blackwood, J. J. Beereboom, H. H. Rennhard, M. Schach von Wittenau and C. R. Stephens, J. Am. Chem. Soc., 85, 3943 (1963).

30. C. R. Stephens, L. H. Conover, R. Pasternack, F. A. Hochstein, W. T. Moreland, P. P. Regna, F. J. Pilgrim, K. J. Brunings and R. B. Woodward, J. Am. Chem. Soc., 76, 3568 (1954).

31. C. W. Waller, B. L. Hutchings, C. F. Wolf, A. A. Goldman, R. W. Broschard and J. H. Williams, J. Am. Chem. Soc., 74, 4981 (1952).

32. R. Pasternack, A. Bavley, R. L. Wagner, F. A. Hochstein, P. P. Regna and K. J. Brunings, J. Am. Chem. Soc., 74, 1926 (1952).

33. R. Pasternack, L. H. Conover, A. Bavley, F. A. Hochstein, G. B. Hess and K. J. Brunings, J. Am. Chem. Soc., 74, 1928 (1952).

34. F. A. Hochstein, C. R. Stephens, L. H. Conover, P. P. Regna, R. Pasternack, K. J. Brunings and R. B. Woodward, J. Am. Chem. Soc., 74, 3708 (1952).

35. F. A. Hochstein, C. R. Stephens, L. H. Conover, P. P. Regna, R. Pasternack, P. N. Gordon, F. J. Pilgrim, K. J. Brunings and R. B. Woodward, J. Am. Chem. Soc., 75, 5455 (1953).

36. R. Huhn and K. Dury, Chem. Ber., 84, 563 (1951).

37. F. A. Hochstein and R. Pasternack, J. Am. Chem. Soc., 73, 5008 (1951).

38. F. A. Hochstein and R. Pasternack, J. Am. Chem. Soc., 74, 3905 (1952).

39. R. Pasternack, P. P. Regna, R. L. Wagner, R. L. Bavley, F. A. Hochstein, P. N. Gordon and K. J. Brunings, J. Am. Chem. Soc., 73, 2400 (1951).

40. L. H. Conover, J. Am. Chem. Soc., 75, 4017 (1953).

41. F. A. Hochstein, P. P. Regna, K. H. Brunings and R. B. Woodward, J. Am. Chem. Soc., 74, 3706 (1952).

42. F. A. Hochstein, C. R. Stephens, P. N. Gordon, P. P. Regna, F. J. Pilgrim, K. J. Brunings and R. B. Woodward, J. Am. Chem. Soc., 74, 3707 (1952).

43. M. Schach von Wittenau, R. K. Blackwood, L. M. Conover, R. H. Glauert and R. B. Woodward, J. Am. Chem. Soc., 87, 134 (1965).

44. C. R. Stephens, L. H. Conover, R. Pasternack, F. A. Hochstein, F. T. Moreland, P. P. Regna, F. J. Pilgrim, K. J. Brunings and R. B. Woodward, J. Am. Chem. Soc., 76, 3568 (1954).

45. C. R. Stephens, L. H. Conover, F. A. Hochstein, P. P. Regna, F. J. Pilgrim, K. J. Brunings and R. B. Woodward, J. Am. Chem. Soc., 74, 4976 (1952).

46. C. W. Waller, B. L. Hutchings, C. F. Wolf, R. W. Broschard, A. A. Goldman and J. H. Williams, J. Am. Chem. Soc., 74, 4978 (1952).

47. C. W. Waller, B. L. Hutchings, A. A. Goldman, C. F. Wolf, R. W. Broschard and J. H. Williams, J. Am. Chem. Soc., 74, 4979 (1952).

48. B. L. Hutchings, C. W. Waller, R. W. Brochard, C. F. Wolf, P. W. Fryth and J. H. Williams, J. Am. Chem. Soc., 74, 4980 (1952).

49. C. W. Waller, B. L. Hutchings, C. F. Wolf, A. A. Goldman, R. W. Broschard and J. H. Williams, J. Am. Chem. Soc., 74, 4891 (1952).

50. C. W. Waller, B. L. Hutchings, R. W. Broschard, A. A. Goldman, W. J. Stein, C. F. Wolf and J. H. Williams, J. Am. Chem. Soc., 74, 4981 (1952).

51. B. L. Hutchings, C. W. Waller, S. Gordon, R. W. Broschard, C. F. Wolf, A. A. Goldman and J. H. Williams, J. Am. Chem. Soc., 74, 3710 (1952).

52. S. Kushner, J. H. Boothe, J. Morton, II, J. Petisi and J. H. Williams, J. Am. Chem. Soc., 74, 3710 (1952).

53. S. Kushner, J. Morton, II, J. H. Boothe and J. H. Williams, J. Am. Chem. Soc., 75, 1087 (1953).

54. V. N. Dobrynin, A. I. Gurevich, M. G. Karapetyan, M. N. Kolosov and M. M. Shemyakin, Tet. Letts., 901 (1962).

55. K. Kamiya, M. Asai, Y. Wada and M. Nishikawa, Experientia, 27, 363 (1971).

56. J. H. Boothe, J. Morton, II, J. P. Petisi, R. G. Wilkinson and J. H. Williams, Antibiotics Annual, 46 (1953-4).

57. P. P. Minieri, M. C. Firman, A. G. Mistretta, A. Abbey, C. E. Brickler, N. E. Rigler and H. Sokol, Antibiotics Annual, 81 (1953-4).

58. J. R. D. McCormick, P. A. Miller, J. A. Growich, N. O. Sjolander and A. P. Doerschuk, J. Am. Chem. Soc., 80, 5572 (1958).

59. J. R. D. McCormick, N. O. Sjolander, U. Hirsch, P. A. Miller, N. H. Arnold and A. P. Doerschuk, J. Am. Chem. Soc., 80, 6460 (1952).

60. M. Schach von Wittenau, F. A. Hochstein and C. R. Stephens, J. Org. Chem., 28, 2454 (1963).

61. J. R. D. McCormick, N. O. Sjolander, U. Hirsch, E. R. Jensen and A. P. Doerschuk, J. Am. Chem. Soc., 79, 4561 (1957).

62. J. S. Webb, R. W. Broschard, D. B. Cosulich, W. J. Stein and C. F. Wolf, J. Am. Chem. Soc., 79, 4563 (1957).

63. J. H. Boothe, A. Green, J. P. Petisi, R. G. Wilkinson and C. W. Waller, J. Am. Chem. Soc., 79, 4564 (1957).

64. J. Keiner, R. Huttenrauch and W. Poethke, Arch. Pharmazie, 300, 840 (1967).

65. F. A. Hochstein, M. Schach von Wittenau, F. W. Tanner, Jr., and K. Murai, J. Am. Chem. Soc., 82, 5934 (1960).

66. M. W. Miller and F. A. Hochstein, J. Org. Chem., 27, 2525 (1962).

67. G. C. Lancini and P. Sensi, Experientia, 20, 83 (1964).

CHAPTER 6

CHEMICAL TRANSFORMATIONS OF THE TETRACYCLINE FAMILY

6.1---Introduction.

Having by now gotten a feeling for the conditions which are too severe for the tetracyclines, the stage is set for a discussion of those reactions which leave the ring system essentially intact and whose products possess a significant chance at biological activity. The presence of a hydroxyl group at C_5 conveys some special properties on tetracyclines which makes their chemistry somewhat different from the others so the two subfamilies will be treated separately. It is convenient, although arbitrary, to discuss individual positions in the tetracycline molecule rather than to organize the chemistry about reaction types. As was pointed out in Chapter 5, 6-deoxy-6-demethyltetracycline (1) is the simplest known tetracycline with essentially complete pharmacological properties so this structure may be regarded as the pharmacophore. Formula 1 recapitulates the numbering system of those centers for which relevant chemistry is available. There are no reactions leading to

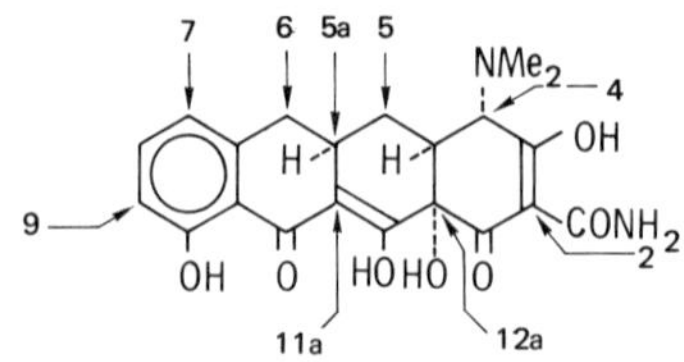

(1)

alterations at carbons 1, 3, 4a, 8, 10, 11 or 12 which have not at the same time altered the whole molecule or led to complete inactivation.

6.2---Chemistry of position 2.

In general, substitutions of other groups for the carboxamide moiety or substituents on the amide nitrogen which do not readily come off in dilute aqueous solutions have resulted in inferior antibiotics. The nature of the substituent at C_2 has a pronounced effect on the water solubility of tetracyclines and this has had considerable practical application.

When tetracyclines (1) are treated with tosyl or mesyl chloride in pyridine, the carboxamide function readily dehydrates to a nitrile moiety (2). In some cases and under some conditions, the C_{10}-sulfonate ester also forms.[1-5] CTC, in particular, shows little tendency to form a tosylate at C_{10}.[2] The nitrile (3) is very poorly water soluble and perhaps in part for this reason has very little antibiotic activity. For reasons which are not clear, the nitriles do not readily epimerize at C_4, a property that was useful in studying this phenomenon.

(1)

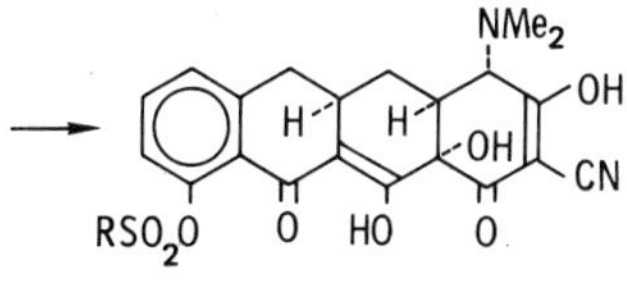

(2)

It has been reported[6] that the nitriles can be converted back to bioactive tetracyclines (1) on treatment with boron trifluoride in acetic acid followed by hydrolysis. The mechanism may be as follows:

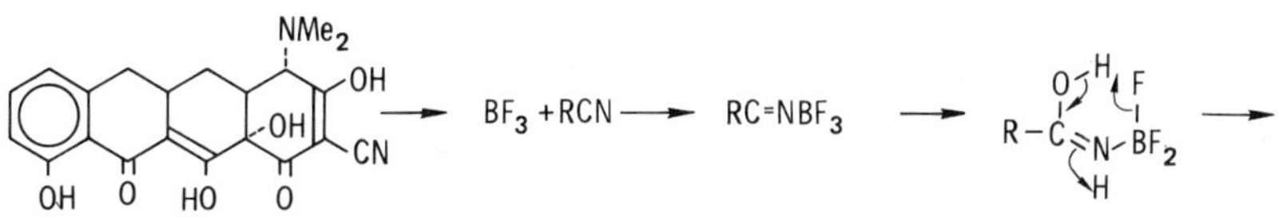

(3)

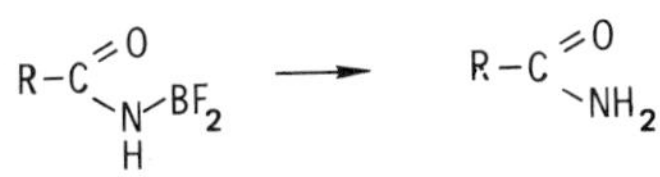

This process might be of some value as a protection-deprotection sequence but would not work if a readily dehydratable OH were present at C_6.

The Ritter reaction, in which the nitrile is treated with isobutylene in sulfuric and acetic acids, converts 3 to the mono N-alkylated amide 4.[4] These derivatives are much more lipophilic than the parent antibiotics* but their antibacterial activity is limited to Gram-positive organisms. Subsequently, the mono N-methyl derivative (7) of

---

* Some derivatives in the 5a,6-anhydro series are even soluble in hexane!

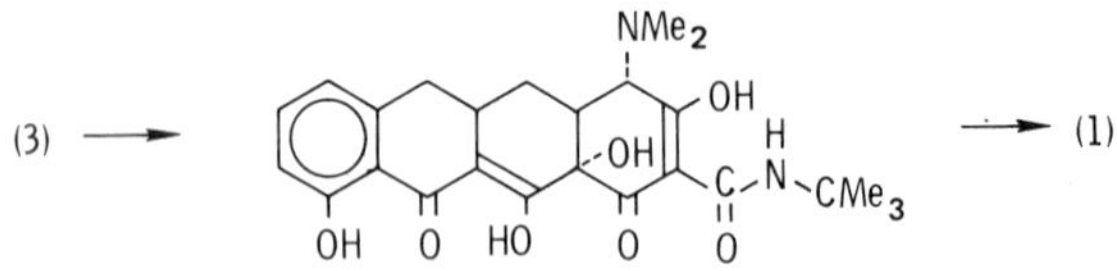

(4)

minocycline (5) was prepared in the hope that a smaller alkyl group would alter the antimicrobial spectrum less.[7] Treatment of 5 with chloromethyl methyl sulfide in strong acid ($MeSO_3H$, *e.g.*) led to the substituted amide (6) which had poor antibiotic activity. Refluxing 6 with Raney nickel in ethanol gave the expected desulfurization product. Compound 7 had an antimicrobial spectrum similar to that of minocycline (5) but the potency was lower.

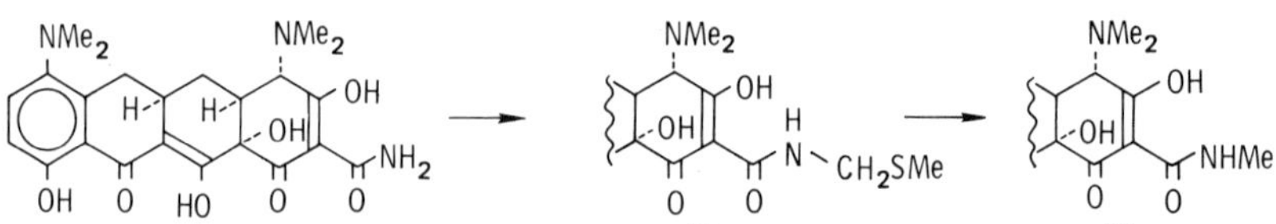

(5) (6) (7)

The oxygen analogs of 6 have been made.[8] Reaction of TC with formaldehyde and methanol at reflux led to 8a in good yield. A number of analogs were made and these derivatives possess from 12-46% of the turbidimetric assay of the parent tetracycline *in vitro* and 6-100% *in vivo*. It was felt, however, that the bioactivity resulted from reversion to the parent antibiotic, a process which could be seen to happen *in vitro*. The acetaldehyde analogs reverted more readily to starting materials and were correspondingly more potent than the formaldehyde derivatives. When formaldehyde alone was used with CTC, the methylol itself

(8b) could be isolated and this was reputed to be better tolerated than CTC itself.[10] Acetone could be substituted successfully for formaldehyde.

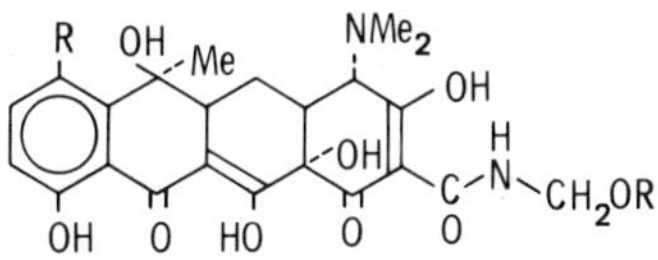

(8) a. $R=CH_3$, R'=H
b. R=H, R'=Cl

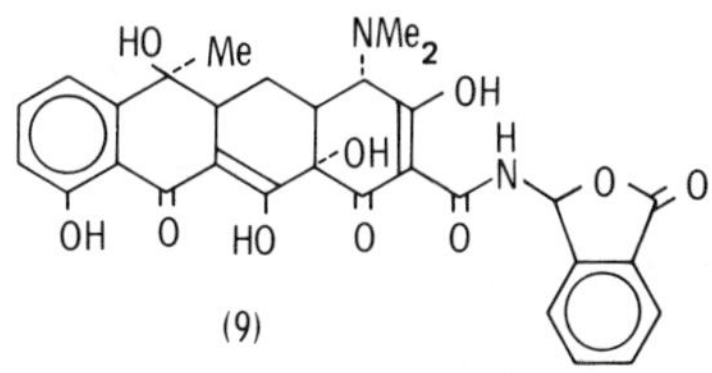

(9)

The N-(3-phthalidyl) analog (9) of TC was obtained under somewhat similar conditions.[9] When TC is warmed with phthalaldehydic acid, 9 precipitates. Its bioactivity *in vitro* against *Micrococcus pyogenes var. aureus* is essentially that contributed by the TC component. The drug is highly soluble in water above pH 9, but not soluble in dilute acid and it gives no blood levels orally or IM in experimental animals.

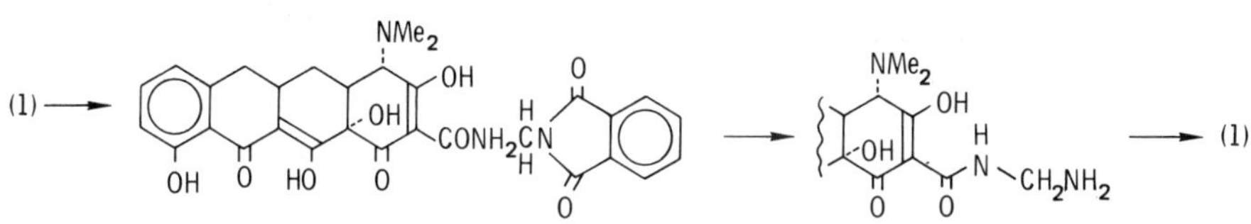

(10) (11)

The aminoanalogs (11) of 6 have been made from the nitriles *via* the Einhorn reaction.[11] Treatment of 1 with a variety of hydroxymethylene amides and imides (the phthalimide is illustrated) in strong acid leads to a Mannich-like condensation to 10, which was inactive as an antibiotic. Hydrolysis was effected by refluxing in methanol containing n-butylamine. Unfortunately, 11 was insufficiently stable for further study, reverting rapidly to 1. The reaction follows quite another course when the carboxamides are used rather than the nitriles. Under these conditions, the D-ring becomes substituted (q. v.).

Formally analogous compounds of significant medicinal value are formed under the conditions of the Mannich reaction. These bases can be as much as 2500 times more soluble in water at physiological pH's than the tetracyclines themselves so they are often preferred for injection or even oral use. They are classical prodrugs in that they rapidly revert in the body to the free tetracycline so their pharmacological properties are essentially equivalent to that of their precursor. Because of the versatility and ease of the Mannich reaction, literally dozens of patents have appeared describing their properties.

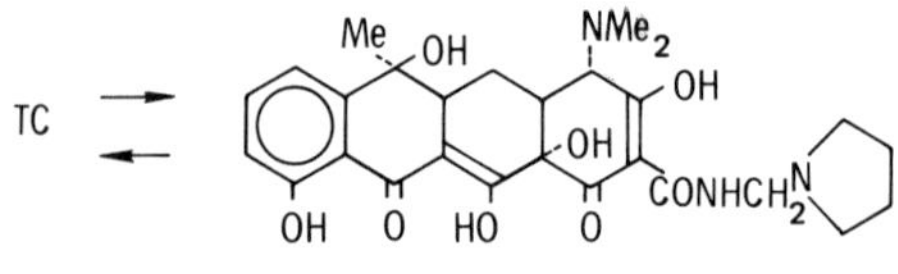

(12)

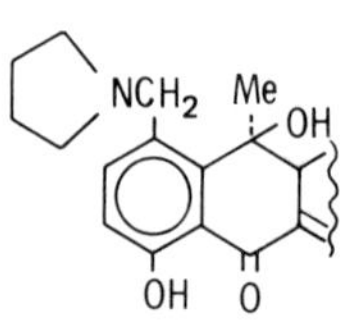

(13)

N-Pyrolidinomethyltetracycline (PMTC, 12) was prepared from TC, pyrolidine and formaldehyde.[12] Phenols also readily undergo the Mannich reaction and the product was initially formulated as 13. Catalytic hydrogenation did not, however, lead to a Ring D methyl tetracycline as formula 13 would require,[13] so the formula was revised to 12. This was confirmed by the comparative studies of the solvolytic behavior of simplified C- and N-Mannich bases[14,15] from which it was shown that C-Mannich bases always solvolyzed to leave the CH_2 attached to the carbon whereas N-Mannich bases came off *via* a β-elimination to liberate the amide. Under identical conditions, lysinomethylenetetracycline went back to TC. Subsequently, it was shown by pmr studies of pure 12 that the methylene peak came at 4.5δ as a two proton doublet (J=6Hz) and the NH at 10.45δ as a one-proton triplet (J=6Hz). Appropriate decoupling studies confirmed this relationship.[16]

The tendency of these prodrugs to revert on standing in solution is supported by paper chromatographic studies[17] and in particular by hplc work.[18] In the latter case, the two are cleanly separated and a T-1/2 of about 3 hr. in water at room temperature was observed.

There is evidence that the Mannich bases may epimerize, in some cases, more readily than the parent tetracycline, although the instability of the prodrug complicates the work.[19] This is especially interesting in light of the effect of the nitrile[3] and the 2-acetyl functions[20] in suppressing epimerization. Obviously, C_2 influences this property, but the rationale has yet to emerge. It has been pointed out that the epimerization tendency increases with an increase in the A-ring dissociation constant and a decrease in the NMe_2 dissociation constant.[21]

It is not possible to list in the space available all of the Mannich bases which have been described. Some idea of the range available can be gotten from the selections in formulae 14-19.

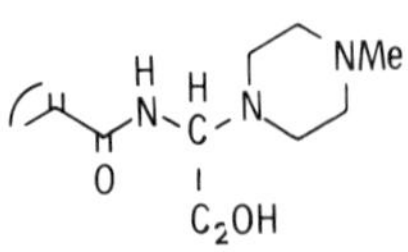

(14)[22]

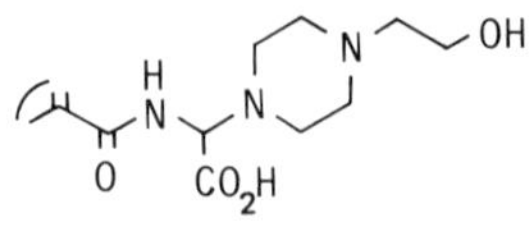

(15)[23]

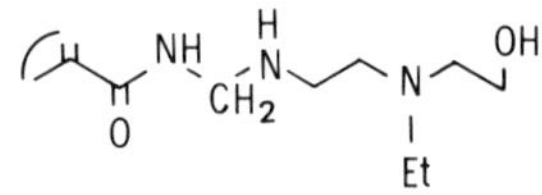

(16)[24]

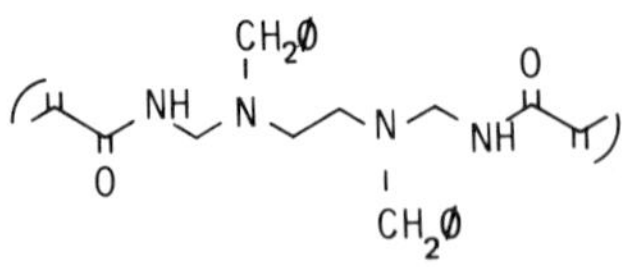

(17)[25]

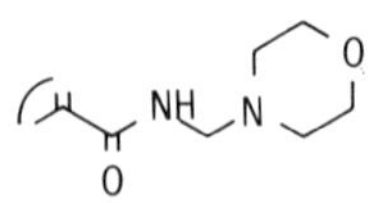

(18)[26]

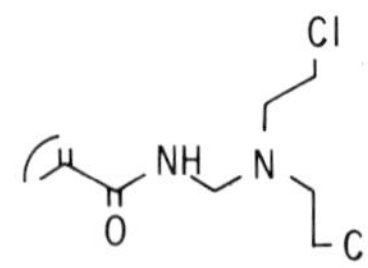

(19)[27]

Compound <u>19</u> represents an interesting attempt to utilize the well-known tendency of tetracyclines to accumulate in tumor cells[28] as a device to deliver a cytotoxic mustard selectively and thus increase the safety margin of such therapy. Unfortunately, the potency was disappointing. It is somewhat daunting for future efforts along these lines to note that mustard <u>19</u> causes such severe inflammation that it has been proposed as a standard irritant to be used in pharmacological studies of antiinflammatory agents.[29]

To complete the record, it will be recalled from Chapter 3 that the 2-acetyl analogs of the tetracyclines are coproduced biosynthetically. In one study, all available commercial samples of tetracyclines contained perceptable quantities of these agents.[30] The analog of OTC,[20,31] TC,[32] and CTC[31] have all been characterized. Their bioactivity is only about 5% of that of the corresponding carboxamide.[32]

6.3---Chemistry of position 4.

The natural α-orientation of the C_4-dimethylamino group is essential for bioactivity. Epimerization to 4-epitetracycline (sometimes called quatrimycins; discussed in Chapter 5) results in loss of potency and 4-epianhydrotetracycline is toxic to the kidneys involving a Fanconi-like syndrome. Concern about the mechanism and detection of these phenomena has engendered a large literature (discussed also in Chapter 4).[33-40]

TC and CTC can be converted to their quaternary ammonium analogs with a variety of alkyl halides, but the resulting products are not useful antibiotics.[41] Interestingly, both C_4-epimers give methiodides which retain their stereochemical integrity and therefore are distinguishable.[34,35] Treatment of either salt with zinc and acid under non-equilibrating conditions leads to the identical dedimethylaminotetracycline (<u>20</u>) which has no antibacterial action. It was subsequently found[42] that photolysis of a methanolic solution of TC methiodide but not 4-epiTC methiodide led to photoreduction to give <u>20</u>. Each quaternary salt also led to a unique anhydrotetracycline quaternary salt and these were converted to the anhydro analog of <u>20</u>. These findings were crucial in locating the position of isomerism, particularly as the only remaining asymmetric centers are those in ring A. Quaternization of TC by heating a solution in tetrahydrofuran with methyliodide in a sealed tube gives the anhydrotetra-

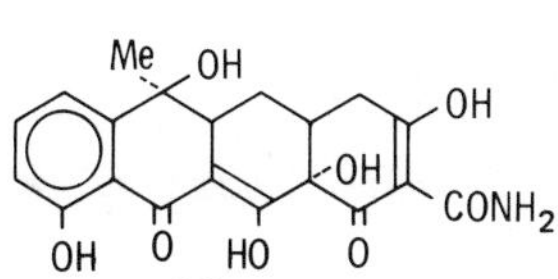

(20)

cycline quaternary salt. Treatment at room temperature for one week avoids dehydration.

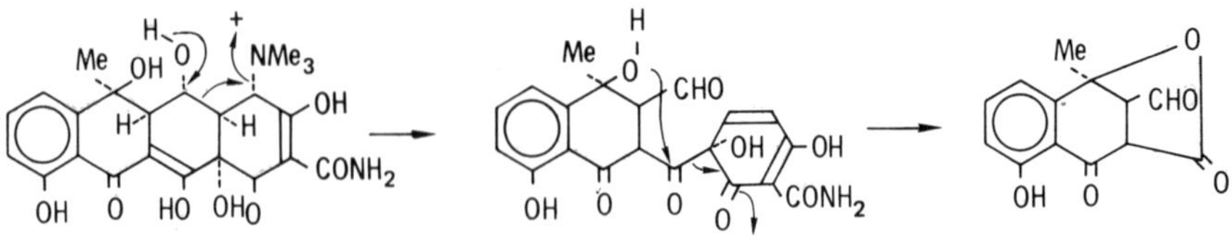

(21) (22) (23)

OTC is quite unstable under either of these conditions, undergoing an interesting fragmentation reaction rationalized as involving the C_5-OH group. Quaternization (<u>21</u>) is thought to preceed fragmentation to <u>22</u> which then undergoes β-diketone cleavage and lactone formation to give <u>23</u>, the product isolated.[43] On the other hand, MOTC and DOOTC form normal methiodides.[44] This is rational as these derivatives have no C_6-OH to participate in the reaction.

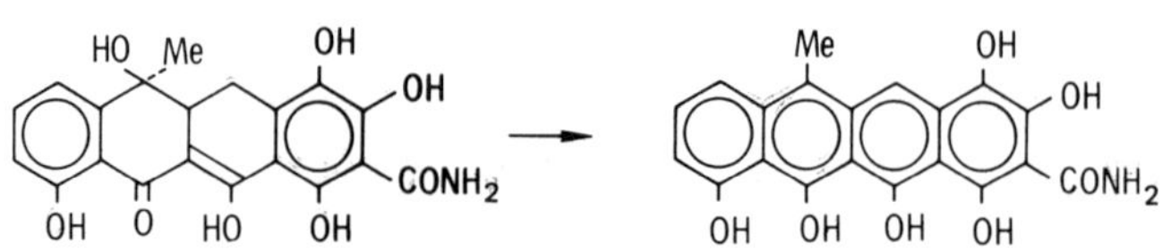

(24) (25)

When tetracycline quaternary salts are dissolved in hydroxylic solvents and the pH raised to near neutrality, the betaines precipitate. It will be recalled from Chapter 3 that heating these in acetonitrile causes elimination of trimethylamine and A-ring rearrangement to the 4-OH analog (<u>24</u>). Dehydration leads to the biosynthetically significant 4-hydroxypretetramides (<u>25</u>).[45-47]

Treatment of the hydrochloride salts of the tetracyclines with a variety of mild oxidizing agents results in enamine formation (26).[48-51] Under certain very special conditions, this highly unstable product can be isolated as its bridged aminohydrin (27). More commonly, the dimethylamino function undergoes hydrolysis to the 4-ketotetracyclines (28). When a C_6-OH is present, as illustrated, hemiketal formation takes place and the product (29) is known as a tetracycloxide. Only one conformation can give this rigid polycyclic structure (30). Although in principle the C_{4a}-hydrogen can epimerize in the 4-keto series, no such reaction has been reported. The cyclic nature of the tetracycloxide molecule preserves the normal geometry at C_{4a}. An unambiguous X-ray study confirmed structure 30.[52] This formula also requires the 11a-hydrogen to be α. Tetracycloxide formation destroys the enolization of the BCD chromophore and shortens the position of the uv max. There is also an IR max at 5.7μ consistent with this.[51]

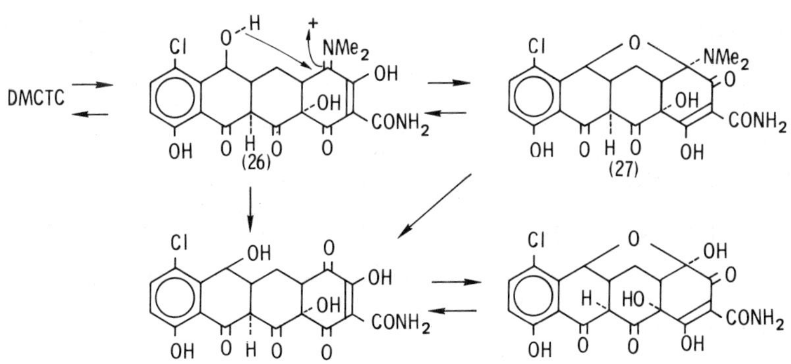

(28) (29)

As might be anticipated from these considerations, enamine forming reactions on 11a-α-chlorotetracycline forms the 11a-chloroanalog of 30.[51]

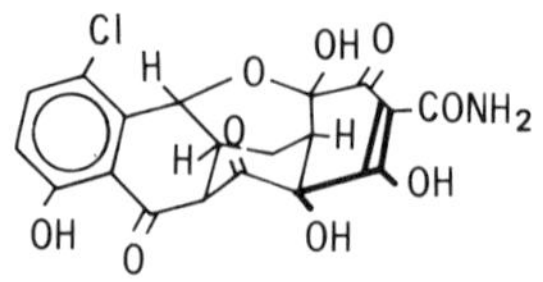

(30)

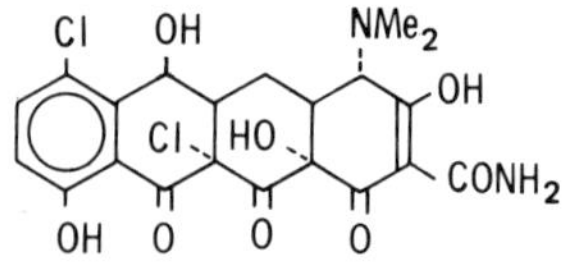

(31)

Among the reagents that will effect these changes are mercuric acetate, cupric acetate, N-chlorsuccinimide in aqueous media (HOBr), sodium hypochlorite, etc. The important role of conditions is illustrated by the finding that N-chlorsuccinimde in nonaqueous solvents (Cl· or Cl+) forms the C_{11a}-Cl analog (31) instead.

Following the discovery that the cyclic enamine (27) could be reduced back to DMCTC with borohydride, this redox sequence has been used to prepare a series of tetracyclines alkylated at C_4 with groups other than methyl.[48,49] The best conditions involved use of deschlorotetracycloxide (29 with H at C_7), and the appropriate primary amine and hydrogenation with palladium-charcoal catalyst. Further reduction in the presence of the appropriate aldehyde led to the tertiary amines in the table while the primary amine was produced by chemical reduction of the oxime or the hydrazone.[50] If methylamine was used in the reductive amination and this was reductively alkylated using formaldehyde, a full circle was accomplished and the parent tetracycline was reformed, although in unspecified yield. It will be recalled from Chapter 3 that fermentation sources will produce bioactive tetracyclines only with dimethylamino, or, when ethionine is added to the fermentation, a small amount of ethylmethyltetracycline can be formed as well. This limitation is overcome by the new reaction sequence, however, the biopotency of the resulting analogs is disappointing (Table 6-1). It would appear that small groups are needed for satisfactory activity. An interesting complication arose in this study in that the products often had the undesired 4-*epi* configuration because the catalyst can more readily approach <u>30</u> from the open α-face and many of the products were unexpectedly difficult to isomerize to the natural configuration. This was, however, not true of the tertiary amino analogs which reverted completely. The wrong stereochemistry at C_4 surely accounts in part for the disappointing bioactivity of some of the products. It

Table 6-1. *In vitro* potency of some N_4 analogs of TC against *Staphylococcus aureus* relative to TC itself.[49]

NRR'		Potency Relative to TC (=100%)
R	R'	
H	H	75%
H	Me	75
H	Et	75
Me	Et	75
H	*n*-Pr	50
Me	*n*-Pr	50
H	*n*-Bu	12
H	*n*-CH_2CH_2OH	12
Me	*n*-CH_2CH_2OH	12
H	*n*-$CH_2CH_2CH_2OH$	25
Et	Et	25

is possible though not likely that some of the problem may lay with isomerism at C_{4a} although this has not been detected. When, for example, the primary amino analog of TC was quaternized, the product isolated was TC betaine.[51] The yield, however, was not quantitative.

Catalytic or chemical reduction of tetracycloxides in the absence of amine[50] or in part in the presence of an insufficient excess of amine[49] led to isolation of the 4-hydroxy tetracyclines of unspecified stereochemistry and unspecified bioactivity.

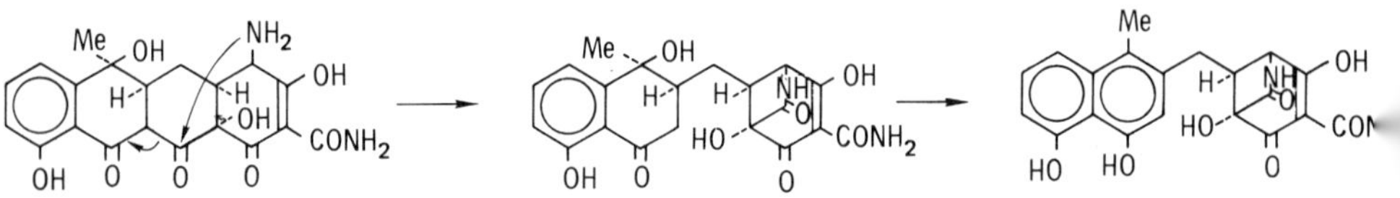

(32) (33) (34)

An interesting consequence of the formation of 4-desdimethylamino-4β-aminotetracycline (32) is its degradation in hot aqueous bicarbonate to lactam 33. This non-basic compound is isomeric with 32 and has an 8-hydroxytetralone ring CD chromophore as well as the A-ring chromophore. Infrared adsorption at 5.7μ agrees with this formulation. Dehydration to anhydro derivative 34 which has a typical 1,8-dihydroxynaphthalene and A-ring uv chromophores as well as lactam IR bands is consistent with the desired structure. The other epimer of 32 is stable to these reaction conditions.[51]

A further example of the practical importance of seemingly trivial variations in conditions is the finding that treatment of TC base, rather than the HCl salt, with mercuric acetate in acetic acid led to 37.[53] This outcome is rationalized by proposing that oxidation occurs to the enamine and that this is rapidly followed by hydrolysis to enol 35. With the liberated base not neutralized by the mineral acid as in the previous tetracycloxide-producing reactions, the alkaline medium leds to participation of the C_6-OH in cleavage of ring B to produce intermediate 37. Driving force for the reaction is gained in part by the aromatization of ring A. Air oxidation leads to the isolated δ-lactone 37 whose identity is attested to by its characteristic benzoquinone uv and lactone ir band at 5.62μ. Lactone 37 is inactive as an antibiotic. Intermediate 36 could be trapped as pentaacetate 38 by treating the reaction mixture with acetic anhydride-sodium acetate. This same acetate could be prepared by reductive ($Na_2S_2O_4$) acetylation of 37.

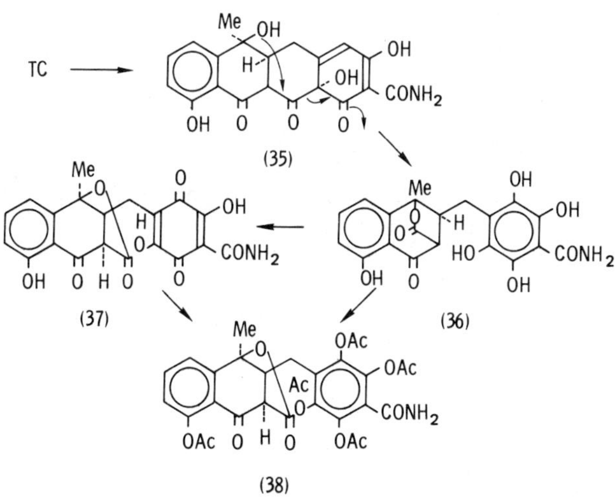

In support of the proposed mechanism, while tetracycloxide was stable in glacial HOAc with or without mercuric acetate, addition of dimethylamine to the solution, however, rapidly led to formation of 37.

A rather similar reaction was observed earlier when tetracycline betaines were heated in CH_3CN, however, in that study 36 was isolated and no mention was made of quinone 37.[45]

6.4---Chemistry of position 4a.

There is none in the literature.

6.5---Chemistry of position 5.

A discussion of the chemistry of position 5 will be deferred to Chapter 7.

6.6---Chemistry of position 5a.

The normal tetracycline stereochemistry at C_{5a} is α. It will be recalled from Chapter 3 that certain blocked mutant cultures elaborate 7-chloro-5a(11a)-dehydrotetracycline (39). Catalytic hydrogenation of 39 produced, besides TC, its 5a-epimer (40).[54] The BCD chromophore was seriously distorted in both the uv[54] and CD spectra.[55] Whereas TC dehydrated to 5a,6-anhydrotetracycline in 1*N* sulfuric acid at 100° in less than 1 minute, isomer 40 took 67 minutes, consistent with the *cis* orientation of the participating H and OH groups. Its *in vitro* potency against *Staphylococcus aureus* is less than 1/50th of that of CTC. A possible

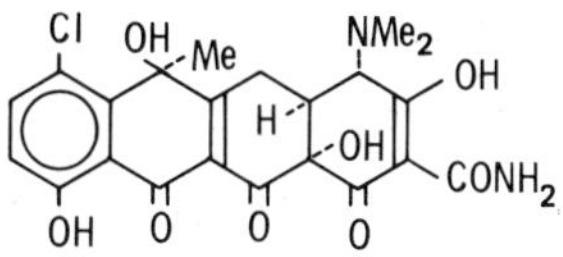

(39)

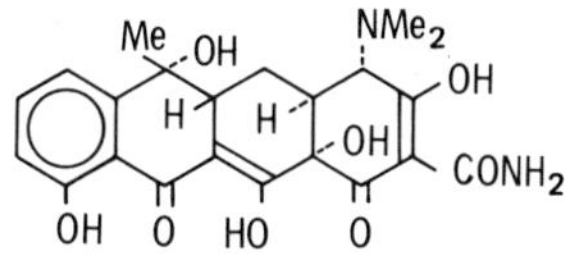

(40)

rationalization is the substantially different solution conformation of 40 as opposed to that of TC.[55]

More recently, a sequence has been found by which treatment of 39 with liquid HF containing two equivalents of water led to inversion of the stereochemistry at C_6 (41) (see Section 6.7).[56] Catalytic reduction once again produces two isomers. Interestingly, one of these (42) has 5a-*epi* stereochemistry but retains 60% of the bioactivity of TC *in vitro*. As might be expected 42 dehydrates upon heating in concentrated HCl for 5 minutes at 60°.

This sequence has not found much practical application because of the relative unavailability (although Section 6.9 details some chemical approaches) and instability of the dehydrotetracyclines.

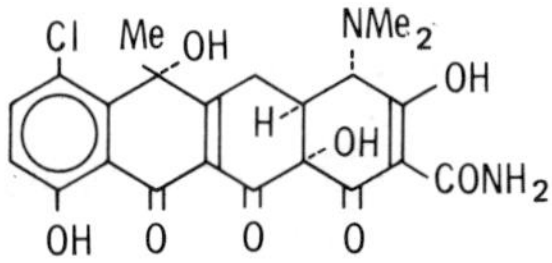

(41)

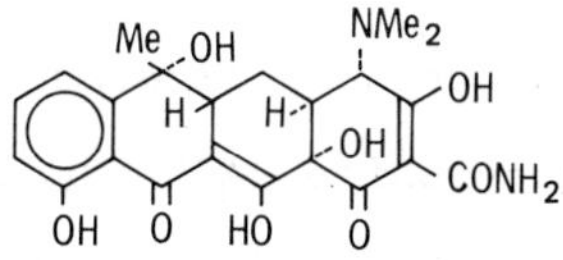

(42)

6.7---Chemistry of position 6.

It will be recalled that a hydroxy group at C_6 contributes instability to acids (with the formation of the 5a,6-anhydrotetracyclines (43)) and to base (with the formation of the isotetracyclines (44)). In the latter regard it is of some interest that a seemingly minor change in conditions, substitution of triethylamine in dioxane for OH^- in water, leads to lactone formation between C_6OH and the C_{12} ketone to give the allotetracyclines (45) rather than the C_6OH to C_{11} ketone reaction which leads to isotetracyclines.[57] This difference is not presently rationalized.

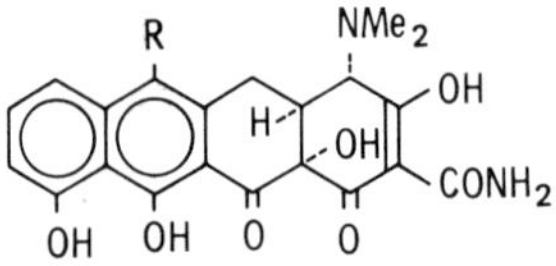

(43)

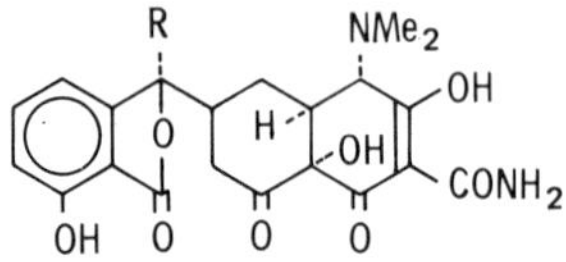

(44)

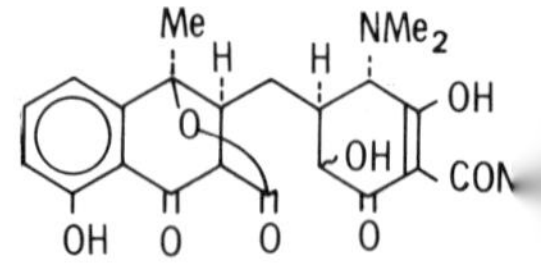

(45)

Neither the iso nor the allo reactions have found synthetic application and they remain a nuisance only.

The anhydrotetracyclines (43), on the other hand, have been reconverted to tetracyclines by photooxygenation followed by reduction. The original report[58] of this biogenetic-like sequence involved passing oxygen through a benzene solution of anhydrochlortetracycline, under the influence of a fluorescent lamp, for six days whereupon the hydroperoxide (46) crystallized. Using recycling techniques, a total of up to 70% could be obtained. Catalytic reduction led to 39, identical with the natural product. Further reduction, of course, led to TC and 5a-epitetracycline. Anhydrotetracycline could only be converted in 1-10% yield directly by this process, apparently, in part, because the product did not crystallize and did not survive the reaction. Subsequently, the t-butyl analogs of anhydrotetracycline, which are so lipophilic that they even dissolve in cyclohexane, were successfully photooxygenated. In this less polar solvent system, especially using 3,4-benzpyrene as a photosensitizer, the desired products are (47, 48) efficiently formed and crystallize in good yields without requiring recycling.

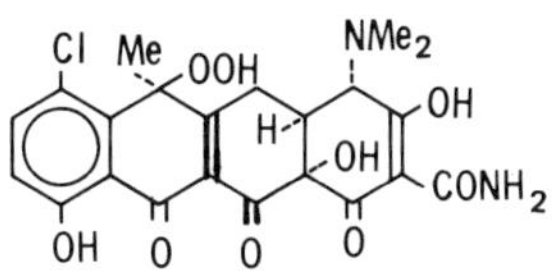

(46)

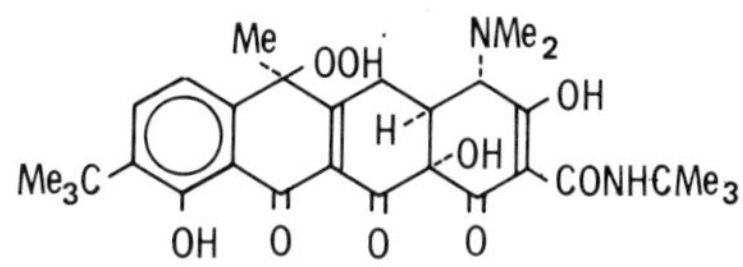

(47)

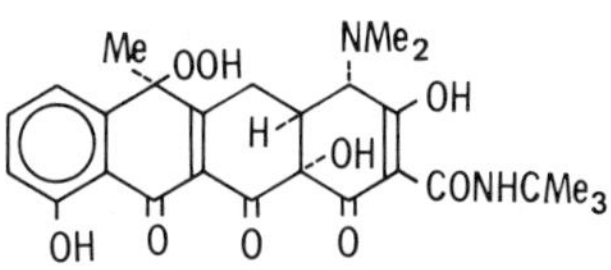

(48)

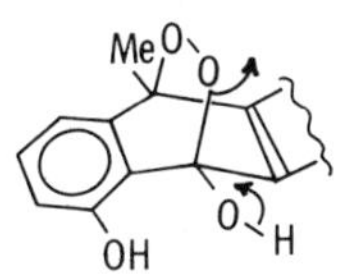

(49)

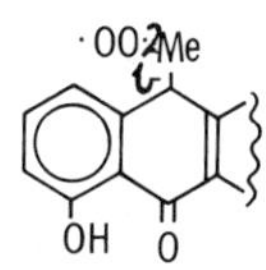

(50)

A variety of mechanisms can be proposed to account in general for the products of these reactions (for example, reaction in enolic form (50) or, more likely, *via* (49) but neither of these formulations provides a wholly convincing rationale for exclusive β-approach.

It has also been reported briefly that anhydrotetracycline will react at C_6 with lead tetracetate under conditions of the Wessely oxidation and with monopersulfuric acid under conditions of the Bamberger reaction. There are no details available and the utility of these processes remains to be established.

These reaction loops were expected to be of great practical value when they were made, but subsequent developments have lessened their impact. Total synthesis (see Chapter 8) no longer is directed toward the intermediacy of the anhydrotetracyclines and the chemistry of the 6-deoxytetracyclines largely avoids their formation.

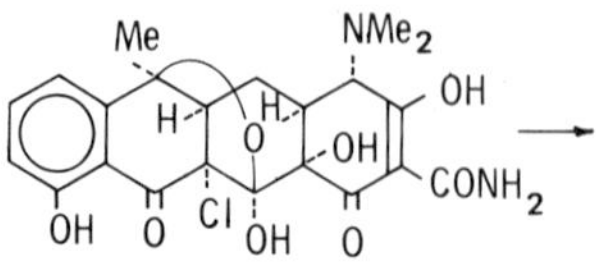

(51)

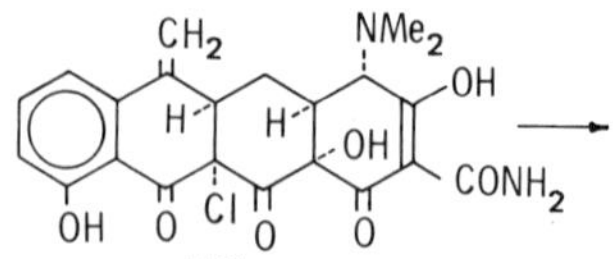

(52)

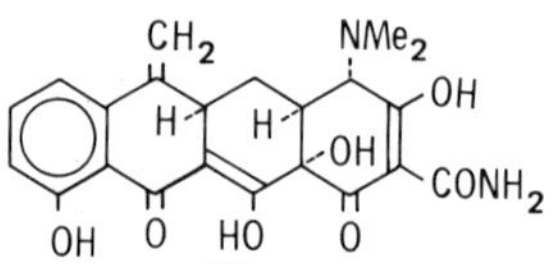

(53)

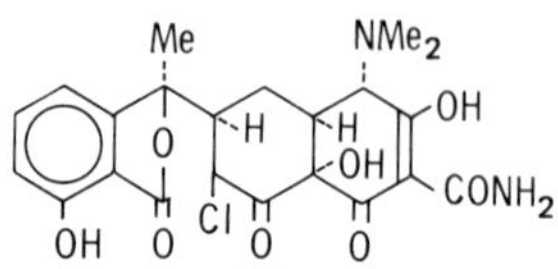

(54)

When the 11a position is blocked by a halogen (see Section 6.8), dehydration takes another course. For example, 11a-chlorotetracycline 6,12-hemiketal (51, formed by treatment of TC with N-chlorosuccinimide in 1,2-dimethoxyethane) is smoothly dehydrated in anhydrous HF to 52.[60] Ozonation of 52 produced formaldehyde in 20% yield, Kuhn-Roth degration gave no acetic acid and the pmr spectrum contains no-CCH_3 group. Sodium hydrosulfite reduction produced 6-methylenetetracycline (53).* On treatment with acids, for example, anhydrous HF, 53 rearranges to 5a,6-anhydrotetracycline. 6-Methylenetetracycline (53) has 1.2 times the *in vitro* bioactivity of tetracycline

---

* Strictly speaking, these derivatives should be named 6-methylene-6-deoxy-6-demethyltetracyclines.

itself. The 7-chloroanalog of 53 was reported in a preliminary communication,[60] but not in a subsequent full paper.[61] Interestingly, use of HCl in hydroxylic solvents, the usual conditions for formation of $C_{5a,6}$-anhydrotetracyclines, leads to cleavage and the apparent formation of a chlorine containing phthalide (54) instead of dehydration. Participation of the 6-11 hemiketal rather than the 6-12 is indicated.

The exocyclic dehydration of 51 is rationalized based upon the inability of 51 to enolyze from C_{11-11a}. This means an aromatic ring C is not achieved in the transition state even if 5a,6-dehydration were to occur. The exocyclic C_6-Me group has 3 hydrogens available for dehydration compared to the one at C_{5a}. Furthermore, the DMTC ketal 55 does not dehydrate in anhydrous HF indicating that the hemiketal bond must open before dehydration can occur.** This would seem to vitiate mechanistic arguments based upon the relative bond angles of the $C_{5a}H$ and C_6-O in the dehydration reaction in 55 as compared to 51.

The availability of the C6-methylene tetracyclines provided a convenient entry into the 6-deoxytetracyclines. The initial preparation of deoxytetracycline was achieved by direct hydrogenolysis of TC.[62,63] The reaction apparently proceeded with inversion unnoticed at the time of publication

---

** In the C_{11a}-Cl derivatives, the equilibrium lies more on the side of ketone than with the C_{11a}-F analogs.

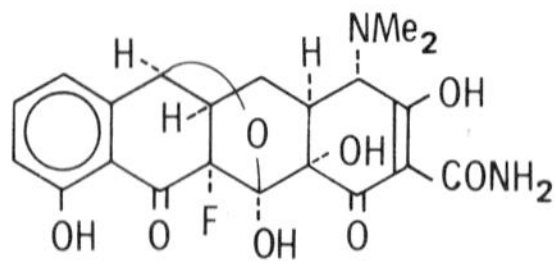

(55)

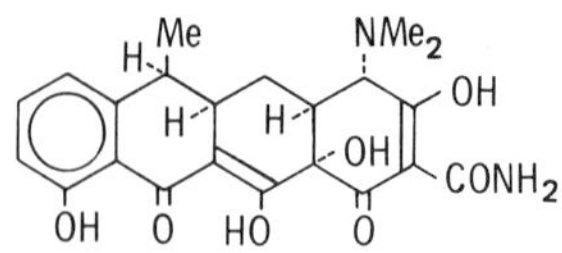

(56)

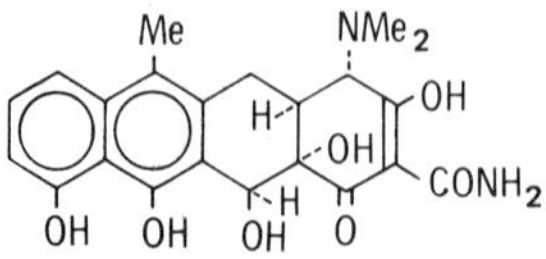

(58)

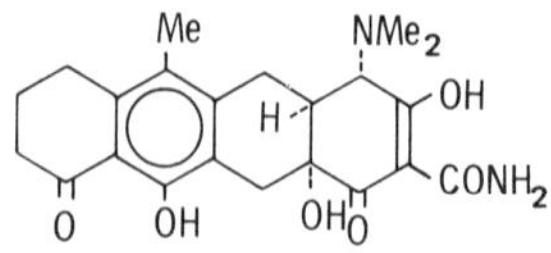

(59)

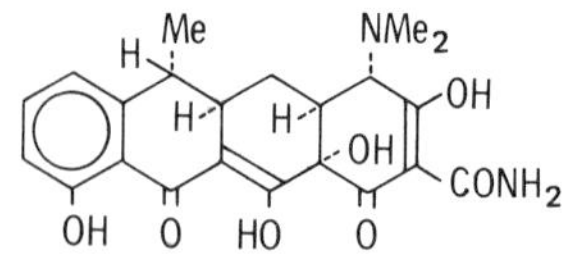

(57)

and the product is now believed to have been 6β-methyl-6-deoxytetracycline (56) which has half the potency of TC *in vitro*. Some uncertainty remains because the yields are poor and there is no information published relating to the possibility of epimerizations occurring in the presence of the catalyst. Under the reaction conditions some anhydrotetracycline is formed which undergoes further reduction to compounds formulated as 58 and 59.[67] These side reactions, occasioned by the acidic reaction medium, are partly avoided by use of boric acid to chelate the BCD system. Subsequently, catalytic reduction of 6-methylene tetracycline gave a 1:1 mixture of 56 and an isomer assigned to be 6α-methyl-6-deoxytetracycline (57).[62] The methyl group in 57 has the same orientation as that in TC itself. Its *in vitro* antibacterial potency is 70% of that of TC, so this derivative is somewhat more active than 56. The same relationship holds *in vivo*. The conformation of the 11a-fluoro analog of 6-methylenetetracycli (52, C_{11a}-F) is convex with the α-side more accessible to reagents (60).

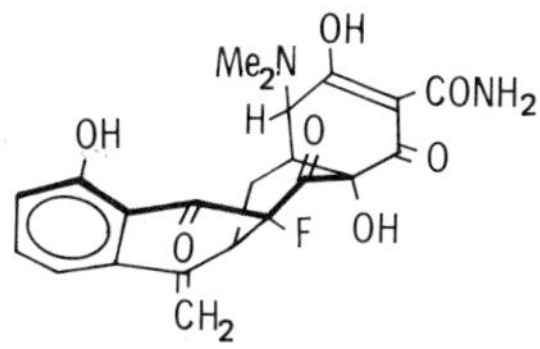

(60)

It is rationalized that catalytic reduction of both groups results in predominant formation of the β-methyl analog 56. This, of course, would require that no prior halogenolysis at C_{11a} took place before saturation of the double bond. A better method was found when it was discovered that benzylmercaptan apparently adds in an anti-Markownikov free radical process to the 6-methylene group to produce a 6α-benzylthiomethylene tetracycline (61). The relative bulk and stability of the benzylic radical accounts for the regio and stereoselectivity to this reaction.[62] Raney nickel desulfuration led to 57 in good yield. The potency of 61 was disappointing. Some other analogs were made. The benzene thiomethylene analog (62) had only 1% of the potency of TC.[65] On the other hand, the acetylthiomethylene (63) and the S-oxide of 61 (64) have 60 and 40%, respectively, of the in vitro potency of TC.[65] Some chemical properties of 64 will be discussed in Sections 6.8 and 6.9. From this, it has been concluded that lipophilicity is of overriding importance. The more fat soluble analogs 61-63 have lower bioactivity, especially against Gram-negatives, whereas they regain much of the loss in potency when treated with peroxide to form 64. The more polar 5-hydroxy analogs (see Chapter 7) lose much less bioactivity.

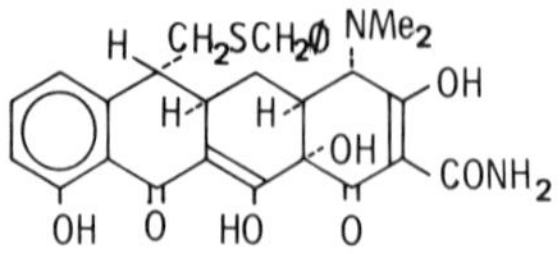

(61)

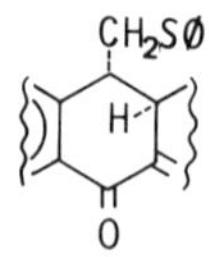

(62)

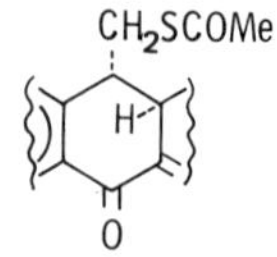

(63)

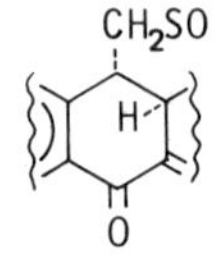

(64)

The 6-deoxytetracyclines (56, 57) are biopotent and dramatically more acid stable than their progenetors,[63] but the competing dehydration and subsequent formation of by-products such as 58 and 59 made the direct process commercially unattractive. The process through the methylene derviatives reached commercial success only in the C_5OH series (Chapter 7). With the other tetracyclines similar commercial and scientific rewards followed studies on the hydrogenolysis of DMCTC.

Hydrogenolysis of DMCTC-HCl in DMF-water at pH 1.8 containing boric acid and palladium-on-carbon led to 6-demethyl-6-deoxytetracycline (65).[63] When assayed turbidometrically against Staph. aureus, 65 was 1.7 times more potent than TC. Against Kl. pneumoniae it is 0.9 times as potent.[65] This compound is the simplest tetracycline known to have essentially the complete microbiological properties of the tetracycline family. The production of undesirable by-products was diminished, but 66 has been isolated as a blue fluorescent contaminant.[64] A rhodium catalyst has been employed to accomplish hydrogenolysis of the benzylic OH group while retaining the C_7-chloroatom.[66]

The comparative stability to acid and base of these 6-deoxy analogs is given in Table 6-2. The stability of

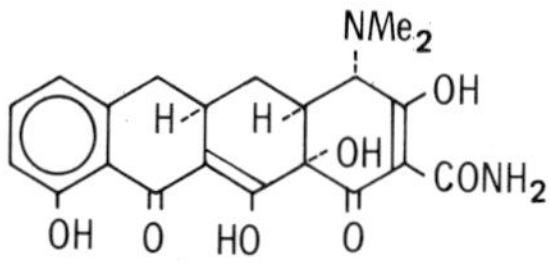

(65)

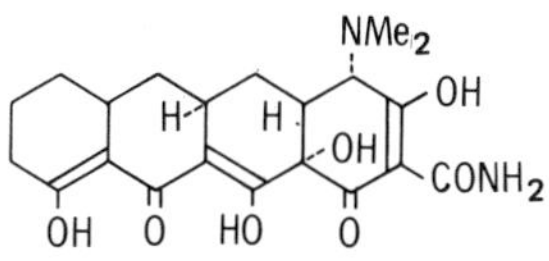

(66)

these agents even extends to recovery essentially unchanged after dissolution in concentrated sulfuric acid. This allowed a range of electrophilic substitution reactions which were hitherto not possible. This chemistry is mostly discussed in Section 6.8.

The reaction of 5a,11a-dehydrochlortetracycline (39) with liquid HF contrasts dramatically with the 11a-halotetracyclines. A carbonium ion is formed at C_6 which, when two equivalents of water are present, recaptures an OH at C_6. This leads to partial inversion, 20-25% yield, of that center to give rise to 41.[56] The derivatives are easily distinguished as the 6β-methyl analog (41) has a C-Me pmr peak at 1.42δ while the 6α-C-Me group in 39 absorbs at 1.82δ. This surely can be attributed to the different degrees of coplanarity of the methyl groups and the D-ring.

Table 6-2. Stability of selected 6-deoxytetracycline analogs.[63]

Antibiotic	T½ 3N HCl, 100°	T½ 0.1N NaOH, 100°
TC	<< 1 min.	6.8 min.
6-DMTC	1.4	32
6β-Me-DOTC (56)	1600	570
6-DO-6-DMTC (65)	1600	200

Perhaps, more importantly, 6-epi-5a,11a-dehydrochlortetracycline (41) is 1.5 times more potent in vitro against Staph. aureus.than TC and is half as active in vivo.

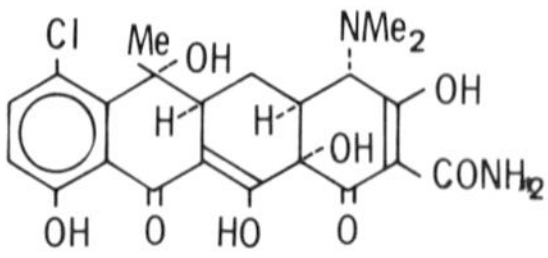
(67)

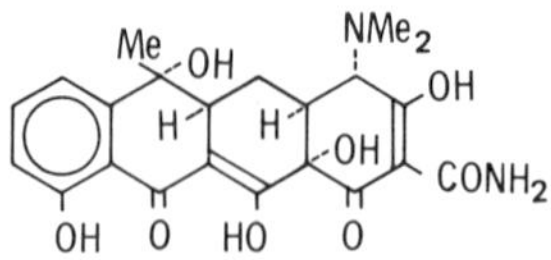
(68)

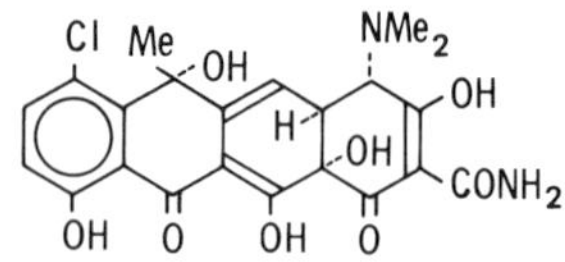
(69)

When 41 is reduced with sodium borohydride at pH 1.5, 6-epiCTC (67) results. No bioresults were given for 67. Catalytic reduction produced 6-epiTC (68) as well as the previously discussed 5a-epi-6-epiTC (42). Compound 68 retained 40% of the bioactivity of TC and 42 retained 60%. These findings - in particular, those dealing with 41 - upset previously held notions of structure-activity relations. Those who retain their faith in the immutable necessity of an intact BCD chromophore extending from C_{10} to C_{12} can rationalize this result as requiring the intervention of tautomer 69. Spectroscopic evidence for the existence of this form with the natural isomer (39) has been presented,[58] but this convenient rationale does not rationalize the almost total lack of activity of 39.

The versatility of liquid HF as a dehydrating agent for tetracyclines is further demonstrated by the results of the reaction of 11a-chloro-6-demethyltetracycline (70) which yielded not dehydration products but rather the substitution products 71 and 72. Mild catalytic reduction produced a mixture of 6β- (73) and 6α-fluoro-6-demethyl-6-

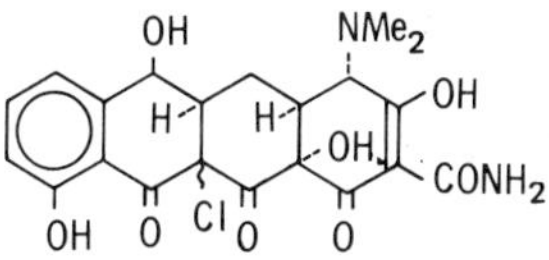
(70)

deoxytetracycline (74) which were separated.[67] Dehydrochlorination of either 71 or 72 with tetraethylammonium bromide produced the identical 6-fluoranhydrotetracycline (75). The geometries of 73 and 74 are not rigorously known, but the one assigned to be 73 loses HF at room temperature to give 6-demethylanhydrotetracycline. The other isomer produced the same 6-demethylanhydrotetracycline, but only under the influence of NaOH. When this sequence was carried out on 7,11a-dichloro-6-demethyltetracycline (76), only the more stable fluoride (77) resulted. Similarly, treatment of 11a-chlorotetracycline (78) with HF gave primarily the 6α-fluoro analog and some of the 6-methylene analog. Careful catalytic reduction produced 79. The 6-F moiety was stable to further reduction.

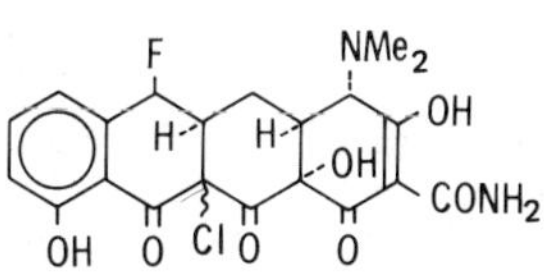
(71)

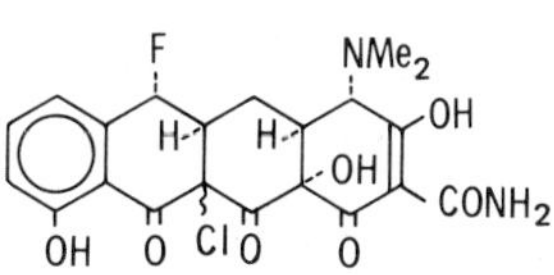
(72)

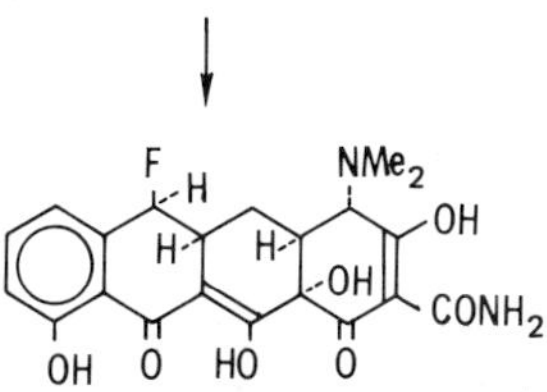
(73)

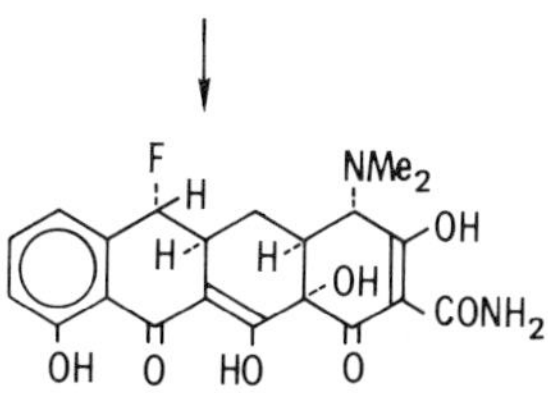
(74)

7α-Fluoro analog 74 is twice as active *in vitro* as TC whereas the β-epimer (73) is only 0.12 times as active. Analog 77 is four times TC while the 6-methyl analog (78) is only 0.3 times as potent. Derivative 79 is 0.13 times as active as TC. Thus, the α-F analogs are more potent and 7-chlorination, as it usually does, further increases activity.

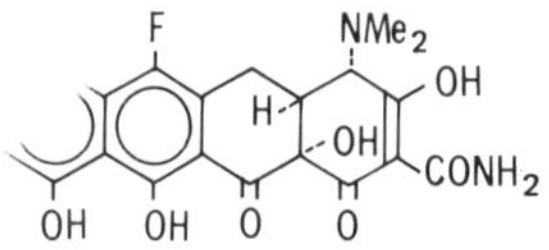

(75)

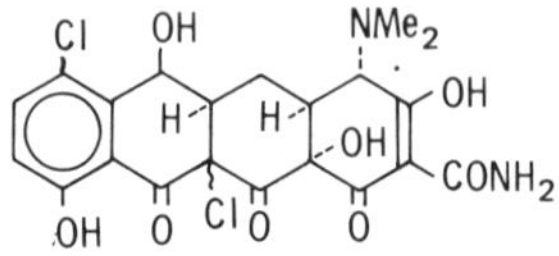

(76)

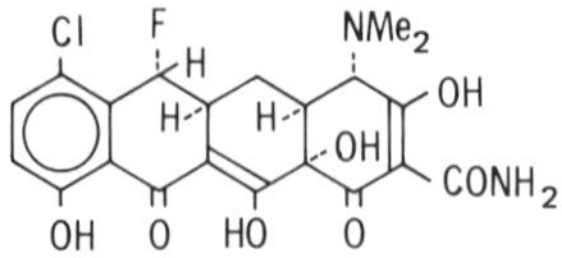

(77)

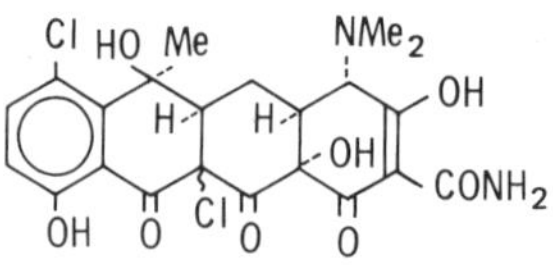

(78)

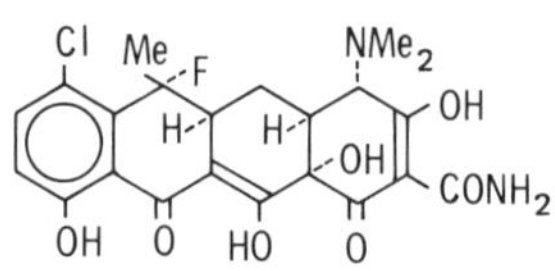

(79)

When 76 was treated with HBr in acetic acid, esterification of C_6 took place with retention of stereochemistry. Careful catalytic reduction led to 6-acetoxy-6-demethylchlortetracycline (80). The deschlor analog (81) was prepared from the analogous reactions with the deschloroanalog of 76. Chloroanalog 80 is 2 times and the deschloroanalog (81) is 0.63 times as potent *in vitro* against *Staph. aureus* as TC.

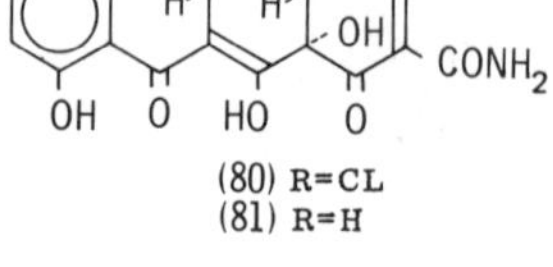

(80) R=CL
(81) R=H

6.8---Chemistry of ring D.

The classic and most important reaction occurring in the tetracycline D ring is the catalytic removal of the 7-chlorine from CTC to give TC. This reaction has been of great commercial importance.

The availability by hydrogenolysis of the 6-deoxytetracyclines and their remarkable, for tetracyclines that is, stability toward strong acids has led to the preparation of a considerable number of new derivatives through the use of electrophilic aromatic substitution reactions which the natural tetracyclines will not survive. The most significant product to emerge from this work is minocycline, the most recent tetracycline to reach the market.

The D ring of 6-DM-6DOTC is activated toward electrophilic substitution by the presence of the phenolic hydroxyl at C_{10}. This, being _ortho-para_ directing, enriches the electron density at C_7 and C_9. This is reinforced by the C_6-CH_2 group. On the other hand, C_8 is deactivated toward substitution by being _para_ to the electron withdrawing C_{11} carbonyl function. Thus, all reactions in the D ring reported to date have involved substitution at C_7 and/or C_9.[68-76] There has never been any report of a substituent being introduced at the C_8 position either chemically or biologically.

Nitration of 6-demethyl-6-deoxytetracycline with sodium or potassium nitrate in concentrated sulfuric acid resulted in a separable mixture of 7- and 9-nitrotetracyclines (_82_, _83_).

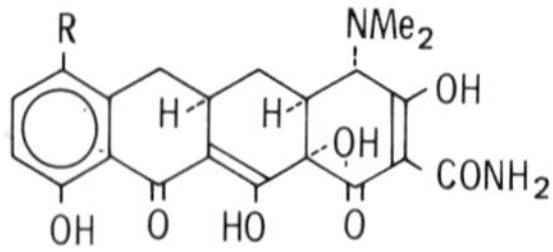

(82) R=NO_2
(84) R=NH_2

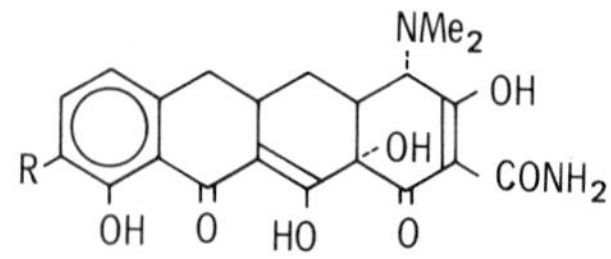

(83) R=NO_2
(85) R=NH_2

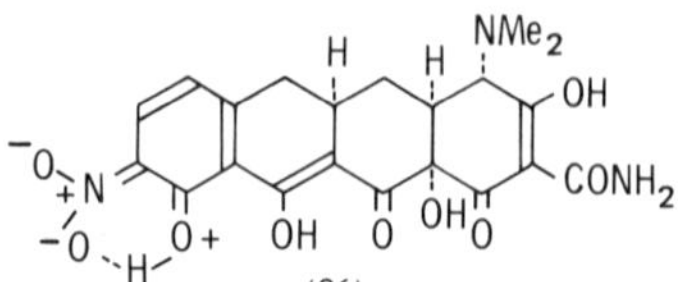

(86)

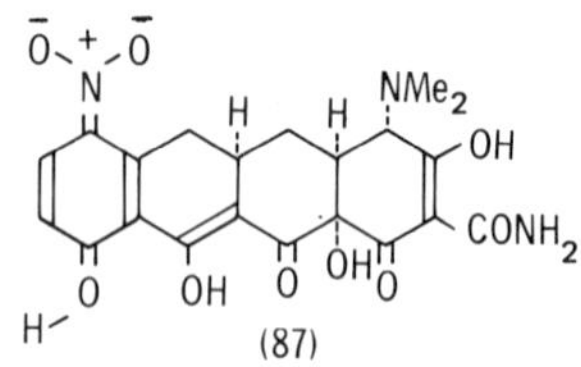

(87)

The nitro group at C_9 interacts with the phenolic hydroxyl at C_{10} so that there is a considerable difference in the ultraviolet absorption spectrum of <u>83</u> as compared with the C_7 nitro derivative of <u>82</u> in which there is only slight interference. Thus, it is easy to distinguish the two isomers. These considerations are illustrated in formulae <u>86</u> and <u>87</u>. Interestingly, the 9-nitro derivative (<u>83</u>) is a very poor antibiotic while the 7-nitro derivative (<u>82</u>) retains considerable activity. This was expected, but a less equivocal proof of structure was desired.[69,71,77] The chlorine atom of DMCTC was removed by catalytic hydrogenolysis using tritium gas and a subsequent "cold" hydrogenation removed the 6-hydroxyl to give 6-DM-6-DOTC-7-^3H where the position of the radioactive atom was unequivocably known. Nitration of this material gave the two products described above (<u>82</u> and <u>83</u>) but in this case the biologically inactive derivative was radioactive while the potent isomer had lost the tritium atom. There is no reasonable doubt as to the structures.

An interesting difference in chemical reactivity was found upon nitration of deoxytetracycline. Whereas demethyldeoxytetracycline gave approximately equal quantities of 7- and 9-nitrotetracyclines, with deoxytetracycline about four times more 9-nitro is formed than 7-nitro. It seems safe to ascribe the difference to a steric effect involving the C_6Me group.[69]

When the 9-nitro derivative is reduced to the amine (85), the peculiarities in the ultraviolet spectrum disappear and antibacterial activity reappears.[69,70] Alkylation or acylation leads to some analogs. Diazotization, for example with butyl nitrite, sets the stage for Sandmeyer replacement with a variety of nucleophiles.[68,69,71,72] Some of the acyloxy and fluoro analogs are prepared by photolysis of the diazonium salts in the appropriate acid.[72] Hydrolysis leads to the 7-hydroxyanalogs. The bromoanalogs can also be made by reaction of the 11a-chloroanalogs with bromonium ion generated from N-bromosuccinimide followed by careful reductive removal of the 11a-halo group. When the C_{11a} halo group is bromine or iodine, the group is quite labile. Solution in concentrated acid[71] or on photolysis[74] rearranges the halo group to the C_7 position. The product is stable, however, in glacial acetic acid. The intermolecular nature of the rearrangement was demonstrated by trapping experiments using 6-deoxytetracycline or, better, α-naphthol as an alternate halogen acceptor. In a separate work[68] the bromo analog could be made conveniently by simply brominating in trifluoroacetic acid and heating the intermediate 7, 11a-dibromo compound in the reaction solution, or by use of N-bromosuccinimide in concentrated sulfuric acid.[71]

In an interesting application directed toward diagnosis of tumors, treatment of 7-diazonium-6-demethyl-6-deoxytetracyclines with potassium ^{131}I led to 7-^{131}I-6-demethyl-6-deoxytetracycline.[78] The different outcome of the halogenation reactions depending upon the acidity of the medium is likely the result of protonation of the BCD chromophore as illustrated in formula 88. This creates an electropositive center near C_{11a} which would diminish the likelihood of a positive halonium ion reacting at that center.[71] Some experimental support for this concept was adduced from uv studies (λ_{max} H_2O = 345 nm; λ_{max} H_2SO_4 = 385 nm). The proton catalyzed rearrangement reaction of the C_{11a}-halo derivatives can also be rationalized in this fashion for protonation followed by ejection of halonium ion would lead to the same intermediate (88).

The biotesting of these various derivatives (Tables 6-3 and 6-4) lead to the general conclusion that C_7 substitution is more favorable for bioactivity than C_9 and that the more electron withdrawing analogs are more potent. Subsequent work has quantitated this qualitative observation.[79,80,81] The 9-nitro analogs did not fit the equations generated, perhaps because the strong *ortho*-effect alluded to earlier in the spectroscopic work.[82]

Broad spectrum activity was retained in many of the derivatives in Tables 6-3 and 6-4 and in a significant number of cases, potency was increased.

Table 6-3. Comparison of the potency of some 7- and/or 9-substituted 6-demethyl-6-deoxytetracyclines with TC and CTC.[60]

TC		100* <u>S. aureus</u>	100* <u>Kl. pneumo.</u>	Ref.
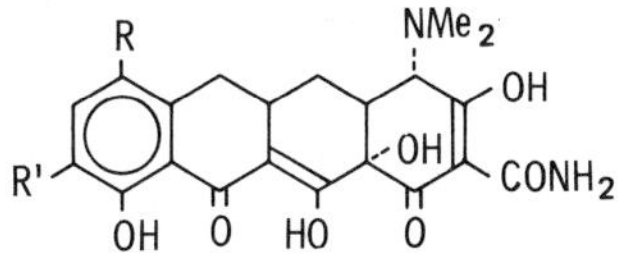				
R	R'			
H	H	160	900	68,71,72
F	H	220		72
Cl	H	300		72
Br	H	200	1300	68,69,71,72
I	H	120		69,71,72
NH_2	H	40	760	68,69,70,71
H	NH_2	160	975	68,69,70,71
N_2	H	20		71,72
H	N_2	17		71
N_3	H	150		71
H	N_3	90		71
Br	NO_2	15	25	68,73
CH_3CO_2	H	120		72
HCO_2	H	32		72
OH	H	23		72
$EtO\overset{S}{\overset{\|}{C}}$-S-	H	50		71
NO_2	H	640	4600	68,69,70
H	NO_2	12	200	68,69,70
HCONH-	H	35	-	70
H	HCONH	225		70
H	$EtO\overset{S}{\overset{\|}{C}}$-S	10		71
NO_2	NO_2	60		73
Cl	NO_2	21		73
Cl	NH_2	525		73
Br	NH_2	320		73
NO_2	NH_2	275		73

*By definition

Table 6-4. Comparison of the potency of some 7- and/or 9-substituted 6-epi-deoxytetracyclines with TC and CTC. Note that these activities would be somewhat higher had the 6α-methyl analog served as the substrate.

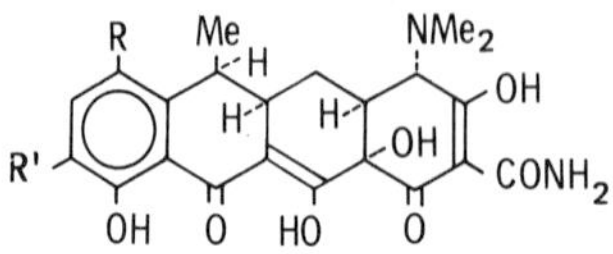

R	R'	*S. aureus*	*Kl. pneumo.*	Ref.
H	H	70*	**	
Br	H	140		69,71
I	H	60		69,71
H	NH_2	60		69,71
H	N_3	10		71
H	EtOC(=S)-S-	"much less active"		71
NO_2	H	240		69,70
H	NO_2	1		69,70
H	AcNH-	24		70
H	NH_2	60		70
Br	NH_2	150		69
NO_2	NH_2	160		69
H	N_2	10		71
Br	CH_3CONH-	75		73
Br	NH_2	140		73
NO_2	NH_2	160		73
NO_2	CH_3CONH-	15		73

*Compared to TC which is 100 by definition.

**Compared to CTC=100, by definition.

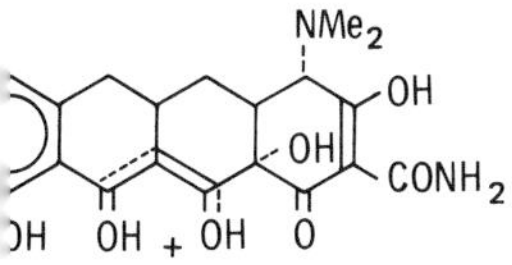
(88)

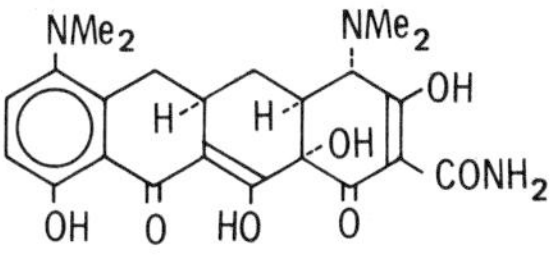
(89)

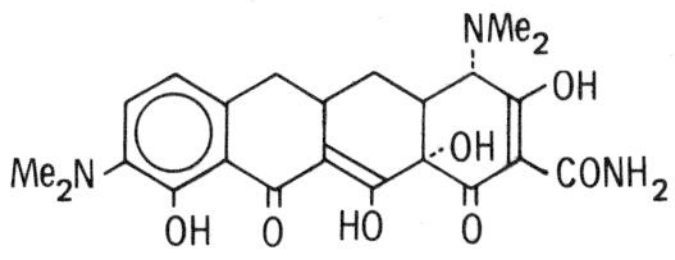
(90)

This work reached clinical fruition when reductive alkylation experiments led to the synthesis of 7-dimethylamino-6-demethyl-6-deoxytetracycline, known more simply as minocycline (89).[75,76] Minocycline has the distinction of retaining the favorable broad spectrum activity of the previously used tetracyclines but also being active against many TC-resistant Staphylococcus aureus strains. This makes minocycline the broadest spectrum of all the tetracyclines and explains its clinical vogue despite its expense. The 7-diethylamino analog of minocycline was less potent than 89 and the 9-dimethylamino analog (90) was devoid of unique antibacterial activity.[75]

The nitration reaction leading to 89, it will be recalled, gave mixtures which had to be separated. The necessity of performing partition chromatography on a very large scale was quite unattractive economically so much subsequent chemical effort was expended in improving the synthesis of 89.

The undesirable 9-nitro-6-demethyl-6-deoxytetracycline (91), which is sometimes produced in excess compared to the 7-nitroanalog, was ultimately used as a precursor for minocycline. The overall yield of nitrated products increased when the reaction was carried out in HF. The separated 9-nitro analog was reduced catalytically to the 9-amino analog (92) which was nitrated to the 7-nitro-9-amino analog (93). Next, this product was diazotized to 94. When 94 was reduced with a palladium catalyst in the presence of formaldehyde, the diazonium group was hydrogenolyzed and the nitro group reductively alkylated to give minocycline in somewhat better overall yield than was accomplished going through the 7-nitro analog, even though that sequence was formally shorter.[82]

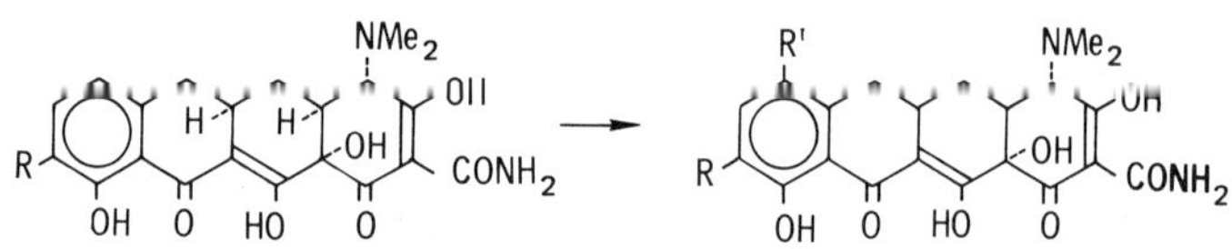

(91) R=NO_2
(92) R=NH_2

(93) R=NH_2, R'=NO_2
(94) R=N_2, R'=NO_2

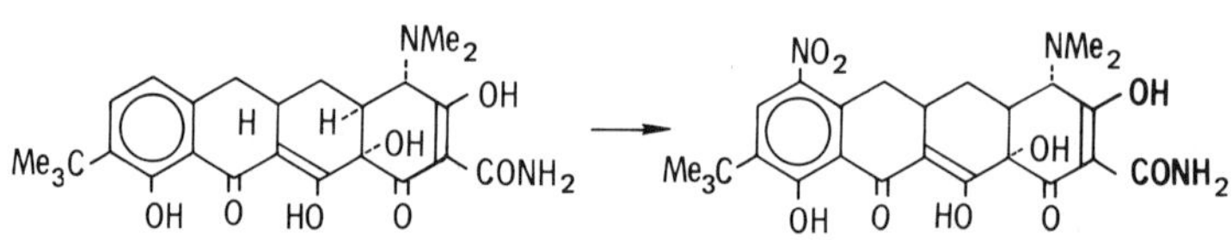

(95)

(96)

Another sequence of interest was published more recently. It will be recalled from Section 6.2 that reaction of C_2-nitriles with isobutylene and strong acid led to the N-t-butyl analogs. The carboxamides, on the other hand, are substituted in ring D. When 6-demethyl-6-deoxytetracycline is treated with t-butanol in methanesulfonic acid, 95 results.[83] Very little C_7 substitution apparently takes place. Reaction of 95 with anhydrous HF regenerates 6-DM-6-DOTC. This, then, represents an interesting blocking group for the C_9 position - particularly so because of the high lipophilicity of 95. Nitration of 95 with a mixture of *t*-butanol, methanesulfonic acid and potassium nitrate gave an excellent yield of 96, especially if 95 was not isolated first. Reduction with platinum catalyst and formaldehyde in acid converted 96 to its dimethylamino analog and then the *t*-butyl protecting group was removed with trifluoromethylsulfonic acid in anisole to produce minocycline in excellent overall yield. Cleavage of the protecting group in the last step required a considerably stronger acid than cleavage of 95 because of the deactivation ring D receives from protonation of the newly introduced dimethylamino function.

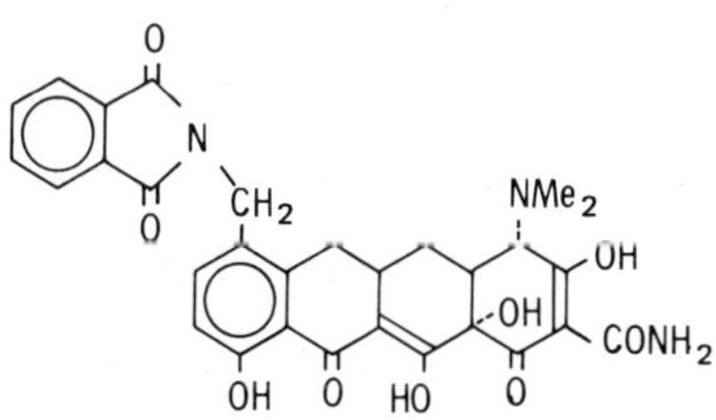

(97)

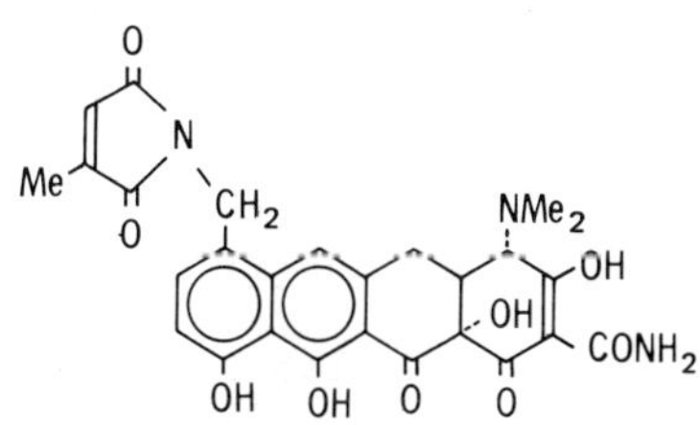

(98)

Another reaction which occurs at C_2 with the nitriles and in ring D with the carboxamides is the Tscherniac-Einhorn.[76] In this case, a N-hydroxyimide in strong acid (presumably in the form of the methylene imide) substitutes predominantly at C_7. For example, N-hydroxyphthalimide reacts with 6-DM-6-DOTC to produce 97 as shown by displacement of tritium from radiolabeled starting material. The product was 3.2 times more potent than TC *in vitro*. Attempts to cleave the imide by partial hydrolysis led to deep-seated decomposition involving loss of the BCD chromophore. Several successful reactions were run and the results are summarized in Table 6-5. Despite the presence of up to 12 times greater activity *in vitro*, these substances are disappointing *in vivo*. The best one was barely equivalent to TC in this respect so its commercialization would be economically unattractive. The reaction was also applied to 6-demethylanhydrotetracycline, whose citraconimide analog (**98**) was about 0.4 times TC *in vitro*. As 6-demethylanhydrotetracycline is only about 0.2 times TC under these conditions, this finding was of some interest. No other substitution reaction of anhydrotetracycline apparently had led to increased potency in Lederle's hands.

An interesting alkylation reaction takes place when 6α-benzylsulfoxymethylene-6-demethyl-6-deoxytetracycline (**99**) is treated with HCl.[65] Protonation of the sulfoxide is followed by nucleophilic attack at C_7 to give intermediate **10**. This undergoes debenzylation to **101** which undergoes a prototropic shift to give pentacyclic dihydrothiophene **102**. An analogous reaction at C_{11a} is described in Section 6.9.

Attempts to introduce oxygen directly onto one of the carbon atoms in ring D have generally failed. For example, reaction of the diazonium salts of the tetracyclines with methanol led to reduction rather than introduction of the desired methoxyl function.[70] Photolysis of the C_7 or C_9-diazo derivatives in acetic acid solution led, in part, to the acetoxy derivatives which could be hydrolyzed

Table 6-5. Bioactivity of various Tscherniac-Einhorn products.

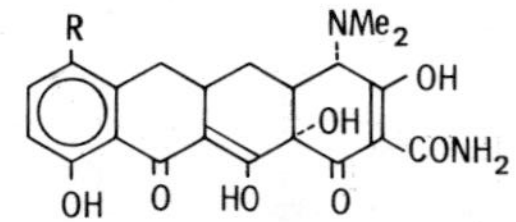

R	Relative Activity *in vitro* against *Staph. aureus* 209P*	Relative Activity *in vivo* against *Staphylococcus aureus* (Smith) in mice.* Oral	IV
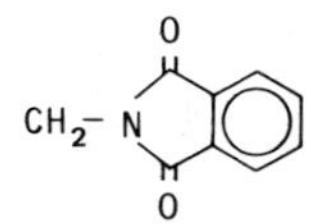	3.2	1	-
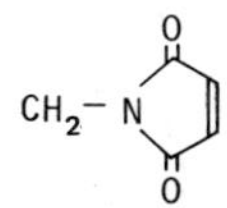	7.0	<0.06	<0.06
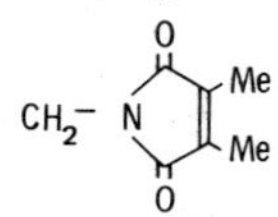	2.3	0.5 -1.0	0.25
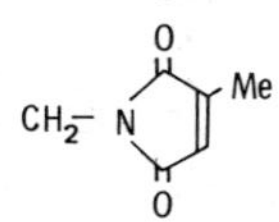	12.0	<0.06	0.25
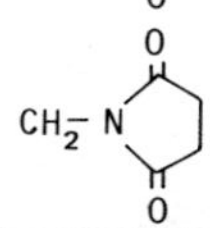	0.4	<0.06	<0.25

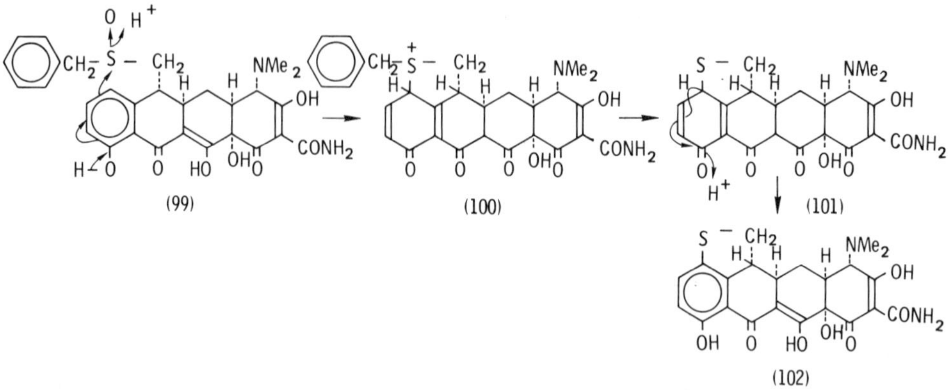

to the free phenol.[72] As seen in Table 6-3, the bioactivity of these compounds was disappointing. This process is limited to 6-DO-6-DM tetracyclines. One other successful experiment utilized a modified Udenfriend reagent;[84] a simulated enzymatic peroxidase containing hydrogen peroxide, iron salts, ascorbic acid and so on, and resulted in hydroxylation of 6-DMCTC at the C_9 position (103).[85] The position of substitution was established by reductive removal of the halogen to give 104 and examination of its nuclear magnetic resonance spectrum wherein a typical A/B quartet was discernible whose coupling constant (J=9Hz) clearly indicated two *ortho*-hydrogens. Analogous reactions on TC and 7-chloro-6-demethyl-6-deoxytetracycline also produced C_9-OH analogs. *In vitro* bioassays against *Staph. aureus* indicated that the derivatives were quite biologically active *in vitro*. The yields were poor, however, and the conditions not conducive to large scale operation, but this does represent an interesting instance of simulated biological oxygenation of the tetracycline D ring.

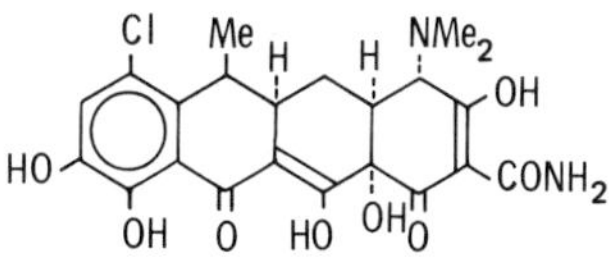

(103)

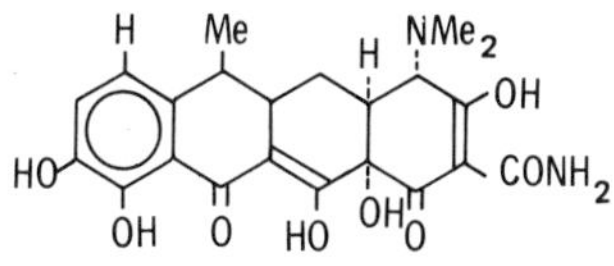

(104)

6.9---Chemistry of position 11a.

Substitution at the C_{11a} position abolishes utility as antibiotics. As has been pointed out in Section 6.8 in discussing the electrophilic substitution of ring D, the C_{11a} position competes with ring D for halogens unless very strong acid is used and, even here, the C_{11a} product probably serves as a labile intermediate. Under milder conditions the C_{11a} position is preferentially attacked. These substances have found considerable utility as blocking agents, particularly for formation of C_6-methylene derivatives.

Among the C_{11a} halo analogs, the bromo and iodo analogs are quite labile to rearrangement in concentrated acid[71] or upon photolysis.[74] Interestingly, photolysis of 11a-bromo-6-demethyl-6-deoxytetracycline (105) in acidic solutions leads to rearrangement to the 7-bromo analog (106) whereas irradiation in acetonitrile led to loss of HBr instead with formation of 6-demethylanhydrotetracycline (107).[74] The chloro and fluoro analogs are not prone to rearrangement.

The C_{11a}-fluoro analogs of the tetracyclines can be formed using perchloryl fluoride.[86] In the 6β-hydroxy series, these compounds exist as the 6,12-hemiketals. This requires that the F be α so that the BC ring juncture be cis and thereby flexible enough for transanular bond formation. The relative stability of the C_{11a}-fluoro analogs and their ease of catalytic removal makes these

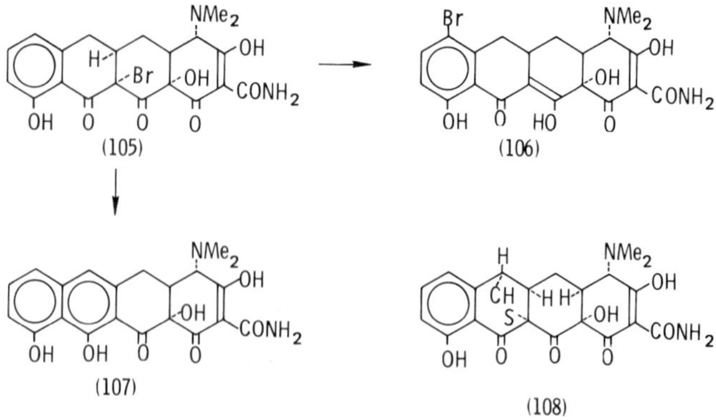

excellent blocking groups. Removal of the blocking halogen is much more difficult with the 6,12-hemiketals. Catalytic hydrogenolysis leads to substantial anhydrotetracycline formation. This side reaction is lessened when zinc and 0.2N HCl is used for deblocking.

Interestingly, treatment of 11a-chloro-7-chlortetracycline with tetraethylammonium bromide takes a different course than the previously described acidic and

Table 6-6. Relative potency of 9-hydroxylated tetracyclines

Antibiotic	Relative bioactivity *in vitro* against *Staph. aureus* 209P
TC	1.0*
9-Hydroxytetracycline	1.2
9-Hydroxy-7-chloro-6-demethyltetracycline (99)	0.7
9-Hydroxy-7-chloro-6-demethyl-6-hydroxytetracycline	1.2
9-Hydroxy-6-demethyltetracycline (100)	0.2

*By definition

photolytic reactions.[87] Instead, loss of HCl occurs and 5a,11a-dehydro-7-chlorotetracycline results.providing a chemical method of preparation of this biosynthetic intermediate.

In addition to the papers previously cited relating to C_{11a} bromination in acidic solutions, there is a report that bromination of TC in pyridine produces the 11a-α-bromo-6,12-hemiketal and that that rearranges to 9-bromoanhydro-tetracycline in a mixture of sulfuric and acetic acids.[88] When sulfuric alone was used some 11a-bromo-6-methylene-6-demethyl-6-deoxytetracycline was also formed and when this was done in a mixture of sulfuric acid and acetonitrile the latter predominated.

A reaction of less present theoretical and practical importance represents one of the condensation pathways which ensues when the sulfoxide of 6-2-benzylthiomethylene-6-demethyl-6-deoxytetracycline is treated with HCl.[65] In addition to cyclization at C_7 (discussed in Section 6.8), the sulfenic acid can be attacked by a carbanion at C_{11a} to give bridged pentacyclic analog <u>108</u>.

6.10--Chemistry of position 12a.

Treatment of the tetracyclines with zinc dust and 15% aqueous ammonia under mild conditions leads to reductive removal of the C_{12a}-OH.[89,90] This function insulates the two chromophoric regions of the molecule and its removal allows them to conjugate with one another. This fact provides the easiest means of detecting this structural change for the ultraviolet absorption is very characteristic. The product has only about 2% of the _in vitro_ bioactivity of TC against _S. aureus_. When measured in alkaline borate solution, the longest wavelength peak is shifted more than 100 nm to longer wavelengths. Formulae have been assigned to a number of these tautomers (109-112).[90]

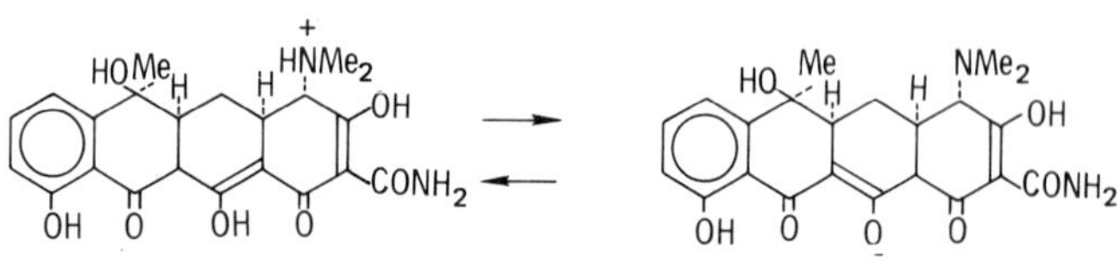

(109) (110)

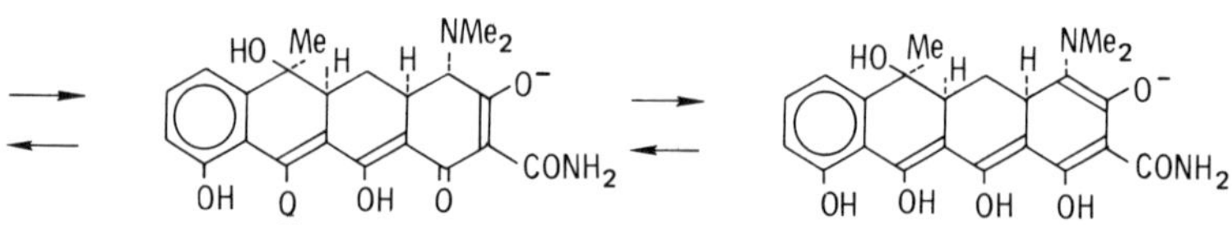

(111) (112)

A great deal of time was spent in the early stages of the studies directed toward total synthesis in searching for methods of reintroducing this function. It was early found that the 12a-position is more reactive than the 11a-position, perhaps because the nitrogen atom at C_4 helps direct the incoming oxidizing agent toward C_{12a} although the same selectivity is observed in the dedimethylamino series. The problem was solved by several groups for it was found that a wide variety of inorganic reagents will oxygenate the 12a-position[91-94] and that certain microorganisms will also carry out this step.[95] Interestingly, none of the normal tetracycline producing Streptomycetes will do this and it has been concluded from several strands of evidence that this function is introduced at an earlier stage in the biosynthesis.

Peracids have been used although the wrong stereochemistry is sometimes obtained.[96] Inorganic reagents such as $MnCl_2$ + oxygen, ceric chloride + oxygen, potassium permanganate, iodine, potassium persulfate, potassium ferrocyanide, and so on, have been used. Catalytic oxygenation in the presence of noble metal catalysts has also been used. Of a number of cultures studied in attempts to use microorganisms, *Curvularia lunata*, *C. pallescens*, and *Botrytis cinerea* were successful hydroxylators at that position.[95] An interesting side observation emerged from the latter study when it was found that an impurity in the nitrate salt used in the culture medium, subsequently identified as sodium nitrite, was responsible for a number of false positive transformations in the exploratory stage of the study!

When the nitrogen atom at C-4 is present, the yields are diminished by competing reactions involving N-oxide formation and tetracycloxide yielding reactions. For example, when 12a-deoxy-7-chlorotetracycline (**113**) is treated with peracids, an aromatic A ring derivative **114** is formed in 20% yield -- perhaps by a Cope-type elimination of the intermediate N-oxide.[97] Further acid treatment led to dehydration to 6-methylpretetramide.

Treatment of tetracycline with acetic-formic anhydride leads to the C_{12a}-*O*-formyl ester (**115**).[98]

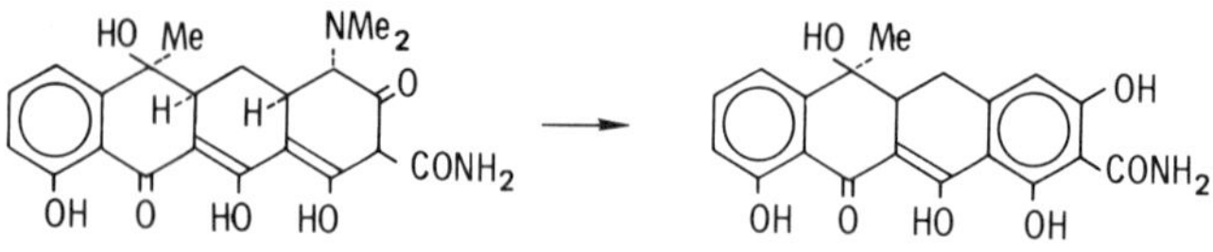

(113) (114)

Catalytic reduction of this product leads to an alternative method for the production of 12a-deoxy tetracyclines (113) whereas heating leads to pyrrolytic removal involving *cis*-loss of the hydrogen at C_{4a} and consequent aromatization of the A ring to give 116. Treatment of 116 with strong acid converts it to 4-dimethyl-amino-6-methylpretetramide.

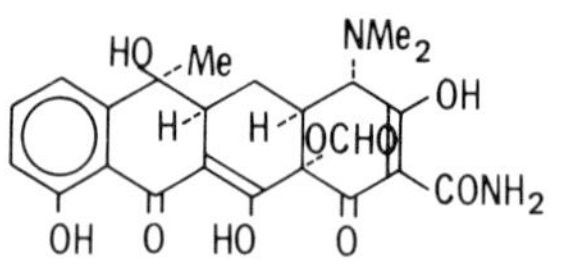

(115)

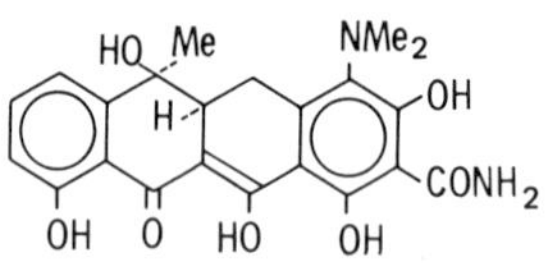

(116)

The formyl ester (115) is markedly unstable toward solvolysis in basic or neutral solution. Solution in methanol for a few minutes is apparently sufficient to cause methanolysis of the ester and liberation of the starting tetracycline. The half life of the formate ester in aqueous buffers is in the order of 5 minutes at pH 7.5 whereas it survives to a half life of 6 hours at pH 2.

TC and 6-demethyl-6-deoxytetracycline behave in an analogous fashion toward formylation-deformylation. Tetracycline $C_{10,12a}$-diacetates, dipropionates and the C_{12a}-phenylcarbamates also readily undergo catalytic loss of the C_{12a} function.

Just as halogen substitution takes place readily under acid conditions at the C_{11a}-position, C_{12a} will also halogenate.[97] In fact, 12a-deoxytetracyclines will react at both C_{11a} and C_{12a} if sufficient halogenating agent is added.[99]

6.11--Summary.

In formula 117 are summarized what is presently known about tetracycline structure-activity relationships. The tetracyclic ring system is required for full bioactivity. Substantial variation in stereochemistry and the nature of substituents is allowed in the hatched area. No irreversible chemical changes are allowed in the clear area or bioactivity is lost. In particular, the free flow of electrons in the BCD chromophore must not be interrupted. No chemistry is available at C_{4a} and C_8.

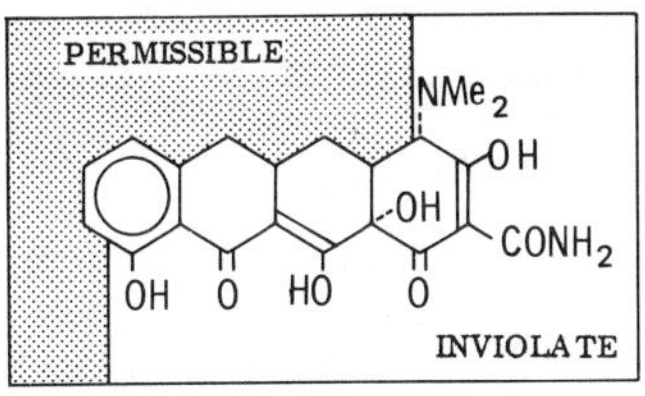

(117)

REFERENCES

1. F. A. Hochstein, C. R. Stephens, L. H. Conover, P. P. Regna, R. Pasternack, P. N. Gordon, F. J. Pilgrim, K. J. Brunings and R. B. Woodward, J. Am. Chem. Soc., 75, 5455 (1953).

2. C. R. Stephens, L. H. Conover, R. Pasternack, F. A. Hochstein, W. T. Moreland, P. P. Regna, F. J. Pilgrim, K. J. Brunings and R. B. Woodward, J. Am. Chem. Soc., 76, 3568 (1954).

3. J. R. D. McCormick, S. M. Fox, L. L. Smith, B. A. Bitler, J. Reichenthal, V. E. Origoni, W. M. Muller, R. Winterbottom and A. P. Doerschuk, J. Am. Chem. Soc., 79, 849 (1957).

4. C. R. Stephens, J. J. Beereboom, H. H. Rennhard, P. N. Gordon, K. Murai, R. K. Blackwood and M. Schach von Wittenau, J. Am. Chem. Soc., 85, 2643 (1963).

5. C. R. Stephens, E. J. Bianco and F. J. Pilgrim, J. Am. Chem. Soc., 77, 1701 (1955).

6. J. J. Beereboom and K. Butler, U. S. Patent 3,069,467 (1962).

7. L. Bernardi, R. DeCastiglione and U. Scarponi, J. Chem. Soc., Chem. Commun., 320 (1975).

8. C. R. Tamorria and R. C. Esse, J. Med. Chem., 8, 870 (1965

9. E. S. Granatek, M. A. Kaplan and F. H. Buckwalter, J. Med. Chem., 6, 202 (1963).

10. E. Tubaro and F. Banci, Arzneimittel-Forsch., 5, 95 (1964)

11. M. J. Martell, Jr., A. S. Ross and J. H. Boothe, J. Med. Chem., 10, 485 (1967).

12. W. Sidel, A. Soeder and F. Lindner, Muench. Med. Wochensch 100, 661 (1958).

13. W. J. Gottstein, W. F. Minor and L. C. Cheney, J. Am. Chem. Soc., 81, 1198 (1958).

14. H. J. Roth and R. Brandes, Arch. Pharm., 298, 34 (1965).

15. C. Bernardelli, G. Bucher, F. Lauria, W. Logemann, G. Tosolini and G. Vita, Ann., 706, 243 (1967).

16. H. Hartung, F. Cavagna, W. Martin and W. Duerckheimer, Arch. Pharm., 307, 651 (1974).

17. A. Brunzell, Acta Chem. Scand., 16, 245 (1962).

18. D. W. Hughes, W. L. Wilson, A. G. Butterfield and N. J. Pound, J. Pharm. Pharmacol., 26, 79 (1974).

19. R. Huettenrauch and J. Keiner, Naturwiss., 53, 552 (1966).

20. F. A. Hochstein, M. Schach von Wittenau, F. W. Tanner, Jr., and K. Murai, J. Am. Chem. Soc., 82, 5934 (1960).

21. R. Huettenrauch and J. Keiner, Arch. Pharm., 301, 97 (1968).

22. U. Valcavi, N. Zonta Bolego, N. Pacini, S. Gorini and M. Del Rosso, Il Farmaco, Ed. Sci., 21, 775 (1966).

23. J. A. Rondalet and P. Froment, Ann. Pharm. Fr., 26, 63 (1968).

24. B. Gradnik, A. Pedrazzoli and E. Ferreo, Pharm. Acta Helv., 35, 529 (1960).

25. O. P. Belazerova, R. S. Potravnova, L. K. Rubtsova, E. I. Eidelshtein and E. N. Lazareva, Antibiotiki, 8, 926 (1963).

26. A. V. Loginov, E. I. Iofina, A. M. Dumova, V. V. Bystrova, Y. E. Strelnikov, T. A. Teterina and O. O. Chirkova, Antibiotiki, 9, 483 (1964).

27. M. A. Kaplan, W. T. Bradner, F. H. Buckwalter and M. H. Pindel, Nature, 205, 399 (1965).

28. R. A. Milch, J. E. Tobie and R. A. Robinson, J. Histochem. Cytochem., 9, 261 (1961).

29. G. Quisnel, J. P. Giroud and H. Schmitt, Therapie, 28, 877 (1973).

30. J. Keiner, R. Huettenrauch and W. Poethke, Arch. Pharm., 300, 840 (1967).

31. M. W. Miller and F. A. Hochstein, J. Org. Chem., 27, 2525 (1962).

32. G. C. Lancini and P. Sensi, Experientia, 20, 83 (1964).

33. A. P. Doerschuk, B. A. Bitler and J. R. D. McCormick, J. Am. Chem. Soc., 77, 4687 (1955).

34. C. R. Stephens, L. H. Conover, P. N. Gordon, F. C. Pennington, R. L. Wagner, K. J. Brunings and F. J. Pilgrim, J. Am. Chem. Soc., 78, 1515 (1956).

35. J. R. D. McCormick, S. M. Fox, L. L. Smith, B. A. Bitler, J. Reichenthal, V. E. Origoni, W. H. Muller, R. Winterbottom and A. P. Doerschuk, J. Am. Chem. Soc., 78, 3547 (1956).

36. J. R. D. McCormick, S. M. Fox, B. A. Bitler, J. Reichenthal, V. E. Origoni, W. H. Muller, R. Winterbottom and A. P. Doerschuk, J. Am. Chem. Soc., 79, 2849 (1957).

37. D. A. Hussar, P. J. Niebergall, E. T. Sugita and J. T. Doluisio, J. Pharm. Pharmacol., 20, 539 (1968).

38. M. A. Kaplan, A. P. Granatek and F. H. Buckwalter, Antibiot. and Chemother., 7, 569 (1957).

39. R. G. Kelly, J. Pharm. Sci., 53, 1551 (1964).

40. E. G. Remmers, G. M. Sieger and A. P. Doerschuk, J. Pharm. Sci., 52, 752 (1963).

41. J. H. Boothe, G. E. Bonvicino, C. W. Waller, J. P. Petisi, R. G. Wilkinson and R. B. Broschard, J. Am. Chem. Soc., 80, 1654 (1958).

42. J. J. Hlavka and P. Bitha, Tet. Letts., 3843 (1966).

43. L. H. Conover, Chem. Soc., (London), Special Publication No. 5 (1956).

44. R. K. Blackwood, J. J. Beereboom, H. H. Rennhard, M. Schach von Wittenau and C. R. Stephens, J. Am. Chem. Soc., 85, 3943 (1963).

45. J. J. Hlavka, P. Bitha and J. H. Boothe, J. Am. Chem. Soc., 87, 1795 (1965).

46. J. J. Hlavka, P. Bitha and J. H. Boothe, J. Am. Chem. Soc., 90, 1034 (1968).

47. J. J. Hlavka, P. Bitha and J. H. Boothe, Tet. Letts., 1139 (1967).

48. R. C. Esse, J. A. Lowery, C. R. Tamorria and G. M. Sieger, J. Am. Chem. Soc., 86, 3874 (1964).

49. R. C. Esse, J. A. Lowery, C. R. Tamorria and G. M. Sieger, J. Am. Chem. Soc., 86, 3875 (1964).

50. R. K. Blackwood and C. R. Stephens, J. Am. Chem. Soc., 86, 2736 (1964).

51. R. K. Blackwood and C. R. Stephens, Can. J. Chem., 43, 1382 (1965).

52. J. H. Van den Hende, J. Am. Chem. Soc., 87, 929 (1965).

53. J. S. P. Schwarz, H. E. Applegate, J. L. Bouchard and F. L. Weisenborn, J. Org. Chem., 32, 1238 (1967).

54. J. R. D. McCormick, P. A. Miller, J. A. Growich, N. O. Sjolander and A. P. Doerschuk, J. Am. Chem. Soc., 80, 5572 (1958).

55. L. A. Mitscher, A. C. Bonacci and T. D. Sokoloski, Antimicrob. Agts. Chemother., 78 (1968).

56. M. Martell, Jr., A. S. Ross and J. H. Boothe, J. Am. Chem. Soc., 89, 6780 (1967).

57. J. S. P. Schwarz and H. E. Applegate, *J. Org. Chem.*, **32**, 1241 (1967).
58. A. I. Scott and C. T. Bedford, *J. Am. Chem. Soc.*, **84**, 2271 (1962).
59. M. Schach von Wittenau, *J. Org. Chem.*, **29**, 2746 (1964).
60. R. K. Blackwood, J. J. Beereboom, H. H. Rennhard, M. Schach von Wittenau and C. R. Stephens, *J. Am. Chem. Soc.*, **83**, 2773 (1961).
61. R. K. Blackwood, J. J. Beereboom, H. H. Rennhard, M. Schach von Wittenau and C. R. Stephens, *J. Am. Chem. Soc.*, **85**, 3943 (1963).
62. M. Schach von Wittenau, J. J. Beereboom, R. K. Blackwood and C. R. Stephens, *J. Am. Chem. Soc.*, **84**, 2645 (1962).
63. J. R. D. McCormick, E. R. Jensen, P. A. Miller and A. P. Doerschuk, *J. Am. Chem. Soc.*, **82**, 3381 (1960).
64. C. R. Stephens, J. J. Beereboom, H. H. Rennhard, P. N. Gordon, K. Murai, R. K. Blackwood and M. Schach von Wittenau, *J. Am. Chem. Soc.*, **85**, 2643 (1963).
65. R. K. Blackwood, J. J. Beereboom, H. H. Rennhard, M. Schach von Wittenau and C. R. Stephens, *J. Am. Chem. Soc.*, **85**, 3943 (1963).
66. U. S. Patent 3,019,260.
67. P. Bitha, J. J. Hlavka and J. H. Boothe, *J. Med. Chem.*, **13**, 89 (1970).
68. J. J. Beereboom, J. J. Ursprung, H. H. Rennhard and C. R. Stephens, *J. Am. Chem. Soc.*, **82**, 1003 (1960).
69. J. H. Boothe, J. J. Hlavka, J. P. Petisi and J. L. Spencer, *J. Am. Chem. Soc.*, **82**, 1253 (1960).

70. J. Petisi, J. L. Spencer, J. J. Hlavka and J. H. Boothe, J. Med. Chem., 5, 538 (1962).

71. J. J. Hlavka, A. Schneller, H. Krazinski and J. H. Boothe, J. Am. Chem. Soc., 84, 1426 (1962).

72. J. J. Hlavka, H. Krazinski and J. H. Boothe, J. Org. Chem., 27, 3674 (1962).

73. J. L. Spencer, J. J. Hlavka, J. Petisi, H. M. Krazinski and J. H. Boothe, J. Med. Chem., 6, 405 (1963).

74. J. J. Hlavka and H. M. Krazinski, J. Org. Chem., 28, 1422 (1963).

75. M. J. Martell, Jr., and J. H. Boothe, J. Med. Chem., 10, 44 (1967).

76. M. J. Martell, Jr., A. S. Ross and J. H. Boothe, J. Med. Chem., 10, 359 (1967).

77. T. Andre and S. Ullberg, J. Am. Chem. Soc., 79, 494 (1957).

78. J. J. Hlavka and D. A. Buyske, Nature, 186, 1064 (1960).

79. A. Cammarata, S. J. Yan, J. H. Collett and A. N. Martin, Mol. Pharmacol., 6, 61 (1970).

80. A. Cammarata and S. J. Yan, J. Med. Chem., 13, 93 (1970).

81. C. Hansch, A. R. Steward and J. Iwasa, J. Med. Chem., 8, 863 (1965).

82. R. F. R. Church, R. E. Schaub and M. J. Weiss, J. Org. Chem., 36, 723 (1971).

83. L. Bernardi, R. DeCastiglione, V. Colonna and P. Masi, Il Farmaco, Ed. Sci., 30, 736 (1975).

84. S. Udenfriend, C. T. Clark, J. Axelrod and B. B. Brodie, J. Biol. Chem., 208, 713 (1954).

85. P. Shu, J. Am. Chem. Soc., 88, 4529 (1966).

86. H. H. Rennhard, R. K. Blackwood and C. R. Stephens, J. Am. Chem. Soc., 83, 2775 (1961).

87. U. S. Patent 3,226,435.

88. D. Bilovic, V. Skaric and S. Djokic, Croat. Chem. Acta, 45, 357 (1973).

89. A. Green and J. H. Boothe, J. Am. Chem. Soc., 82, 3950 (1960).

90. R. K. Blackwood, H. H. Rennhard and C. R. Stephens, J. Am. Chem. Soc., 82, 5194 (1960).

91. C. E. Holmlund, W. W. Andres and A. J. Shay, J. Am. Chem. Soc., 81, 4748 (1959).

92. H. Muxfeldt and A. Kreutzer, Chem. Ber., 94, 881 (1961).

93. H. Muxfeldt and A. Kreutzer, Naturwiss., 46, 204 (1959).

94. R. B. Woodward, Pure and Applied Chem., 6, 561 (1963).

95. C. E. Holmlund, W. W. Andres and A. J. Shay, J. Am. Chem. Soc., 81, 4750 (1959).

96. H. Muxfeldt, G. Buhr and R. Bangert, Angew. Chem., Internat. Ed., 1, 157 (1962).

97. A. Green and J. H. Boothe, J. Am. Chem. Soc., 82, 3950 (1960).

98. R. K. Blackwood, H. H. Rennhard and C. R. Stephens, J. Am. Chem. Soc., 82, 5194 (1960).

99. A. Green, R. G. Wilkinson and J. H. Boothe, J. Am. Chem. Soc., 82, 3946 (1960).

CHAPTER 7

CHEMICAL TRANSFORMATIONS OF THE OXYTETRACYCLINE FAMILY

7.1---Introduction.

It is amply clear from the information in Chapters 5 and 6 that the C_6OH group in the tetracyclines is responsible for a number of degradative reactions toward acids and bases which destroy antibiotic activity and that manifold opportunities for molecular manipulation became possible only when practical routes to the C_6-deoxytetracyclines became available. The C_5OH moiety of the OTC subfamily also plays a significant role in the chemistry of that family. No practical means has ever been developed for removal of that function, so means have had to be found whereby successful manipulation of the molecule could be carried out in its presence. Two semi-synthetic antibiotics have found commercial acceptance as a consequence of this work and this chapter is devoted to this body of knowledge.

7.2---Chemistry of position 2.

Dehydration of OTC to the C_2-CN analog (1) was accomplished by treating the antibiotic with benzenesulfonyl chloride in pyridine.[1] The nitrile had the expected absorption band at 2220 cm^{-1} in the ir spectrum. It is interesting that the secondary hydroxyl group at C_5 did not esterify. Regeneration of 1 to a tetracycline has not been reported, probably because of the strong acid this would require.

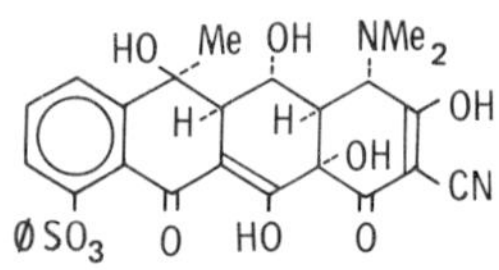

(1)

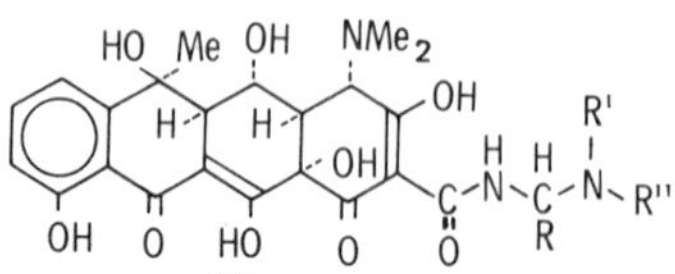

(2)

The Mannich bases (2) of the OTC family have been prepared, but have not found the clinical acceptance of the TC products. They are clearly prodrugs as they rapidly degrade to the parent antibiotic when dissolved in hydroxylic solvents.[2]

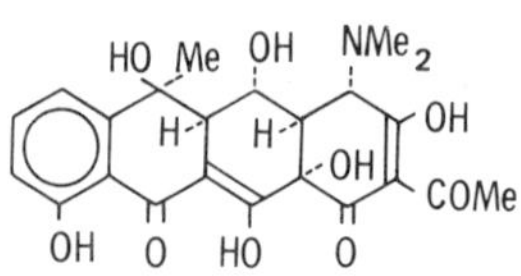

(3)

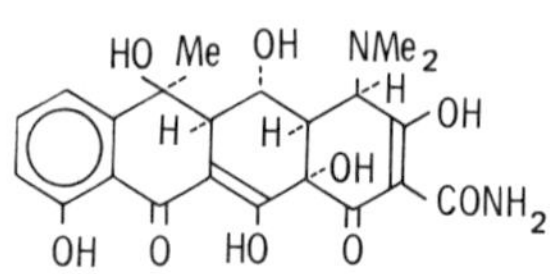

(4)

The C_2-acetyl analog of OTC (3) has been isolated from mutants and cultures producing OTC itself.[3,4] This product has only 10% of the activity of TC. One chromatographic study[5] has in fact found perceptible quantities of 3 in every commercial sample examined -- samples obtained from 15 different lands.

7.3---Chemistry of position 4.

As might be expected, epimerization of OTC to 4 takes place with substantially complete loss of biopotency.[6,7] OTC does this at a slower rate and to a lesser extent than TC or CTC, an effect which has been attributed to hydrogen bonding between the C_5-OH and C_4-NMe_2 groups.[8] MOTC and DOOTC would be expected to behave similarly. This hydrogen bonding is not possible with TC or CTC. As was found with the other tetracyclines, the nature of the C_2 substituent affects the ease of epimerization of OTC derivatives. The results are somewhat conflicting regarding the influence of the Mannich bases. In one study, the OTC Mannich base cleaved more completely than the TC and the OTC produced was more epimerized.[9] This finding is apparently at variance with other work showing a lesser epimerization tendency for OTC.[8] The result has been rationalized by pointing out that acetic acid is present in the one study[9] and not the other.[8] Presumably this hydrogen bonds with the C_5OH group and removes its protecting influence. This could perhaps successfully explain the lack of protection by the C_5OH in the one study, but not why more isomer was formed than would have occurred with OTC alone. This point would seem to need further clarification in light of studies showing the equilibrium point to favor OTC.[10]

The 2-acetyl-2-decarboxamidooxytetracycline (3) shares many chemical properties with OTC, however, it does not appreciably epimerize under the conditions examined.[3,4]

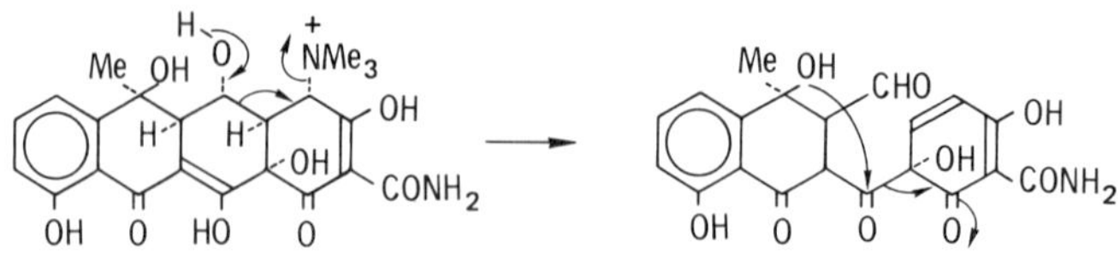

(5) (6)

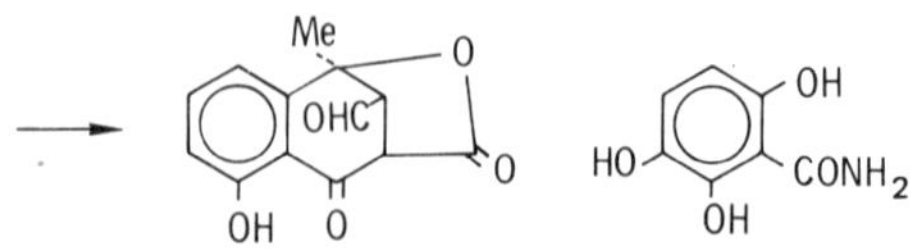

(7) (8)

In the case of OTC, attempted quaternization with methyl iodide leads to fragmentation instead.[11] Presumably after quaternary salt 5 is formed, a 1,5-fragmentation ensues triggered by the C_5OH group. This leads to 6 and expulsion of trimethylamine. The C_6OH then attacks the C_{12} carbonyl cleaving the molecule into lactone 7 and phenol 8. The C_5OH is obviously important, but the C_6OH is also essential because MOTC and DOOTC, both lacking a C_6OH, form normal methiodides.[11] Careful treatment of OTC with zinc and acid leads to 4-dedimethylaminooxytetracycline.[1] This substance has some intriguing biological properties. It has rather good and broad antibacterial potency *in vitro* but, disappointingly, is not useful *in vivo*.[12]

7.4---Chemistry of position 4a.

There is no record of a reaction at C_{4a} in the literature.

7.5---Chemistry of position 5.

As might be expected, esterification is characteristic of the C_5OH group. The sequence of acylation is C_{12a} and then C_5, so consumption of two equivalents leads to the C_{12a},C_5-diacetate.[1] The structure and conformation of this product has been settled by X-ray.[13] The C_{12a}-formyl group is readily solvolyzed providing a convenient means for making a substantial number of mono and diesters. Unfortunately, this depresses bioactivity.[12] Such activity as is seen is believed to be the result of deacylation back to the parent antibiotic. When OTC is esterified in the presence of strong acids, such as HF and CH_3SO_3H, the C_5 esters are formed, possibly via intermediacy of the C_{12a} esters which would not survive the reaction conditions in this view.[14] These esters showed decreased activity against Gram-positive, but increased activity against TC-resistant strains. The C_5-formyl ester was reported to be better absorbed after oral administration than OTC itself and therefore to give an improved therapeutic response.

A method of introducing a C_5 oxygen substituent via the intermediacy of the 5a,11a-dehydrotetracyclines has been found, although the reaction proceeds at the cost of aromatization of the C ring. When 5a,11a-dehydro-7-chlortetracycline (9) is treated with acid in the presence of the appropriate alcohol, an alkoxy group appears at C_5.[15] There has been considerable speculation about the position of the double bond in the dehydrotetracyclines.[15,16] In fact, two tautometric forms have been isolated, one showing a carbonyl band at 1715 cm^{-1} while the other shows the customary TC lack of absorption above 1660 cm^{-1}. These two forms are assigned structures 9 and 10, respectively. Clearly the molecule is capable of a tautomeric equilibrium

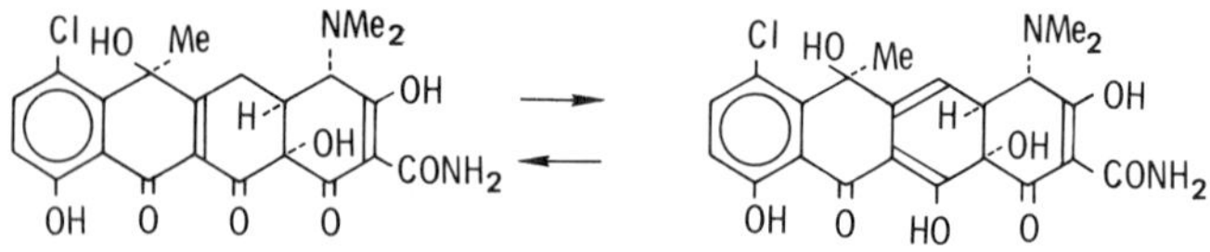

(9) (10)

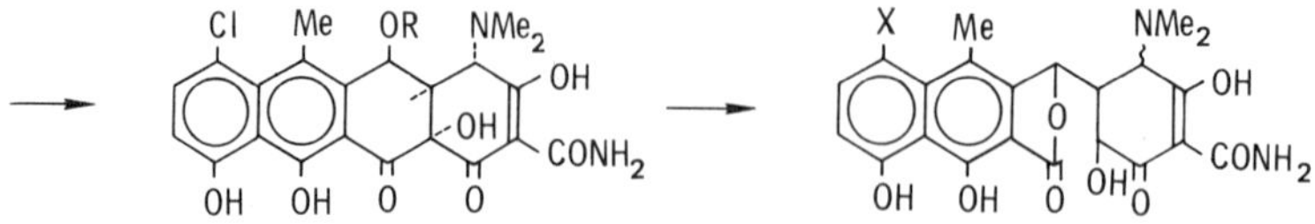

(11) (12)

depending upon the conditions. The conversion of 10 to 11 can conveniently be envisiaged as the consequence of an S_N2' process following proton attack on the C_6OH group. Accordingly, the stereochemistry of the entering group has been arbitrarily assigned to be β (11) although there is no experimental evidence upon this point. These compounds in common with most other anhydrotetracycline derivatives, are active *in vitro*, but not *in vivo*.[12] The processes used for rehydration of the C ring which were discussed in the previous chapter have not apparently been applied to 11.

The relative stability of 11 contrasts to the situation when R=H. This structure is available upon heating 9-10 with aqueous acid.[11] Its deschloro-C_5 epimer arises when OTC is treated with anhydrous acid. In the presence of aqueous acid, the C_5OH of 11 (R=H) and its C_5 epimer attacks the C_{12} keto group across the ring to form the apoterramycins (12) (X=Cl or H).[1] This does not appear to happen when R in 11 is alkyl, presumably because alkoxide cannot form as an attacking species.

No practical application of these studies has been made.

7.6---Chemistry of position 5a.

The rearrangement and tautomerism of $C_{5a,11a}$-dehydrotetracyclines has been described in Section 7.5. The analogous derivative in the OTC class (13) was encountered in biosynthetic studies and partially purified by paper chromatography.[17] It (13) was too unstable for more extensive experimentation. In this case (13) participation of the $C_{5,5a}$-tautomeric form would convert ring B to a dione (14). Subsequent epimerization at C_{4a} would be followed by dehydration at $C_{4a,12a}$ to produce an unstable hydroquinone which could readily decompose further. This speculation might account for the difficulty of working with 13.

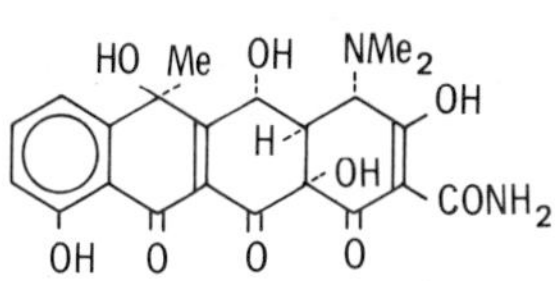

(13)

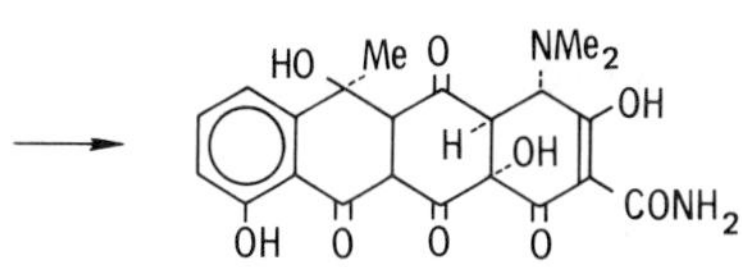

(14)

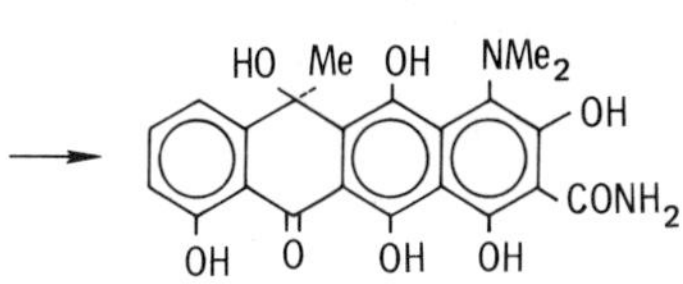

(15)

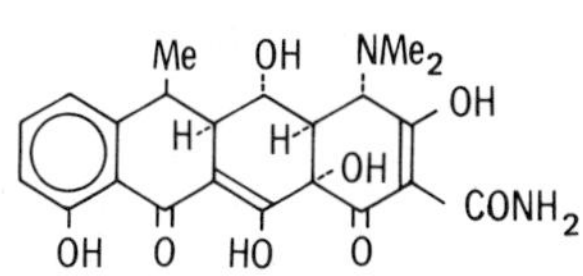

(16)

7.7---Chemistry of position 6.

Learning how to remove the C_6OH group has been the key to the preparation and introduction of two new semisynthetic OTC analogs into commercial use. No culture or mutant has ever been found which omits the C_6 methyl of OTC so other means of effecting C_6OH removal than those used in the non-5-hydroxylated series had to be developed.

Direct hydrogenation of OTC with a noble metal catalyst in acidic media results in some decomposition <u>via</u> dehydration and overreduction, but a compound assigned to be C_6-<u>epi</u>-deoxyoxytetracycline (<u>16</u>) was isolated.[18-22] When tested <u>in vitro</u>, <u>16</u> was found to be only 0.36 times as active as OTC itself. It will be recalled that the loss of potency in the TC series was not nearly as great.

With the discovery that C_{11a}-halogenation-dehalogenation constituted a valuable protection deprotection scheme, a route to the C_6-methylene and thence C_6-deoxy series was developed.[23] Fluorination, chlorination, etc., produces the C_{11a}-haloanalog as the 6,12-hemiketal.[27] Evidence is that the newly introduced group is α (<u>17</u>) in order to allow for hemiketal formation. Reduction of <u>17</u> regenerates OTC.

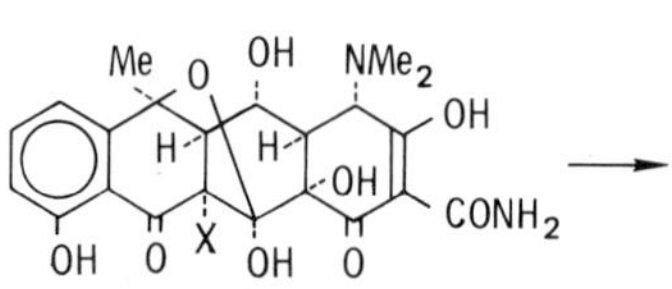

(17)

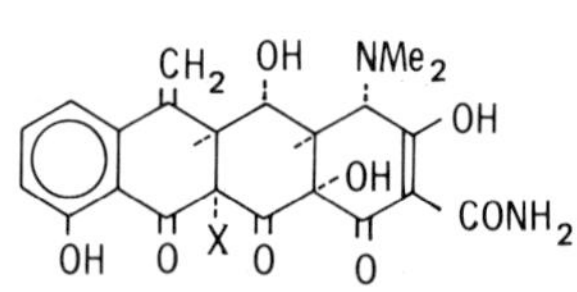

(18)

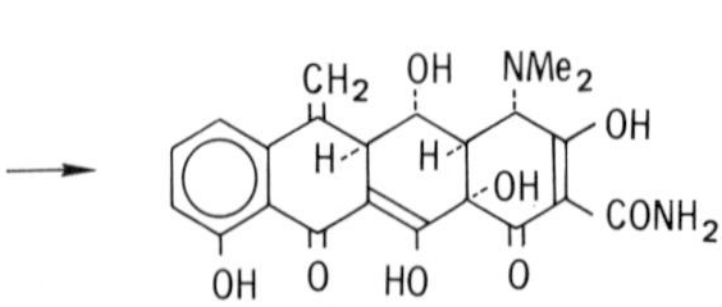

(19)

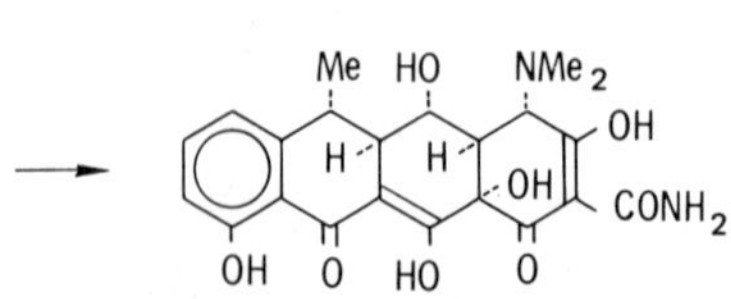

(20)

Dehydration of 17 by anhydrous HF or with 85% sulfuric acid proceeds exocyclicly to give 18 because 17 cannot enolize toward C_{11a} to provide driving force for endocyclic dehydration. Careful reduction leads to 6-methyleneoxytetracycline (MOTC) (19). An alternate method involves treatment of OTC with pyridine-SO_3 to give an intermediate sulfuric acid ester (21) which goes to 19 on treatment with HF.[27] The yield is low in this sequence. Compound 19 is 2.3 times more active in vitro against Kl. pneumonia than TC. This potency advantage carried over to in vivo and clinical tests and 19 has been on the U.S. market since 1966 under the name, methacycline. Further reduction leads to 6-deoxyoxytetracyclines (20) and (16). When catalytic reduction is carried out on 19, an approximately 1:1 ratio of 20 to 16 is obtained, whereas reduction of 18 (R=F) gives a preponderance of what is assigned to be 16 because of presumed absorption to the catalytic surface from the convex α-face of the molecule.[25,26] This view requires that reduction of the double bond precede reduction of the halogen atom. DOOTC (20), in contrast to 16, is more active (ca 1.4 fold vs Kl. pneumoniae) than OTC in vitro and retains high activity in vivo and was marketed in the U.S. in 1967 as doxycycline.

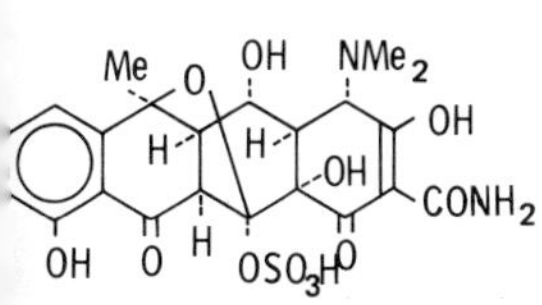

(21)

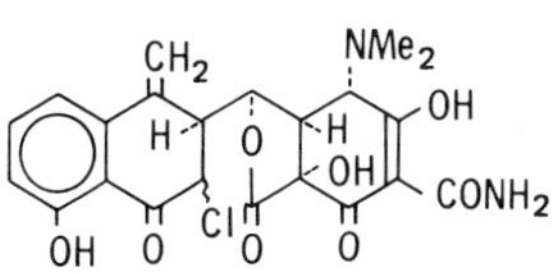

(22)

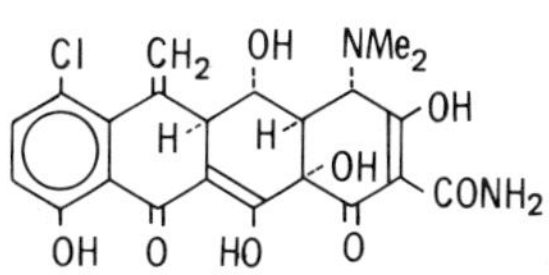

(23)

When a C_5OH is present, as in 18, the C_{11a}-halo analogs are somewhat unstable at neutral or basic pH's and trans-anular cleavage to 22 is observed. Under more acidic conditions, 18 is sufficiently stable to allow electrophilic substitution reactions. For example, treatment with NCS in liquid HF followed by careful deblocking with hydrosulfite produces the 7-chloro analog (23) which is 6.3-fold more potent *in vitro* than MOTC (19) itself.

Mercaptans add in an anti-Markownikov sense under free radical conditions to 19 to produce alkylthioanalogs (24) of 20.[26,27] The more acidic mercaptans give substantial amounts of anhydro byproducts. Under the influence of peroxides and peracids, these are converted to sulfoxides (25). Although in principle diastereomers could result, no mention has been made of this in the literature. Reduction of the alkylthiomethylene analogs (stereochemistry assigned as in 24) with Raney nickel provides an alternate route to DOOTC. Production of the simple C_6-CH_2SH analog is accomplished by strong acid hydrolysis of the CH_3COSCH_2 analog.[26,27]

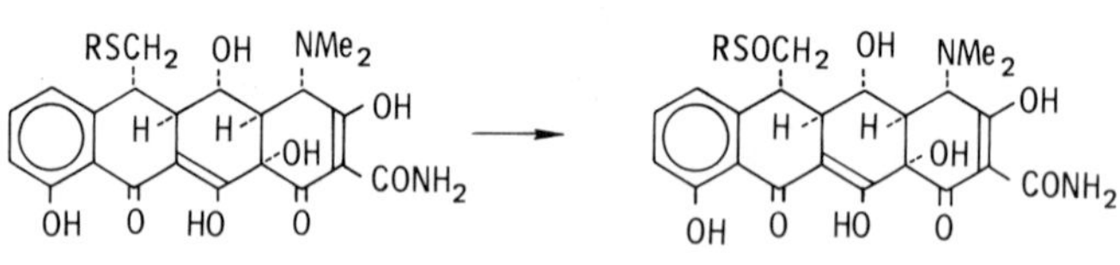

(24) (25)

The increased lipophilicity of 24, where R is phenyl or benzyl, apparently is responsible for somewhat depressed potency against Gram-negative bacteria -- although the loss is not as dramatic as is encountered in the C_5 deoxy analogs. Some support for this argument comes from the observation that the sulfoxides are rather more potent than the sulfides in the non C_5OH series. These considerations are illustrated by the data in Table 7-1.

Finally, just as in the non-C_5OH series, when OTC is refluxed with triethylamine in dioxane, allooxytetracycline (26) is produced in small yield along with non-basic decomposition products.[28] A fragmentation reaction analogous to that seen when OTC is reacted with methyl iodide (see Section 7.3) may be responsible for the non-basic products whereas 26 probably arises via the 6,12-hemiketal.

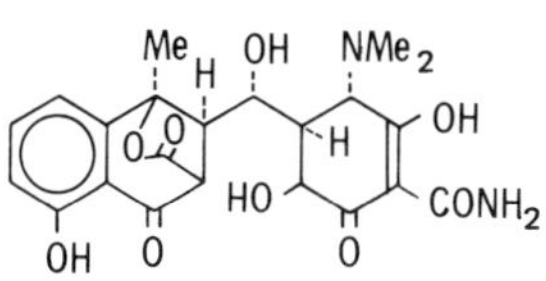

(26)

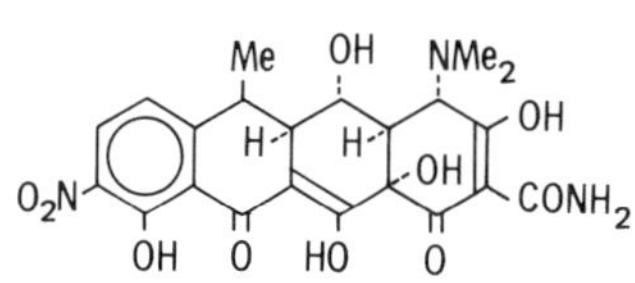

(27)

7.8---Chemistry of ring D.

While the C_6 methylene analog of OTC (19) is much more stable to acid than OTC itself, nonetheless it is not sufficiently inert to allow the wide range of eletrophilic reactions possible in the non-C_5OH series. As a consequence, only the 7-chloro analog 23 has been reported.[27] Its potency enhancement suggests this to be a fruitful area of chemistry to explore if this barrier can be overcome. Treatment of 6-deoxy-6-epioxytetracycline (16) with nitrating agents produced the C_9 nitro analog (27).[29]

Table 7-1. Relative activity of several OTC derivatives modified at C_6.[12]

Antibiotic	Relative Activity *in vitro vs Kl. pneumo.* (OTC = 1.0)	Subcutaneous Activity *vs Staph. aureus* 5 in Mg/kg
OTC	1.0	-
16	0.4	-
20	1.4	1.0
24, R = H	0.06	-
24, R = C_6H_5	0.2	>25
24, R = $CH_2C_6H_5$	0.26	>12
24, R = CH_3CO	0.4	>25
19	2.3	1.19
23	6.3	-

This substance was inactive and no further use of it in making analogs is given in the chemical literature.

7.9---Chemistry of position 11a.

The significant chemistry of C_{11a} involves halogenation and deblocking. In the C_6OH series, a 6,12-hemiketal (17) forms whereas in the C_6-desoxy-C_6-epi series, the C_{12} carbonyl is free. The hemiketal is more difficult to reduce back to the unblocked tetracycline. The fluoro analogs are made with perchloroylfluoride.[11,24] The chloro analogs are made with a variety of reagents especially N-chlorosuccinimide in fairly strong acid.[23,27] The iodo and bromo analogs are less stable than the chloro and fluoro analogs and are more easily removed reductively.

7.10--Chemistry of position 12a.

The $C_{12a}OH$ group esterifies easily and esters at this function are easily solvolyzed.[1,13,30] Direct removal of the $C_{12a}OH$ group with zinc and acid was discovered during the structure elucidation days.[1] Catalytic reduction of the C_{12a} formyl ester will also serve.[31]

REFERENCES

1. F. A. Hochstein, C. R. Stephens, L. H. Conover, P. P. Regna, R. Pasternack, P. N. Gordon, F. J. Pilgrim, K. J. Brunings and R. B. Woodward, J. Am. Chem. Soc., 75, 5455 (1953).
2. A. Brunzell, Acta Chem. Scand., 16, 245 (1962).
3. F. A. Hochstein, M. Schach von Wittenau, F. W. Tanner, Jr. and K. Murai, J. Am. Chem. Soc., 82, 5934 (1960).
4. M. W. Miller and F. A. Hochstein, J. Org. Chem., 27, 2525 (1962).
5. J. Keiner, R. Huettenrauch and W. Poethke, Arch. Pharm., 300, 840 (1967).
6. J. R. D. McCormick, N. O. Sjolander, U. Hirsch, E. R. Jensen and A. P. Doerschuk, J. Am. Chem. Soc., 79, 4561 (1957).
7. A. P. Doerschuk, B. A. Bitler and J. R. D. McCormick, J. Am. Chem. Soc., 77, 4687 (1955).

8. D. A. Hussar, P. J. Niebergall, E. T. Sugita and J. T. Doluisio, J. Pharm. Pharmacol., 20, 539 (1968).

9. R. Huettenrauch and I. Keiner, Naturwiss., 53, 552 (1966).

10. J. R. D. McCormick, S. M. Fox, L. L. Smith, B. A. Bitler, J. Reichenthal, V. E. Origoni, W. H. Muller, R. Winterbottom and A. P. Doerschuk, 79, 2849 (1957).

11. R. K. Blackwood, J. J. Beereboom, H. H. Rennhard, M. Schach von Wittenau and C. R. Stephens, J. Am. Chem. Soc., 85, 3943 (1963).

12. R. K. Blackwood and A. R. English, Adv. Appl. Microbiol., 13, 237 (1970).

13. R. E. Hughes, H. Muxfeldt and R. B. Von Dreele, J. Am. Chem. Soc., 93, 1037 (1971).

14. L. Bernardi, R. DeCastiglione, V. Colonna, P. Masi and R. Mazzoleni, Farmaco, Ed. Sci., 29, 902 (1974).

15. M. Schach von Wittenau, F. A. Hochstein and C. R. Stephens, J. Org. Chem., 28, 2454 (1963).

16. A. I. Scott and C. T. Bedford, J. Am. Chem. Soc., 84, 2271 (1962).

17. P. A. Miller, Developments in Industrial Microbiology, 8, 96 (1967).

18. C. R. Stephens, K. Murai, H. H. Rennhard, L. H. Conover and K. J. Brunings, J. Am. Chem. Soc., 80, 5324 (1958).

19. J. R. D. McCormick, E. R. Jensen, P. A. Miller and A. P. Doerschuk, J. Am. Chem. Soc., 82, 3381 (1960).

20. H. Muxfeldt, Angew. Chem., Intnl. Ed., English, 1, 372 (1962).

21. H. Muxfeldt, W. Rogalski and K. Striegler, Chem. Ber., 95, 2581 (1962).

22. H. Muxfeldt, E. Jacobs and K. Uhlig, Chem. Ber., 95, 2901 (1962).

23. R. K. Blackwood, J. J. Beereboom, H. H. Rennhard, M. Schach von Wittenau and C. R. Stephens, J. Am. Chem. Soc., 83, 2773 (1961).

24. H. H. Rennhard, R. K. Blackwood and C. R. Stephens, J. Am. Chem. Soc., 83, 2775 (1961).

25. M. Schach von Wittenau, J. J. Beereboom, R. K. Blackwood and C. R. Stephens, J. Am. Chem. Soc., 84, 2645 (1962).

26. C. R. Stephens, J. J. Beereboom, H. H. Rennhard, P. N. Gordon, K. Murai, R. K. Blackwood and M. Schach von Wittenau, J. Am. Chem. Soc., 85, 2643 (1963).

27. R. K. Blackwood, J. J. Beereboom, H. H. Rennhard, M. Schach von Wittenau and C. R. Stephens, J. Am. Chem. Soc., 85, 3943 (1963).

28. J. S. P. Schwarz and H. E. Applegate, J. Org. Chem., 32, 1241 (1967).

29. J. J. Beereboom, J. J. Ursprung, H. H. Rennhard and C. R. Stephens, J. Am. Chem. Soc., 82, 1003 (1960).

30. Neth. Appl. 6,602,413 (1966) via Chem. Abs., 67, 32522w (1967).

31. R. K. Blackwood, H. H. Rennhard and C. R. Stephens, J. Am. Chem. Soc., 82, 5194 (1960).

CHAPTER 8

TOTAL SYNTHESIS

8.1---Introduction.

The art of total synthesis of complex organic natural products of biological interest has flowered in this generation. The challenge of the tetracyclines has attracted many groups and a substantial literature has grown up about the subject with the result that all of the major tetracyclines have now been conquered. The magnitude of the accomplishment can be appreciated in part from considering that in OTC, for example, there are six contiguous asymmetric centers, and that the molecule is unstable to acids and bases.

At first, several ultimately unsuccessful approaches were tried as model studies in attempts to solve specific conceptual and practical problems. Next, a number of successful syntheses were accomplished and, finally, the present phase was entered -- that of application of this body of knowledge to the synthesis of novel tetracyclines which would not be accessible by partial synthesis or by directed biosynthesis.

All of the successful syntheses have started from the aromatic D ring and advanced from there through the aliphatic regions to the A ring with its sensitive β-tricarbonyl moiety and appended asymmetric centers. While this is the most sensible approach, it is limiting in that the region that experience indicates can be most successfully modified with retention of useful bioactivity is that involving rings C and D. The early incorporation of these rings into linear syntheses requires a separate total synthesis for each analog. A solution to this practical dilemma lies in the future.

The following account details those syntheses which result in products which are complete or substantially so. A fairly large number of model studies in which major elements of the tetracyclines were left off have not been covered unless the results were particularly relevant to later complete syntheses. Fortunately, a detailed review of this work exists.[1]

8.2---Model studies failing to reach bioactive tetracyclines.

Muxfeldt began his studies by examining some reaction loops whereby he hoped to simplify the task somewhat.[2,3] His first objective was the synthesis of 4-dedimethylamino-12a-deoxyanhydro-7-chlorotetracycline (1) which was available from degradation of CTC. If 1 could be converted back to CTC, then a formal total synthesis would be achieved by the preparation of 1 which has only a single asymmetric center to contend with.

The reintroduction of the C_{12a}-OH group promised to be the easier of the tasks and, indeed, treatment of 4-dedimethylaminoanhydrotetracycline (4) with diazomethane led to the C_{10}-methoxy derivative (2), which was separated from the $C_{10,11}$-dimethoxy analog, and 2 could be reconverted to 4 with strong acid. For reasons of convenient availability, these studies were carried out in the TC series. Treatment of 2 with zinc and acetic acid removed the C_{12a}-OH and produced 3. As was well known by this time, β-dicarbonyl compounds could frequently be oxygenated on the α-carbon, and treatment of 3 with peracids gave a mixture from which 2 could be isolated, completing the reaction loop.[4]

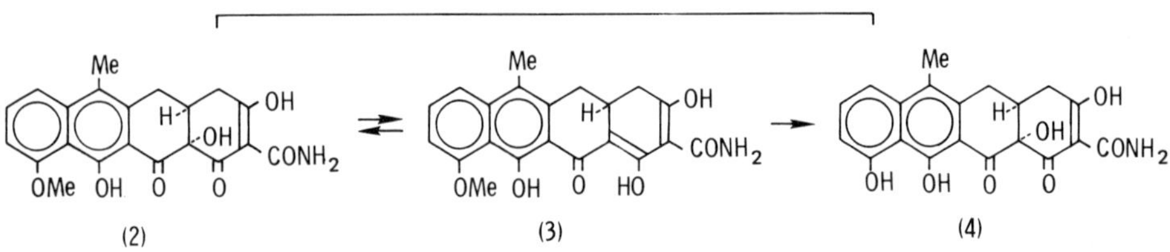

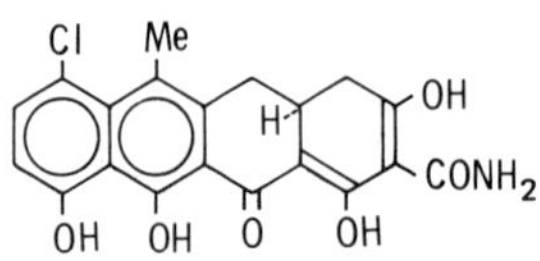

(1)

The next phase of the study encompassed the total synthesis of 1.[5-8] Starting with m-methoxybenzoic acid (5), conversion to the acid chloride and condensation with the magnesium salt of ethylmalonate was followed by decarboxylative hydrolysis with HCl to produce m-methoxy-acetophenone. A Stobbe condensation produced an E and Z mixture of monoesters from which 6 could be separated by fractional crystallization. On treatment with sodium acetate in acetic acid, the Z analog cyclized *para* to the OCH_3 group while the *E* isomer (6) was recovered unchanged. In order to effect cyclization in the desired sense, each isomer was hydrogenated separately. When dihydro 6 was treated with one equivalent of chlorine and then polyphosphoric acid, *trans* tetralone 7 was obtained. The same sequence of reactions on the Z isomer produced the isomeric *cis* tetralone 8.* Each tetralone could be aromatized to 9 by photocatalyzed free radical bromination followed by dehydrobromination with NaOH. Confirmation of the success of this process was achieved by treatment of 9 with HI which saponified the ester, cleaved the OMe group and removed the chlorine to give terranaphthoic acid, obtained earlier by degradation of OTC. Next 9 was methylated with dimethyl sulfate in acetone, reduced with lithium alumnium hydride, converted to the benzyl bromide with PBr_3 and then reacted with di*tert*butylethoxycarbonylmethylmalonate to give 10. Careful hydrolysis proceeds preferentially at the less hindered ethyl ester and Friedel-Crafts cyclization followed by saponification and heating produced tricyclic derivative 11 in high yield. Homologation *via* the Arndt-

---

* The pmr and uv properties of these two analogs were instrumental in suggesting that hydrogenolysis of TC had led to epimerization at C_6 (see Chapter 6).

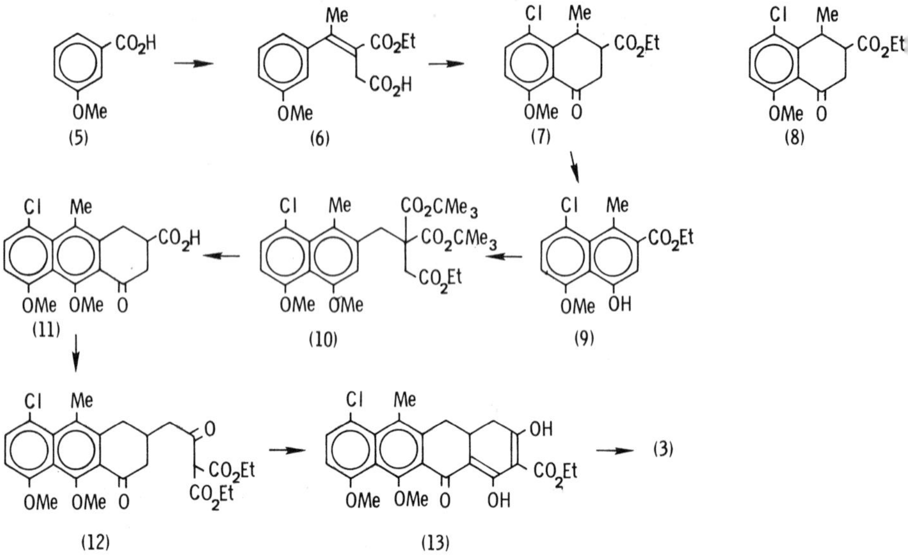

Eistert procedure was followed by acylation, as the acid chloride, of the magnesium salt of diethylmalonate to give acylmalonate 12. Strong non-nucleophilic base (NaH) ultimately succeeded in cyclizing 12 to 13. Conversion of the ethyl ester to carboxamide 1 was accomplished only in poor yield on treatment with methanolic ammonia, catalyzed by methoxide, followed by ether cleavage with HCl/HOAc.

The reaction loop described above (2-4) was next effected on 3 itself by use of peracid whereby, after ether cleavage, the desired 7-deschloroanalog of 4 and its C_{12a} epimer were obtained.[7] The ethers were used to help with the solubility of the products. Ultimately, a considerable improvement in yield and stereoselectivity was obtained using Pt catalyzed oxygenation of deschloro 1 itself.[7,9] This work followed that of a Lederle group who had accomplished the same transformation in poorer yield using sodium nitrite.[10]

Utilization of 13 as a synthon for tetracycline requires the development of methods of introducing a hydroxy group at C_6, a process which had been accomplished in other laboratories by photooxygenation,[11,12] and the development of means of reintroducing the C_4-NMe_2 group, which remains to be done. This approach has not, therefore, led to finished tetracyclines.

Another relatively successful entry utilizing an anhydrotetracycline pathway was developed by a Lederle group.[13-17] Starting with 4-chloro-3-methylanisole (14), a Wohl-Ziegler reaction with NBS and peroxide produced the benzylbromide which was used to alkylate sodiomalonic ester to give 15. Bishomologation was achieved by reduction with lithium aluminum hydride to the 1,3-diol mesylation of both primary OH groups, and then displacement with KCN and saponification to give 16. Polyphosphoric acid served to close ring C to give tetralone 17. Next, 17 was converted to the acid chloride with oxalylchloride and Rosenmund reduction converted this to the aldehyde. Condensation with excess cyanoacetamide under the influence of piperidine gave a dicyanodiamide and this was followed by decarboxylative hydrolysis in HCl/HOAc to give 18. The strenuous hydrolysis also cleaved the ether function. This was reprotected as the benzyl ether and the product was esterified under Fischer conditions (HCl/MeOH). Dieckman cyclization with NaH then gave tricyclic 19.

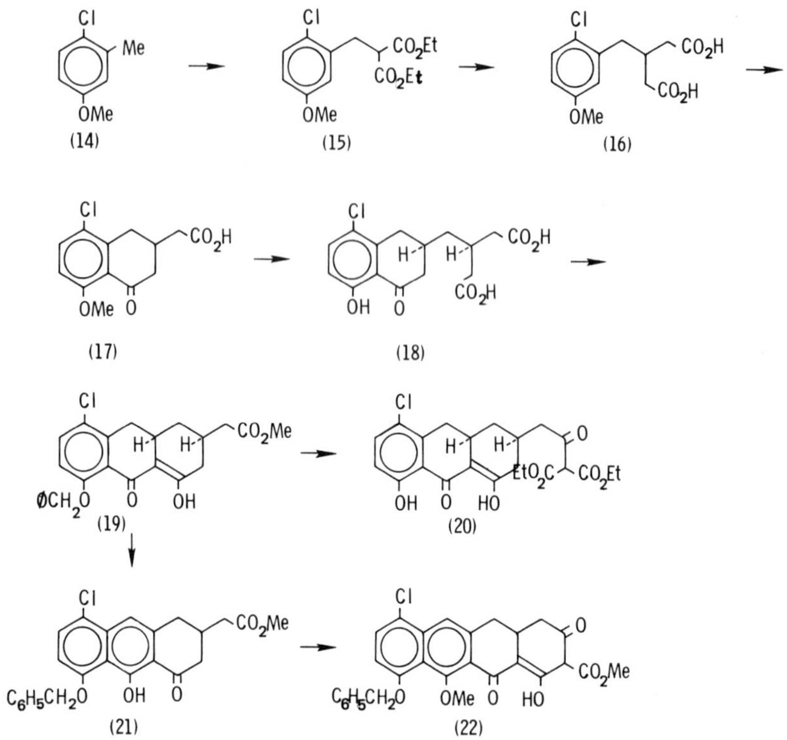

The cis-product is favored because of the lack of 1,3-diaxial interactions in the transition state. Unfortunately, 19 could not be converted to the free acid, so the benzyl ether was removed catalytically. Saponification was then successful and homologation to 20 was accomplished by reaction of the acid chloride with the magnesium salt of ethyl malonate. Unfortunately, 20 would not cyclize with NaH. The synthesis was then diverted to the anhydro series by brominating 19 and dehydrohalogenating to produce naphthalene 21. The phenolic OH was protected with dimethyl sulfate and the substituted acyl malonate was generated as before on 19, only cyclization to 22 was now successful. In this case, as opposed to 20, enolization to the desired position is now required on structural grounds. Fusion with ammonium formate converted the ester to the amide and deblocking with HCl/HOAc produced the desired (±)-7-chloro-4-dedimethylamino-6-demethyl-12a-deoxyanhydrotetracycline (23) where this approach stopped.[13,16] Compound 23 was identical, except for optical activity, with a sample prepared by degradation of DMCTC. No chemical means are yet available for reintroduction of a C_6OH group in the C_6-demethyl series so this work has not been extended.

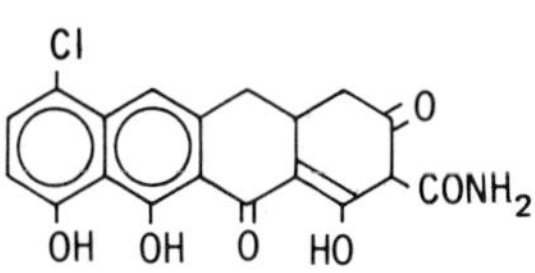

(23)

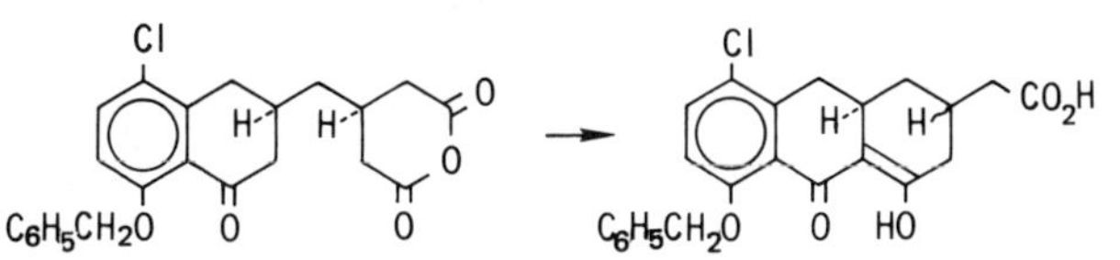

(24) (25)

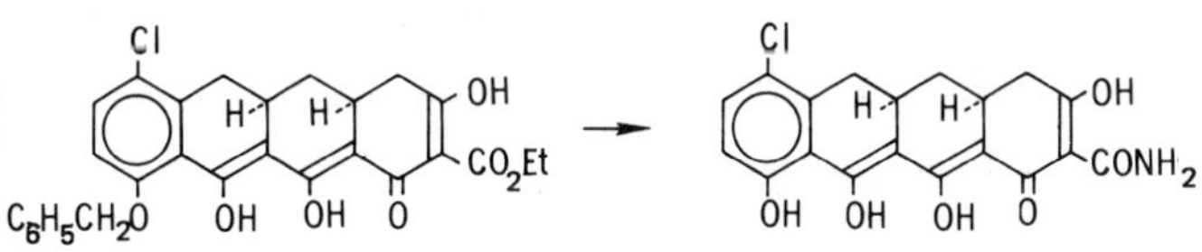

(26) (27)

Success with the partial synthesis of 6-deoxytetracyclines and their retention of bioactivity led to attempted total synthesis of these easier objectives. The Lederle group was able to overcome some of the limitations inherent in their first scheme by modifications which allowed production of 19 directly as the free acid, thereby avoiding facile base β-diketone cleavage. Compound 18 was refluxed with acetic anhydride leading to conversion to glutaric anhydride 24. Addition of one equivalent of sodium methoxide led to the monoester-monoacids which were cyclized to separable mixture 25 with NaH. Diethylmalonate was then acylated by 25, using the mixed anhydride method and the product, in contrast, to 20, cyclized to tetracyclic 26 with NaH. Hydrogenolysis of 26 removed the benzyl group and fusion with ammonium formate completed the synthesis of (±)-7-chloro-4-dedimethylamino-6-demethyl-6-deoxy-12a-deoxytetracycline (27) whereupon this group ceased their work on total synthesis.[13,15]

The initial Muxfeldt synthesis has also been modified to approach 6-deoxytetracyclines with a reduced C ring.[1,18-20] Compound 7 was ketalized with ethylene glycol, the ester group was converted to a primary alcohol with lithium aluminum hydride, this was mesylated and replaced by a nitrile using KCN. Reduction with lithium triethoxyalumnium hydride produced aldehyde 28. This was condensed with malonic ester using piperidine acetate to give 29. Michael addition-Dieckman condensation of 29 with ethyl acetoacetate and KOMe produced 30. The ketal was removed using tosic acid and acetone and hydrogenolysis produced 31 which underwent Dieckman cyclization to produce tetracyclic 32 after deblocking. Detailed uv analysis of 33, produced by a simple variant of this scheme, in comparison with a degradation product (34) obtained at Lederle following hydrogenolytic removal of the C_6OH group showed that the configuration at C_6 could not be the same. The C_6-CH_3 and C_7-Cl groups of 33 interact

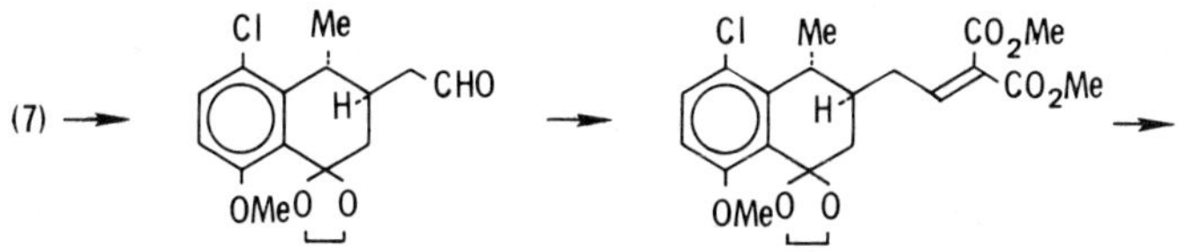

(28) (29)

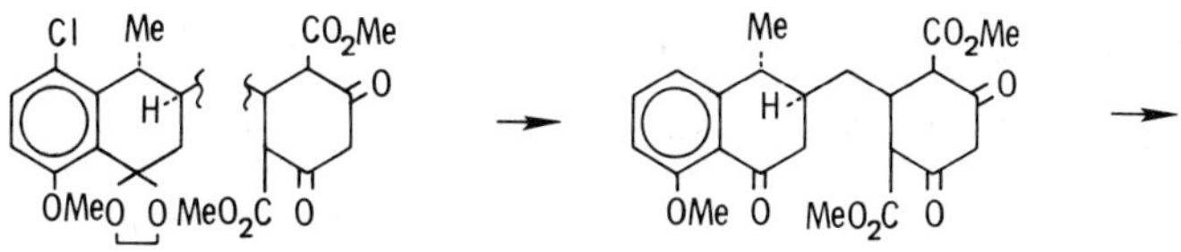

(30) (31)

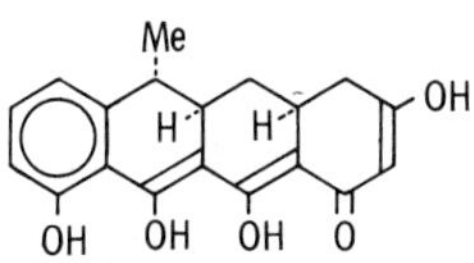

(32)

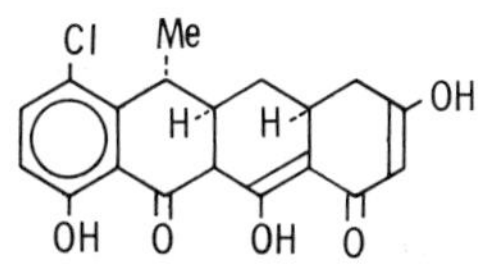

(33)

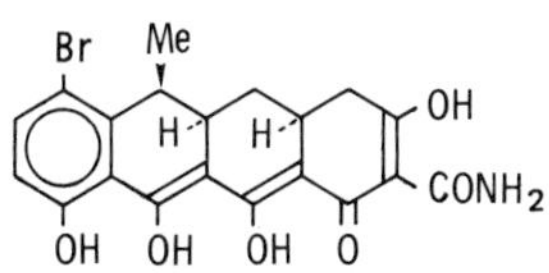

(34)

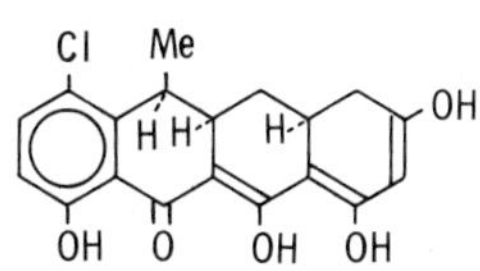

(35)

sterically to prevent easy enolization toward C_{11a} in 33.[18,20] This meant that the synthesis would have to be recast if compounds identical to those produced at Lederle were to result and suggested that the hydrogenolysis products be assigned C_6-epi geometry (34). Experimental details relating to the synthesis of 34 have never been published so the weight of this argument is lessened. Repetition of the sequence starting with 8 rather than 7 led to 35.[19]

The problems associated with uncertainty of the configuration to be sought at C_6 were avoided by synthesis of the demethyldeoxy system.[19] First, m-methoxybenzaldehyde (36) was condensed with methylsuccinate, and the Stobbe product was saponified and reduced to give 37. This was chlorinated with an iodine catalyst and cyclized with polyphosphoric acid to give decalin 38. Compound 38 was ketalized and reduced with lithium alumnium hydride to give 39 which was mesylated and solvolyzed with KCN and then reduced by lithium triethoxyaluminum hydride to aldehyde 40. Condensation with methyl malonate with the aid of piperidine/acetic acid gave 41. Condensation with methyl acetoacetate, as before, led to 42. Deketalization, cyclization with NaH and deblocking with HBr led to the final product in this sequence, 7-chloro-4-dedimethylamino-6-deoxy-6-demethyl-12a-deoxytetracycline (43).

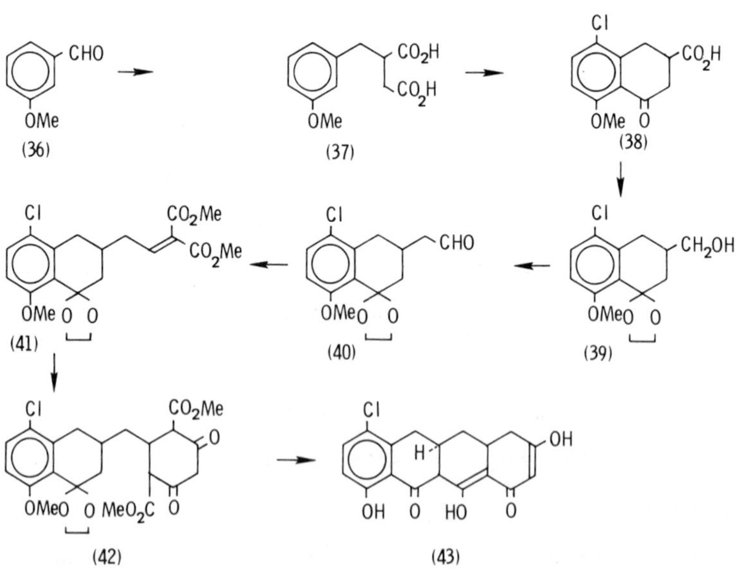

Barton and his school undertook extensive experiments designed to lead to tetracyclines through intermediates with rings A and D both aromatic and then to reduce ring A at a late stage.[21-33] Much novel chemistry was uncovered but 6-methylpretetramide is the only natural tetracycline which emerged from this imaginative undertaking. The overall research plan[21] is illustrated in formulae 44-47. Selection of a suitable strategy for joining C_{11a} to C_{12} is essential as is the judicious choice of blocking and activating groups.

The first sequence reported utilized latent functionality to avoid side reactions.[24] A Friedel-Crafts condensation of 1,5-dihydroxynaphthalene (48) with benzoic acid and zinc chloride produced 49, apparently by p-acylation as expected, followed by hemiketal formation with the peri-OH group and then dehydration involving the p-H to give the furan. This protects the phenolic OH and allows further selective transformations on the future ring C. The double bond is reduced with Raney nickel to give 50 which is condensed at the activated methylene with ring A precursor 51, using sulfuric acid in acetic acid as catalyst. Compound 51 is prepared from 3,5-dihydroxytoluene via methyl orcinol-p-carboxylate (57) which, in a Gattermann reaction, forms a carboxaldehyde. This is converted to the oxime which is itself converted to isoxazole 58 on heating in acetic anhydride. Thiele oxidation ($Ac_2O/HOAc/H_2SO_4/CrO_3$) gave the desired 51 in which one aldehyde group is masked as the diacetate

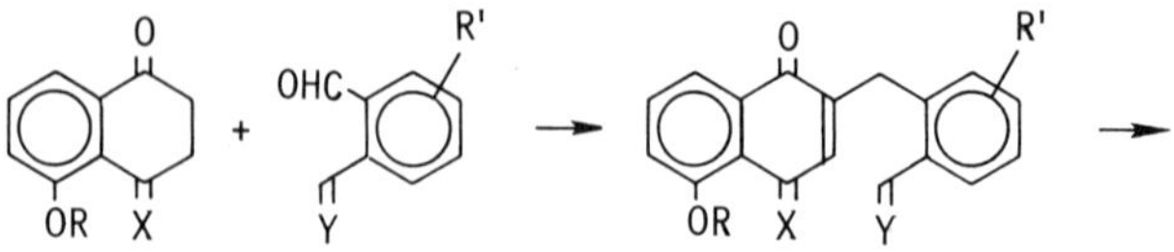

(44) (45) (46)

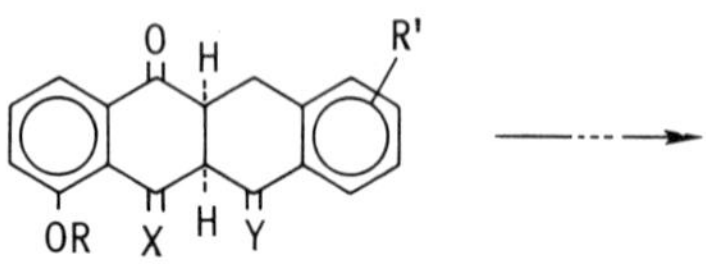

(47)

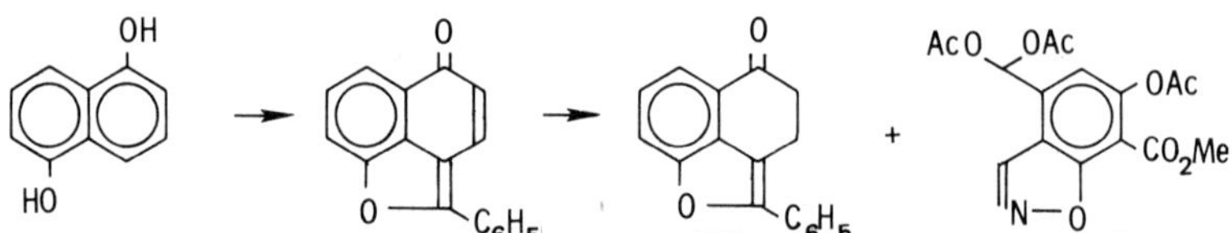

(48) (49) (50) (51)

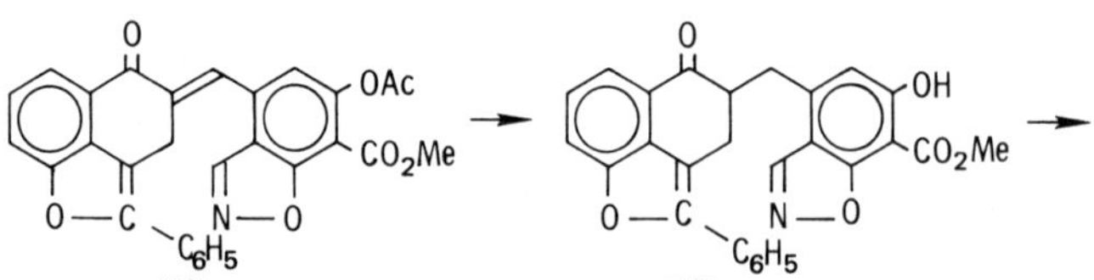

(52) (53)

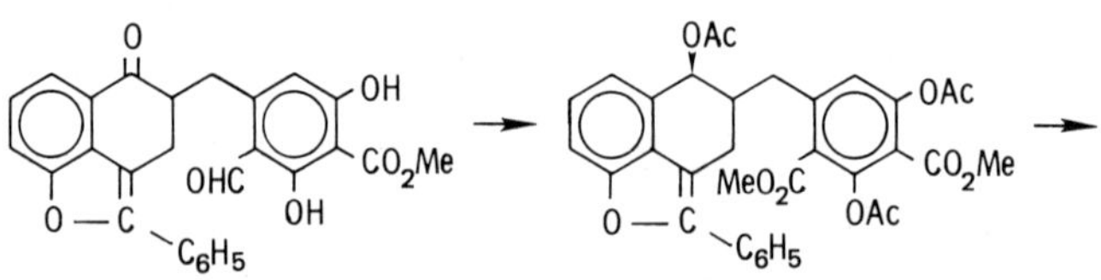

(54) (55)

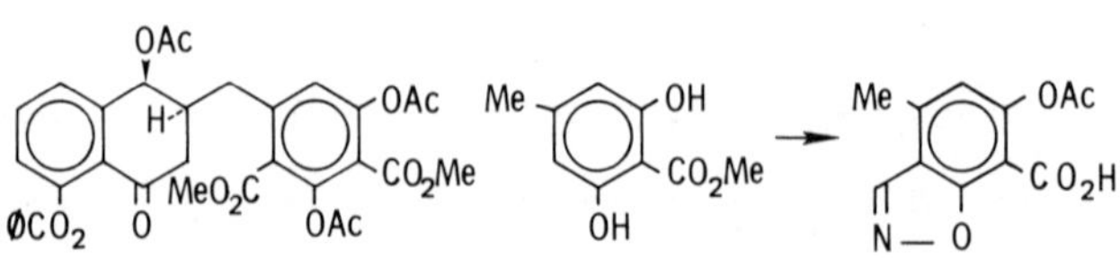

(56) (57) (58)

and the other latent carbonyl could be dehydrated to a nitrile or reduced to an aldehyde as needed. The condensation product of 50 and 51 (52) was reduced to 53 only after some trouble as the isoxazole reacted preferentially under a number of conditions. Finally, in an unusual reaction, dry HI finally gave 53. Hydrogenation cleaved the isoxazole ring to give aldehyde 54 which was prepared for cyclization by chromium trioxide oxidation to the acid which was esterified and the molecule was reduced with potassium borohydride and then acetylated to give 55. The latent functionality in the furan ring of 55 was unmasked by ozonization and 56 resulted. Unfortunately, 56 failed to cyclize and this approach was dropped.

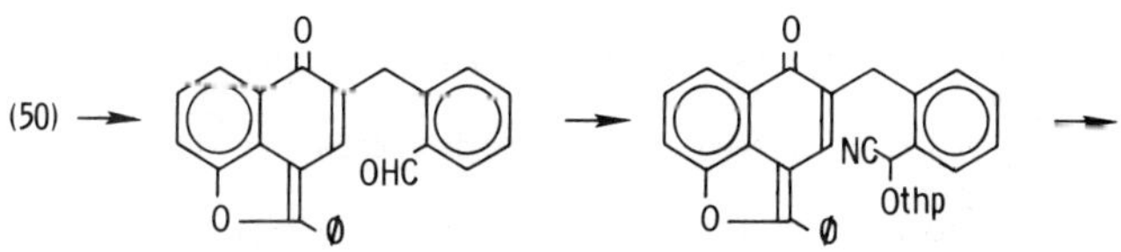

(59) (60)

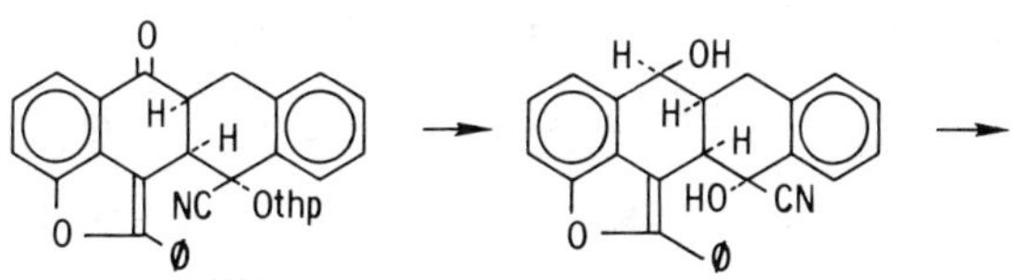

(61) (62)

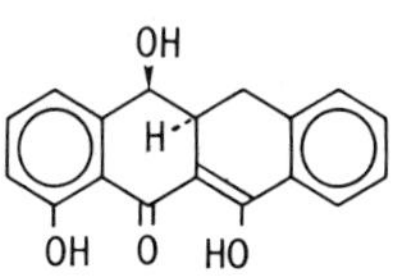

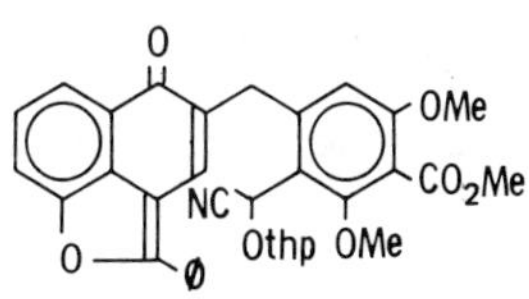

(63) (64)

The next variation utilized an umpolung reaction of a nucleophilic carbonyl synthon in an attempt to get a Michael addition to close ring B.[25] The furan described previously (50) was condensed with o-phthaldehyde using triethylamine and 59 resulted. In order to reverse the normal polarity of the aldehyde carbonyl, a variety of derivatives were investigated. Finally, treatment of 59 successively with KCN and dihydropyran in acid gave 60 which had the desired properties. When 60 was treated with sodium t-butoxide, Michael addition occurred to give tetracyclic 61. Brief treatment with acid converted 61 to the unprotected cyanohydrin and Meerwein-Ponndorf reduction led to 62. Ozonolysis generated the target model 63. Unfortunately, when the sequence was repeated utilizing an elaborated A ring synthon, the synthesis failed when key intermediate 64 refused to cyclize. The substantial peri-buttressing effects present in the cyclization product of 64 and absent in 63 may play an important role in this. In any event, this approach was terminated at this point.

Since it was known that nitrones added readily to conjugated double bonds in a 1,3-dipolar sense, an attempt was made to make use of this property.[26] Aldehyde 65, the immediate precursor of synthon 64, was reacted with phenylhydroxylamine to form a nitrone (66) which does not survive the reaction but adds in a 1,3-dipolar sense to the conjugated double bond to give 67. Reductive cleavage of the N-O bond was finally achieved with Cr(II)Cl_2. The resulting α-ketol (68) was deoxygenated with zinc and acid to give 69, which epimerized to the desired α-isomer (70) on alumina chromatography. Hydride reduction and acetylation gave 71. Despite numerous attempts with various reagents and with various analogs of 71, the aniline could not be converted to a C_{12} ketone and this approach had to be dropped.

The next, and most successful sequence, involved a radical coupling reaction to join together ring B.[27] The lessons learned in a model study[27] were successfully applied to the total synthesis of 6-methylpretetramid (79), a fully aromatic biogenetic intermediate (Chapter 3).[29] Compound 65 was prepared by an improved route and then converted to the dioxolane 72. Photolysis under benzoic acid catalysis gave a 35% yield of tetracyclic ketal 76. The formation of 76 is rationalized as passing through several intermediate stages. The acid is necessary to protonate the dioxolane and form 1,3,5-triene 73 which undergoes a conrotatory photocyclization to 74 whereupon prototropic shifts and readdition of oxygen (75) results in the isolated product (76). Saponification to the acid was followed by treatment with methyl lithium to give 77. Ozonolysis freed the C_{10} and C_{11} functions and HI cleaved the various ether bonds and dehydrated the intermediate 78 to 6-methylpretetramid (79).

An attempt to extend this synthesis to the preparation of 4-hydroxy-6-methylpretetramid (81) failed when the

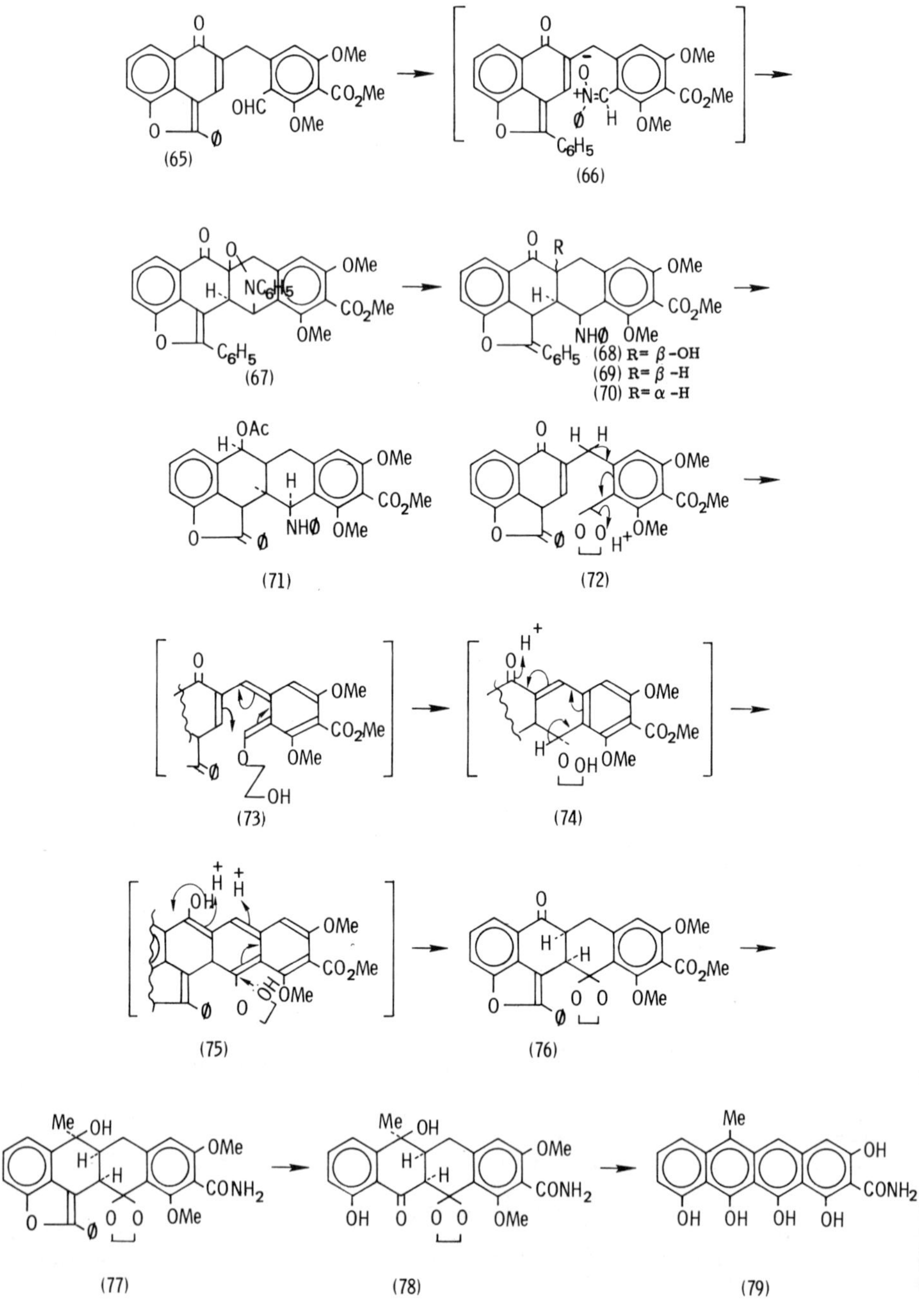
(65)
(66)
(67)
(68) R= β-OH
(69) R= β-H
(70) R= α-H
(71)
(72)
(73)
(74)
(75)
(76)
(77)
(78)
(79)

requisite analog of 78 (80) underwent more extensive reaction with HI than planned and 6-methylpretetramid (79) was the isolated product.[30]

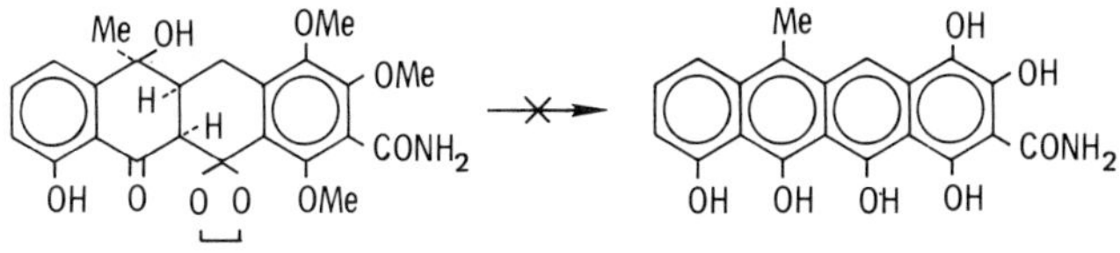

(80) (81)

An Indian group under Kulkarni has also been involved over an extended period of time in attempts to synthesize tetracyclines and related naphthacene analogs in which the A and D rings are aromatic.[34-40]

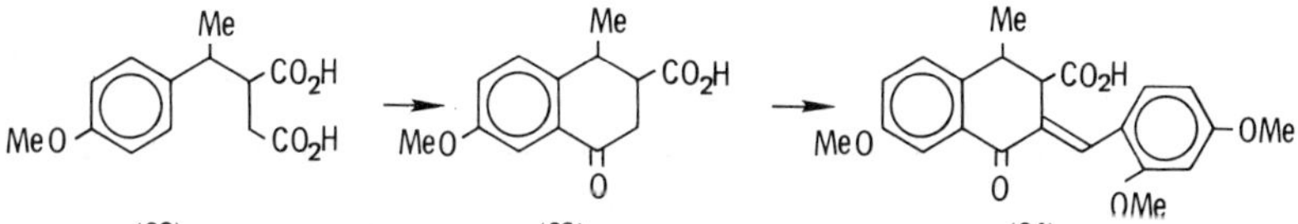

(82) (83) (84)

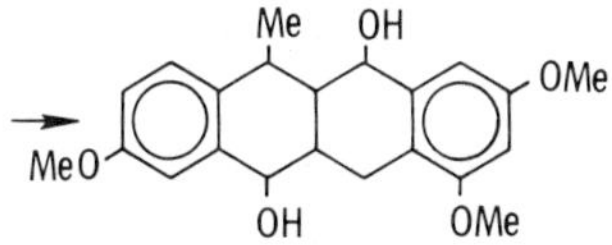

(85)

The approach of this group is illustrated by their recent synthesis of 1,3,9-trimethoxy-6-methyl-5,6a,6,11,11a,12-hexahydronaphthacene-5,11-diol (85).[34] Stobbe condensation of p-methoxyacetophenone and succinate led to a mixture of 3 major isomeric olefins all of whom could be converted to 82 on hydrogenation. Reaction with acetyl chloride produced the substituted succinic anhydride which cyclized to 83 on treatment with aluminum chloride. Base catalyzed condensation of 2,4-dimethoxybenzaldehyde led to 84 which was hydrogenated, cyclized with P_2O_5 and reduced with sodium borohydride to give the final product (85). Considerable elaboration of this route will be required before these model studies can produce bioactive tetracyclines.

8.3---Total synthesis of anhydrotetracyclines.

The anhydrotetracyclines are not clinically useful, nevertheless, they possess significant in vitro bioactivity which justifies interest in their synthesis.

A Russian team under the leadership of Akademician Shemyakin spent about ten years studying this problem and ultimately synthesized C_{12a}-deoxyanhydrotetracycline which they regarded as tautamount to a total synthesis of tetracycline itself.[41-53]

The ultimately successful route[44,51] starts with the benzyl ether of juglone (86) which undergoes a Diels-Alder reaction with 1-acetylbutadiene to give 87. It is of more than passing interest that Muxfeldt and his group found a very closely analogous reaction to proceed in the opposite regio sense.[62,64] Nevertheless, 87 was reported to undergo selective reduction to 88 which was converted to tertiary alcohol 89 by methyl magnesium iodide. The acetate ester was cleaved concomitantly. The remaining acetyl group was saponified

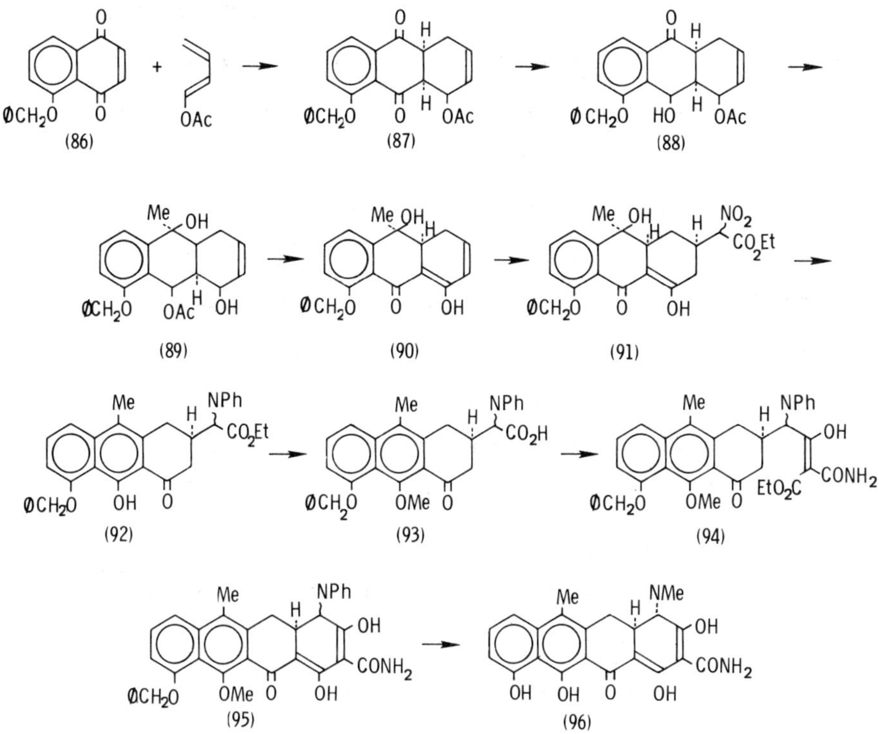

with KOH and then Jones oxidation and silica gel chromatography produced the enolized diketone 90. Michael addition of nitroacetic ester produced 91 in which the future C_4-NMe_2 group is foreshadowed. Treatment with hydrochloric acid aromatized the future C ring and zinc and HOAc reduced the nitro group to give the α-amino acid which was protected as the phthalimide (92) on reaction with N-carboethoxyphthalimide. The phenolic function was converted to the methyl ether with methyl iodide and silver oxide and then the ethyl ester was saponified to give acid 93. Conversion to the acid chloride with phosphorous pentachloride was followed by treatment with the magnesium salt of β-carboxamidoethyl acetate to give β-tricarbonyl 94. Dimsyl sodium treatment led to closure of ring A to give tetracyclic 95. The sequence concluded with hydrobromic-acetic acid removal of the blocking agents and alkylation of the liberated primary amine with methyliodide to give 96. Compound 96 was said to be identical to the degradation product of the same formula prepared from TC. If one allows the precedented reconstruction of ring C and C_{12a} hydroxylation, this would constitute a total synthesis of both anhydrotetracycline and TC. The last step, rehydration of ring C, only goes well, however, when C_7 is chlorinated or other highly lipophilic functions are present in the molecule.

More recently, Muxfeldt reported an alternate synthesis of anhydrochlortetracycline.[54] This synthesis starts with racemic nitrile 97[55] which is reduced to the aldehyde with diisobutylaluminum hydride followed by careful acid treatment. Condensation with hippuric acid, lead acetate and acetic anhydride leads to oxazolidone 98. Reaction with 99 (formed from 3-ketoglutaric acid monomethyl ester and t-butylamine in boiling dioxane and tosic acid) catalyzed by one equivalent of sodium hydride led to formation of 100 in which much of ring A is present. Further treatment with sodium hydride closed ring B to give the mixture of C_4 and C_{4a} epimers (101). These could be resolved by chromatography and crystallization. The uv spectra of the two pairs of C_{4a} epimers differed

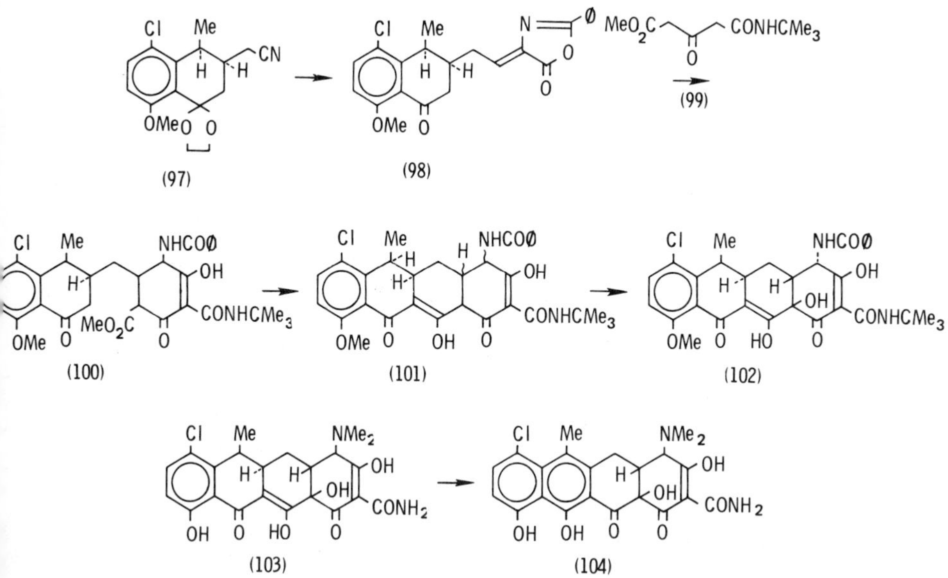

dramatically allowing ready differentiation. The $C_4\alpha$-NMe_2, $C_{4a}\beta$-analog was cis-hydroxylated at C_{12a} by careful treatment with oxygen in DMF-triethyl-phosphite and t-BuOK to give 102 in good yield. The C_4-benzamide function was cleaved by alkylation to the iminoethyl ether with Meerwein's reagent and converted to the primary amine with dilute HCl, but the yield was poor so special conditions were developed whereby proton free solvolysis could be performed (1,8-bis-dimethylaminonaphthalene and anhydrous methanol). Reductive methylation with Huenig's base (diisopropyl-ethylamine), formaldehyde and sodium cyanoborohydride gave cleanly the tertiary amine. Heating in 48% HBr removed the protecting groups to give 103. Treatment of 103 with dicyanodichlorobenzoquinone in dioxane led to aromatization of ring C and production of anhydrochlortetracycline (104 --

illustrated as the enantiomer). With the work of Scott and Bedford,[11] this constitutes a formal total synthesis of CTC also.

8.4---Total synthesis of 6-demethyl-6-deoxytetracycline.

The first successful total synthesis of a major bioactive tetracycline was that of Woodward and a Pfizer group.[56-58] This synthesis proceeded in a linear fashion from ring D adding each ring in turn until A was finished. Base catalyzed condensation of methyl 3-methoxybenzoate (105) with methyl succinate led to active ester 106. The same product (106) could be obtained by sequential base catalyzed condensation of 105 with ethyl acetate and this product with methyl chloroacetate. Michael condensation of 106 with methyl acrylate and Triton B gave triester 107. This product was also obtained from 105 by condensation with methyl glutarate followed by base catalyzed condensation with methyl bromoacetate. Next, the C ring was constructed. Acid hydrolysis of 107 resulted in loss of the tertiary ester group as CO_2. The intermediate was esterified with diazomethane and then hydrogenolyzed with Pd-C, possibly *via* intervention of the δ-lactone. Saponification of the remaining ester group and chlorination in acetic acid led to 108. Freidel-Crafts cyclization

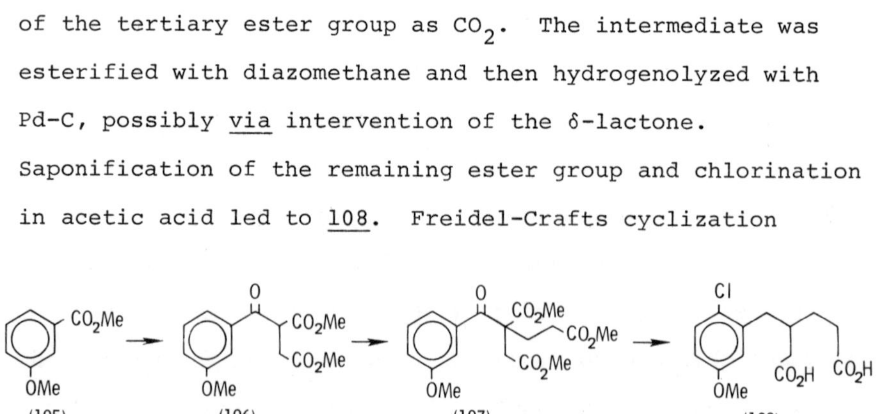

(105) (106) (107) (108)

with anhydrous HF followed by Fischer esterification produced bicyclic 109. Chlorination assured regioselectivity and 6-membered ring formation took precedence over 7. Although the carbonyl group had been removed from 107, it could in principle serve as a means of further elaborating ring C provided that it did not lead to fragmentation reactions in subsequent steps. The oxalate insertion reaction utilizing ethyl oxalate and base to give 110 required much experimentation to achieve.

Hydrolysis with hot aqueous acid removed the superfluous carbomethoxy group of 110 and the resulting trione was condensed with *n*-butyl glyoxylate using magnesium methoxide to give 111. Michael addition under carefully controlled conditions led to placement of the needed NMe_2 function for the future ring A. Borohydride reduction to 112 was needed to stabilize the product as otherwise a

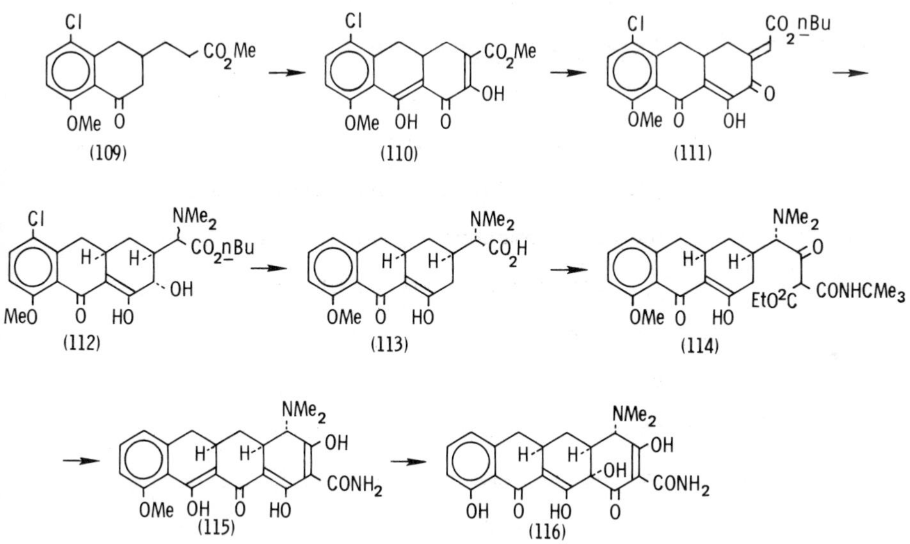

reverse Michael reaction back to 111 occurred on attempted isolation.

Removal of activating and protecting groups was accomplished by tosic acid treatment which lactonized the 12_aOH group with the C_{4a}-amino acid moiety with concomitant expulsion of the n-butyl group. Zinc and acid reductively removed the C_{12a} oxygen and hydrogenolysis led to α-aminoacid 113. Unfortunately, the n-butyl ester could not be cleaved by more direct methods so its removal required concomitant loss of the future C_{12a}OH which, then, had to be reintroduced later. Acid 113 was activated as the mixed anhydride for further condensation by treatment with isopropylchlorocarbonate and then reacted with ethyl N-t-butylmalonamate using magnesium ethoxide in acetonitrile to give 114. This product cyclized with NaH in DMF containing a trace of methanol. Heating with HBr cleaved protecting groups to give 115. The C_{12a}-OH was introduced under carefully controlled conditions using cerous chloride in buffered DMF-methanol. Adjustment of the stereochemistry at C_4 was accomplished by forming the calcium chelate at pH 8.5. This led to 6-demethyl-6-deoxytetracycline (116). Adjustment of C_4 stereochemistry with chelating salts at elevated pH's had been worked out previously with a variety of tetracyclines and is discussed in Chapter 4.

This remarkable synthesis is characterized at several stages by the extreme care with which experimental conditions had to be devised and adhered to. Thus, it is not only a great intellectual feat, but also a first-rate experimental achievement. These factors do, however, at the same time diminish its applicability to commercial scale preparations of novel tetracyclines.

More recently the Muxfeldt group has completed its own total synthesis of 6-DM-6-DO by quite a different path.[59-63] One feature of special interest about this work is the facile attainment of the tetracyclic framework in relatively high yield and in few steps.

This synthesis proceeds from the bicyclic aldehyde elaborated previously (40) (although a new route involving several improvements was developed in this paper) and involves a novel application of the azlactone synthesis for reintroduction of the desired nitrogen in the A ring. Aldehyde 40 was subjected to the azlactone synthesis using hippuric acid and lead acetate and this was followed by careful acid treatment to give 117. Condensation with methyl N-t-butyl-3-oxoglutaramate (99) under careful base (NaH) catalyzed conditions led to establishment of rings A and B simultaneously (118). The C_4 epimers could be separated and the benzoyl group was removed *via* the Meerwein process followed by aqueous acetic acid. Hot HBr/HOAc cleaved the protecting groups to give 119. Reductive alkylation with formaldehyde, hydrogen, Pd-C and triethylamine gave the requisite C_4-NMe_2 group and removed the C_7Cl group. The C_{12a} OH group was introduced with Pt and oxygen to give 6-demethyl-6-deoxytetracycline (116).

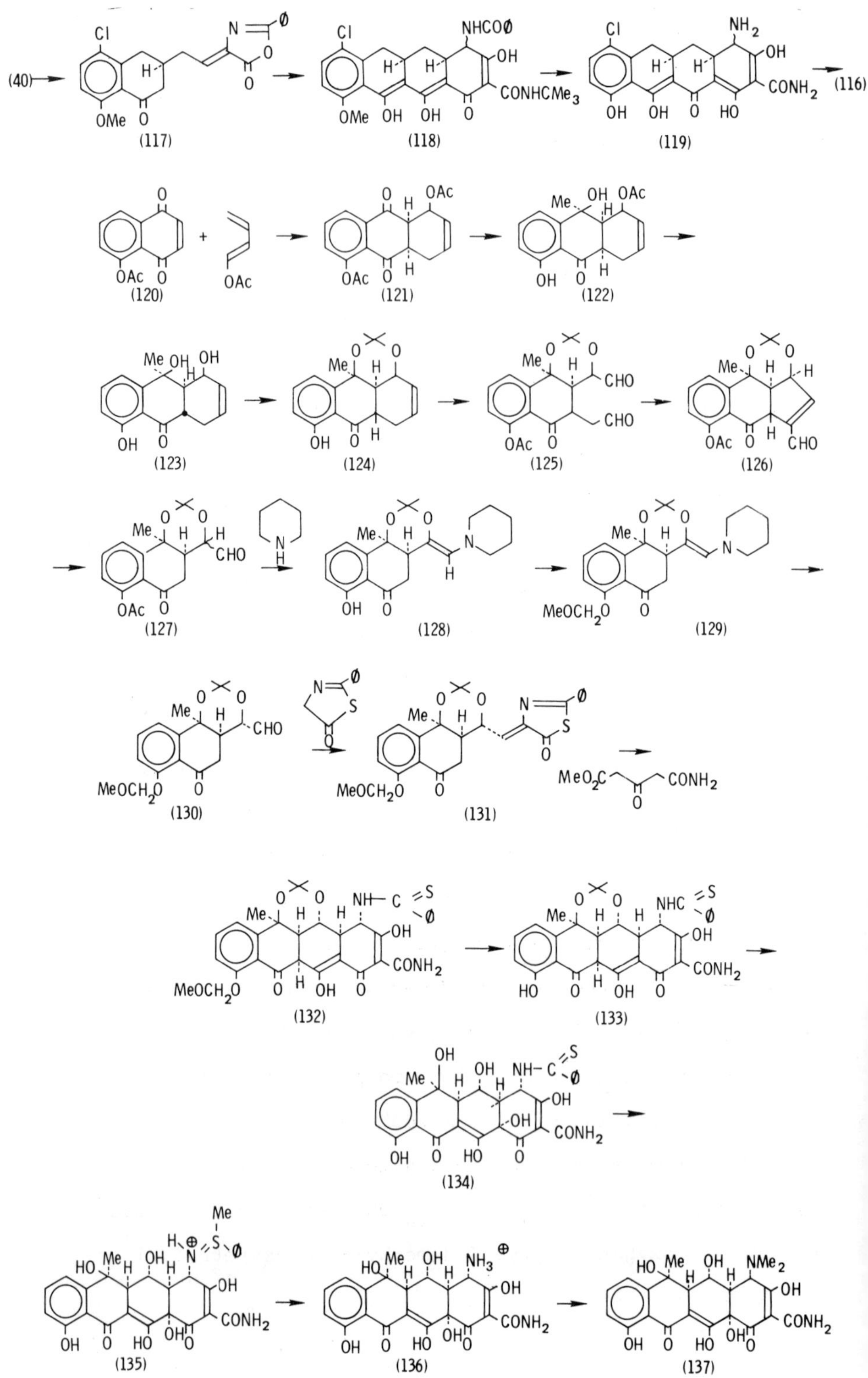

(40)
(117)
(118)
(119)
(116)
(120)
(121)
(122)
(123)
(124)
(125)
(126)
(127)
(128)
(129)
(130)
(131)
(132)
(133)
(134)
(135)
(136)
(137)
NHCOØ
CONHCMe3
CONH2
MeOCH2O
MeO2C

8.5---Total synthesis of oxytetracycline.

The Muxfeldt total synthesis of OTC is unquestionably the supreme synthetic achievement in this area to date.[64-66] The diabolical collection of acid and base sensitive functional groups and the presence of 6-contiguous asymmetric centers which characterize the OTC molecule presented obstacles which were finally overcome by the development of novel reactions and use of specially selected protecting groups.

In Muxfeldt's hands, Diels-Alder reaction of acetyljuglone (120) and 1-acetoxybutadiene went in the opposite regiosense as had Shemyakin's benzyljuglone (87 vs 121). Grignard reaction goes stereospecifically to 122 possibly by the intermediacy of an orthoester salt. The remaining acetyl group of 122 is saponified with concomitant isomerization of the ring juncture and the *peri*-1,3-diol system is protected as the acetonide (124). Acetylation and hydroxylation of the double bond with osmium tetroxide, catalyzed by potassium chlorate, leads to the glycol which is cleaved with periodate to give the dialdehyde 125. Tetraethylammonium acetate resulted in self condensation to give 126. Ozonolysis and bicarbonate treatment led to the isolation of diastereo-isomeric aldehydes 127. Piperidine and acid produced the identical enamine from each isomer and concurrently hydrolyzed the acetyl ester. The sodium phenolate was then reacted with chloromethylmethylether and this underwent selective hydrolysis when adsorbed on deactivated silica gel to give key intermediate 130. Thioamides are much easier to cleave than normal amides, so 130 was reacted with the sulfur analog of an oxazolidine (a thiazolone) in the presence of lead acetate to give thiazolidone 131. This latter was condensed with methyl 3-ketoglutaramate using a mixed base of t-BuOK and BuLi to close both rings A and B simultaneously and produce tetracyclic 132. Acetic acid treatment freed the C_{10}-phenolic OH and the C_{12a} α-OH was introduced by oxygen in a basic solution. Acid treatment removed the acetonide and 134 was isolated. Treatment with methyl iodide led to S-methylation (135) and the blocking group was easily solvolyzed with HCl to give 4-dedimethyloxytetracycline (136). Methylation using methyl iodide and Huenig's base produced dl-OTC (137). The product had half the biopotency of natural OTC.

This work represents the first total synthesis of a natural bioactive tetracycline.

8.6---Total synthesis of unnatural tetracyclines.

While much valuable and elegant synthetic chemistry resulted from these experiments, medicinal chemists have been additionally interested in the possibility of utilizing the technology developed in order to prepare novel tetracyclines that could not be made by either directed biosynthesis (Chapter 3) or partial chemical syntheses (Chapters 5 and 6). Recently, workers at Hoechst A.G. have begun to publish their work in this area.[67-69] The advantages of shortness and ease of purificatio

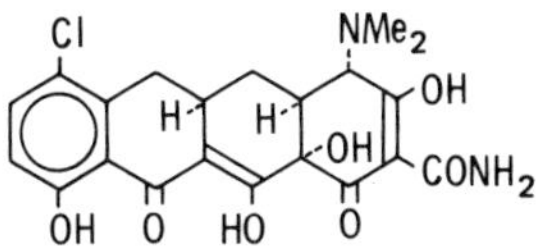
(138)

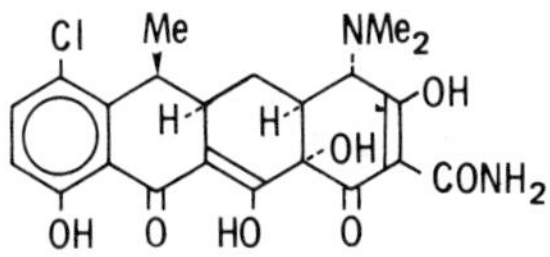
(139)

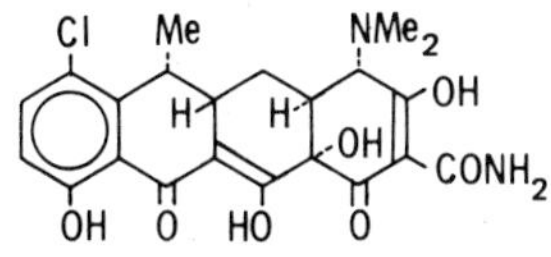
(140)

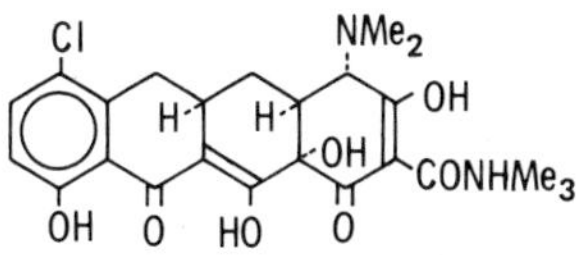
(141)

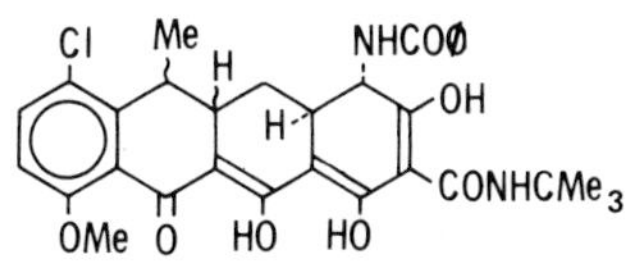
(142)

of intermediates without chromatography attracted this group to modifications of the Muxfeldt approach. Reaction of oxazolidone 117 or its pro 6β-methyl and pro 6α-methyl analogs with the appropriately N-substituted 3-oxoglutaramates and deblocking, etc., led to novel tetracyclines 138-141. Omission of N-methylation step leads to the corresponding C_4-NH_2 analogs of 138, 139, 140 and 141 as well. As had been noted by Esse in his tetracycloxide work, the primary amino analogs did not epimerize at C_4. These compounds were highly active *in vitro*, especially against TC resistant strains, an effect attributed to their enhanced lipophilicity compared to other tetracyclines. When serum was added to the culture media, *in vitro* potency decreased and animal protection tests were disappointing.

Nevertheless, one hopes that these initial disappointments do not prevent further exploration of this area and one awaits details of the completion of syntheses, such as that of 142, briefly recorded as under way.[67]

REFERENCES

1. G. C. Barrett, J. Pharm. Sci., 52, 309 (1963).
2. H. Muxfeldt, Angew. Chem., Intl. Ed., English, 1, 372 (1962).
3. H. Muxfeldt, Angew. Chem., 74, 443 (1962).
4. H. H. Inhoffen, H. Muxfeldt, H. Schaefer and H. Kraemer, Croat. Chem. Acta, 29, 329 (1957).
5. H. Muxfeldt, Mitt. Braunschweig. Wiss. Ges., 10, 1 (1958).
6. H. Muxfeldt and A. Kreutzer, Naturwiss., 46, 204 (1959).
7. H. Muxfeldt and A. Kreutzer, Chem. Ber., 94, 881 (1961).
8. H. Muxfeldt, Chem. Ber., 92, 3122 (1959).
9. H. Muxfeldt, G. Buhr and R. Bangert, Angew. Chem., 74, 213 (1962).
10. C. E. Holmlund, W. W. Andres and A. J. Shay, J. Am. Chem. Soc., 81, 4748 (1959).
11. A. I. Scott and C. Y. Bedford, J. Am. Chem. Soc., 84, 2271 (1962).
12. M. Schach von Wittenau, J. Org. Chem., 29, 2746 (1964).
13. J. H. Boothe, A. S. Kende, T. L. Fields and G. R. Wilkinson, J. Am. Chem. Soc., 81, 1006 (1969).
14. T. L. Fields, A. S. Kende and J. H. Boothe, J. Am. Chem. Soc., 83, 1250 (1960).
15. R. G. Wilkinson, T. L. Fields and J. H. Boothe, J. Org. Chem., 26, 637 (1961).
16. A. S. Kende, T. L. Fields, J. H. Boothe and S. Kushner, J. Am. Chem. Soc., 83, 439 (1961).

17. T. L. Fields, A. S. Kende and J. H. Boothe, *J. Am. Chem. Soc.*, *83*, 4612 (1961).

18. H. Muxfeldt, W. Rogalski and K. Striegler, *Angew. Chem.*, *72*, 170 (1960).

19. H. Muxfeldt, E. Jacobs and K. Uhlig, *Chem. Ber.*, *95*, 2901 (1962).

20. H. Muxfeldt, W. Rogalski and K. Striegler, *Chem. Ber.*, *95*, 2581 (1962).

21. D. H. R. Barton, *Chem. Brit.*, 301 (1970).

22. D. H. R. Barton, *Proc. Royal Soc.*, *A*, *319*, 145 (1970).

23. D. H. R. Barton and P. D. Magnus, *J. Chem. Soc.*, *C*, 2164 (1971).

24. D. H. R. Barton, B. Halpern, Q. N. Porter and D. J. Collins, *J. Chem. Soc.*, *C*, 2166 (1971).

25. E. Aufderhaar, J. E. Baldwin, D. H. R. Barton, D. J. Faulkner and M. Staytor, *J. Chem. Soc.*, *C.*, 2175 (1971).

26. J. E. Baldwin, D. H. R. Barton, N. J. A. Gutteridge and R. J. Martin, *J. Chem. Soc.*, *C*, 2184 (1971).

27. D. H. R. Barton, D. L. J. Clive, P. D. Magnus and G. Smith, *J. Chem. Soc.*, *C*, 2193 (1971).

28. D. H. R. Barton, L. Bould, D. L. J. Clive, P. D. Magnus and T. Hase, *J. Chem. Soc.*, *C*, 2204 (1971).

29. D. H. R. Barton, P. D. Magnus and T. Hase, *J. Chem. Soc.*, *C*, 2215 (1971).

30. D. H. R. Barton, P. D. Magnus and M. J. Pearson, *J. Chem. Soc.*, *C*, 2225 (1971).

31. D. H. R. Barton, P. D. Magnus and M. J. Pearson, *J. Chem. Soc.*, *C*, 2231 (1971).

32. D. H. R. Barton, J. A. Challis, P. D. Magnus and J. P. Marshall, J. Chem. Soc., C, 2241 (1971).

33. D. H. R. Barton, P. D. Magnus, G. Smith, G. Streckert and D. Zurr, J. Chem. Soc., Perkin I, 542 (1972).

34. B. D. Hosangadi and A. B. Kulkarni, Ind. J. Chem., 13, 218 (1975).

35. A. D. Mahajan and A. B. Kulkarni, Ind. J. Chem., 13, 1254 (1975).

36. B. R. Samant, B. D. Hosangadi and A. B. Kulkarni, Ind. J. Chem., 12, 916 (1974).

37. B. D. Hosangadi, N. S. Amonkar and A. B. Kulkarni, Ind. J. Chem., 7, 561 (1969).

38. A. L. Pandit and A. B. Kulkarni, Ind. J. Chem., 2, 327 (1964).

39. B. D. Hosangadi, A. L. Pandit and A. B. Kulkarni, Ind. J. Chem., 2, 235 (1964).

40. V. L. Barkshi and A. B. Kulkarni, Ind. J. Chem., 1, 215 (1963).

41. I. G. Bolesov, M. N. Kolosov and M. M. Shemyakin, Izv. Acad. Nauk SSSR, Ser. Khim., 1039 (1965).

42. M. N. Kolosov, V. V. Onoprienko and M. M. Shemyakin, Zh. Obshch. Khim., 35, 659 (1965).

43. A. I. Gurevich, M. G. Karapetjan, M. N. Kolosov, V. G. Korobko and M. M. Shemyakin, Zh. Obshch. Khim., 35, 668 (1965).

44. A. I. Gurevich, M. G. Karapetjan, M. N. Kolosov, V. G. Korobko, V. V. Onoprienko, S. A. Popravko and M. M. Shemyakin, Tet. Letts., 131 (1967).

45. A. I. Gurevich, M. N. Kolosov, V. G. Korobko and S. A. Popravko, Zh. Obshch. Khim., 38, 57 (1968).

46. M. N. Kolosov, S. A. Popravko and M. M. Shemyakin, Dokl. Akad. Nauk SSSR, 150, 1285 (1963).

47. I. G. Bolesov, M. N. Kolosov and M. M. Shemyakin, Tet. Letts., 1631 (1963).

48. M. N. Kolosov, S. A. Popravko and M. M. Shemyakin, Ann., 668, 86 (1963).

49. A. I. Gurevich, M. G. Karapetyan, M. N. Kolosov, V. G. Korobko, V. V. Onoprienko and M. M. Shemyakin, Tet. Letts., 877 (1964).

50. M. M. Shemyakin, M. N. Kolosov and A. I. Gurevich, Angew. Chem., 76, 791 (1964).

51. A. I. Gurevich, M. G. Karapetyan, M. N. Kolosov, V. G. Korobko, S. A. Popravko and M. M. Shemyakin, Dokl. Akad. Nauk. SSSR, 174, 358 (1967).

52. A. I. Gurevich, M. G. Karapetyan, M. N. Kolosov, V. G. Korobko, V. V. Onoprienko and S. A. Popravko, Zh. Obshch. Khim., 38, 50 (1968).

53. A. I. Gurevich, M. N. Kolosov and L. N. Nametkina, Zh. Obshch. Khim., 38, 1240 (1968).

54. H. Muxfeldt, H. Doepp, J. E. Kaufman, J. Schneider, P. E. Hansen, A. Sesaki and T. Geiser, Angew. Chem., 85, 508 (1973).

55. H. Muxfeldt, E. Jacobs and K. Uhlig, Chem. Ber., 95, 2901 (1962).

56. L. H. Conover, K. Butler, J. D. Johnson, J. J. Korst and R. B. Woodward, J. Am. Chem. Soc., 84, 3222 (1962).

57. R. B. Woodward, Pure and Appl. Chem., 6, 561 (1963).

58. J. J. Korst, J. D. Johnson, K. Butler, E. J. Bianco, L. H. Conover and R. B. Woodward, J. Am. Chem. Soc., 90, 439 (1968).

59. H. Muxfeldt and W. Rogalski, J. Am. Chem. Soc., 87, 933 (1965).

60. H. Muxfeldt, W. Rogalski, F. G. Kathawala, G. Grethe and J. Behling, Angew. Chem., 76, 791 (1964).

61. H. Muxfeldt, G. Grethe and W. Rogalski, J. Org. Chem., 31, 2429 (1966).

62. H. Muxfeldt, Antimicrob. Agts. Chemother., 977 (1965).

63. H. Muxfeldt, Angew. Chem., 74, 825 (1962).

64. H. Muxfeldt, G. Hardtmann, F. Kathawala, E. Vedejs and J. B. Mooberry, J. Am. Chem. Soc., 90, 6534 (1968).

65. H. Muxfeldt and G. Hardtmann, Ann., 669, 113 (1963).

66. H. Muxfeldt, J. Behling, G. Grethe and W. Rogalski, J. Am. Chem. Soc., 89, 4991 (1967).

67. W. Martin, H. Hartung, H. Urbach and W. Duerckheimer, Tet. Letts., 3512 (1973).

68. H. Urbach, H. Hartung, W. Martin and W. Duerckheimer, Tet. Letts., 4907 (1973).

69. W. Duerckheimer, Angew. Chem., Intnl. Ed., English, 14, 721 (1975).

CHAPTER 9

RELATED NATURAL PRODUCTS

9.1---Chelocardin (Cetotetrine).

Chelocardin (1) was isolated from fermentations of *Nocardia sulphurea* and its general properties were described in 1962.[1,2] Its structure determination was reported in 1970[3,4] and some reactions in 1975.[5] Chelocardin is a broad-spectrum antibiotic differing substantially from most other tetracyclines in being more active against Gram-negative than Gram-positive organisms (Table 9-1). Chelocardin protected mice against experimentally induced *E. coli* and *Proteus* infections at intermuscular doses ranging from 2 to 20 mg/Kg, even against TC resistant strains. The LD_{50} was found to be 88 mg/Kg i.v., 140 i.p. and 2500 orally. Against *Staphylococcus aureus* infections from 5 to 100 mg/Kg i.m. were required to achieve a cure. The drug is bacteriostatic and cross resistance to TC resistant strains was seen with Gram-negative, but not Gram-positive organisms. Subsequently, a report appeared that the drug caused drug-induced intrahepatic cholestasis in rhesus monkeys[6] and a brief report that chelocardin is efficaceous orally and subcutaneously in mice with acute experimental ascending pyelonephritis infections caused by *E. coli*, *P. mirabilis*, *P. vulgaris* and *Ps.*

Table 9-1. *In vitro* antimicrobial spectrum of chelocardin (cetotetrine).[1,2]

Culture	m.i.c.*
A. aerogenes	6.1 mcg/ml
B. subtilis	12.3
C. albicans	>256
Cl. perfringens	9.0
D. pneumoniae	12.3
E. coli ATCC 6880	1.5
Kl. pneumoniae	0.6
M. tuberculosis	>100
P. multocida	0.07
Pr. mirabilis	1.5
Pr. morganii	1.5
Pr. rettgeri	1.5
Pr. vulgaris ATCC 6897	0.77
Ps. aeruginosa	49
N. catarrhalis	0.38
S. typhimurium	1.5
S. lutea	0.77
Sh. sonnei	1.5
S. aureus 209P	6.1
S. faecalis	6.1
S. pyogenes	1.5

*24 hr.

aeruginosa.[7] Extensive *in vitro* studies on chelocardin (renamed cetotetrin) against 1300 clinical strains confirmed potency at 3.1 mcg/ml against most Enterobacteriaceae and Haemophilis strains and at 0.2 mcg/ml or less for Neisseria. Pseudomonas was less responsive. Cetotetrine retained potency against a majority of TC-resistant strains, however, when TC was tested concomitantly, it antagonized the potency of cetotetrine.[8]

Structure 1 contains several chemical features unusual among the clinically useful tetracyclines, but which can be accommodated readily within biogenetic hypothesis. The drug has a C_2COCH_3 group, a feature which usually decreases bioactivity, it has a C_4-βNH_2 group, which one expects to decrease bioactivity when compared to precedent tetracyclines, and belongs to the anhydrotetracycline family of which no member has found clinical use. The C_9-methyl group has not been encountered previously, although more examples are given in this chapter, so its presence could not be evaluated based on prior experience with major tetracyclines. On balance, one would probably have anticipated low activity so the relatively high potency of chelocardin against Gram-negative pathogens is seemingly anomalous.

The molecular formula was established as $C_{22}H_{21}NO_7$ based upon high resolution electron impact mass spectrometry (M^+=411; M^+-H_2O=393.1273) and the uv spectrum [λ_{max}^{MeOH} 226, 276 and 437 nm (log ε 4.51, 4.70 and 3.91)] was typical of anhydrotetracyclines bearing a 2-acetyl-1,3-dione system in ring A. Confirmatory of this was the presence of an ir band at 1684 cm^{-1}. Confirmation of the general features of the structure were seen upon chemical ionization mass spectrometry whereupon, in addition to the intense protonated molecule ion (MH^+=412), only the two retro-Diels-Alder fragments (3 and 4) were present.[9] The single nitrogen atom was isolable as ammonia on strong alkaline treatment and was basic, because treatment with methyl iodide and Huenig's base led to dimethylchelocardin (2) or its quaternary analog. On standing chelocardin (1) and 2 both epimerized to $C_{4\alpha}$ analogs. Furthermore, acetic anhydride or carbobenzyloxychloride readily and selectively acylate the nitrogen so there is no real doubt about it being a basic primary amine and not a carboxamide. The majority of the carbon framework as well as the oxygens are encompassed in the anhydro-tetracycline formulation the uv spectrum requires. This

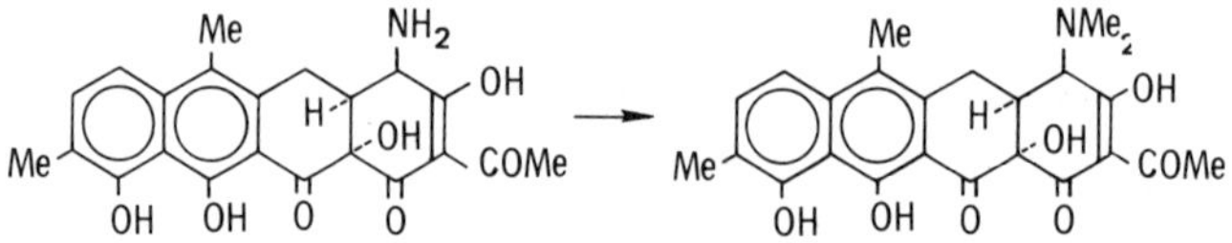

(1) (2)

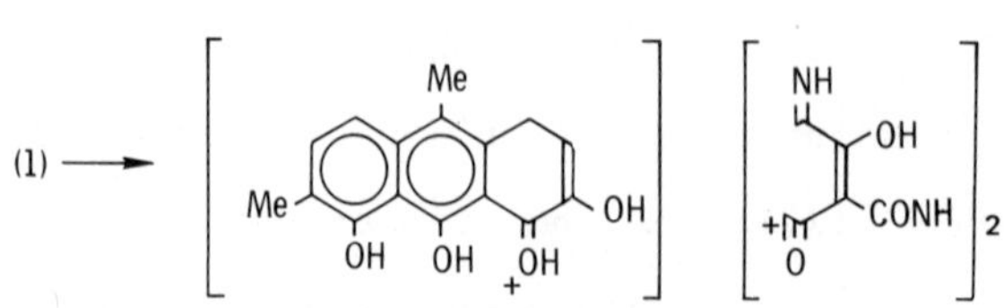

(3) (4)

found further support upon zinc dust distillation which gave anthracene and naphthacene derivatives.

The pmr spectrum was strongly supportive of the assigned structure. The N-acetate of 1 gave the best resolved spectra in acetone-d_6. Four methyl singlets were seen (2.10δ=NAc, 2.31=C_6Me, 2.34=C_9Me and 2.50=C_2COMe. H_4 was a one proton doublet (J=4.2Hz), H_{4a} a doublet of triplets ($J_{4,4a}$=4.2Hz; $J_{4a,5}$=12.3; $J_{4a,5'}$=4.4) at 3.08δ, H_5 a doublet of doubets ($J_{5,5}$=16.4H_z) at 2.72δ and $H_{5'}$ also a doublet of doublets at 3.53δ. The aromatic protons were particularly revealing, resonating at 7.32 and 7.50δ as mutually coupled doublets, J=8.5Hz, showing their ortho-relationship to one another. Furthermore, simultaneous irradiation of both aromatic Me resonances gave a strong nuclear Overhauser effect (H_7=16.5%; H_8=11.5%) showing that each hydrogen was adjacent to a Me group. This finding ruled out the alternate possibility, a 6,7-dimethyl structure.

The absolute configuration and solution conformation were established by circular dichroism and pmr shift measurements. The cd spectrum of chelocardin tracked reasonably closely that of 4-epianhydrotetracycline while that of 4-epichelocardin was a close match for anhydrotetracycline. In all known cases, H_4 of anhydrotetracyclines is more deshielded when its orientation is β as contrasted to α. This relationship also holds for chelocardin and 4-epi-chelocardin.

It is known that C_2-acetyl-1,3-cyclohexanediones hydrolyze in dilute acid to give acetic acid and the 1,3-dione. When chelocardin HCl was reacted in benzene with a large excess of ethylene glycol and tosic acid, a 1,3-bisdioxolane resulted which had lost the C_2-acetyl group by ir and pmr (5).[5] This was more readily visible with its N-carbobenzyloxy derivative 6. Hydrolysis of 5 in HCl/Me_2CO gave C_2-desacetylchelocardin itself. The formation of 5 requires the presence of a free amino group and a 1,2-glycol. Some mechanistic speculations have been made encompassing the fact that 2-acetyldimedone itself does not undergo this reaction.

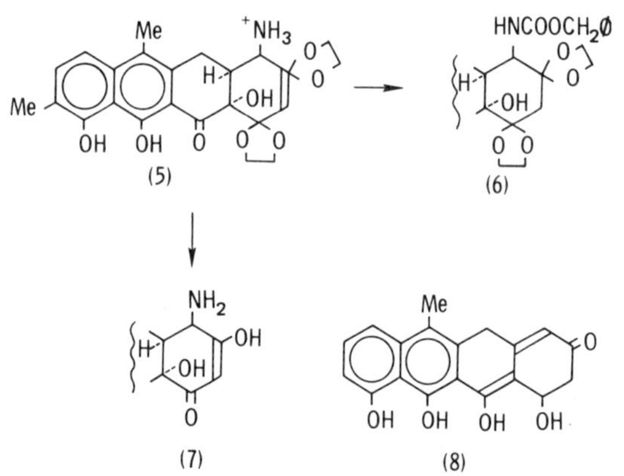

Unfortunately, all attempts to acylate or alkylate the now free C_2 position in 7 led to O-alkylated/acylated products. No biological properties were presented for these compounds.

9.2---X-340.

Antibiotic X-340 was isolated from an unidentified Streptomycete sp. in 1957[10] and formulated as 8 based upon a variety of spectroscopic and simple chemical properties.[11]

The molecule solvated readily but a molecular formula of $C_{19}H_{16}O_5$ was settled upon. The compound formed a monoacetate at room termperature and a triacetate at reflux. Likewise, a monomethyl ether formed with diazomethane and a trimethyl ether with dimethylsulfate. The compound produced naphthacene on zinc dust distillation accounting for almost all of the carbons. Kuhn-Roth oxidation gave only acetic acid showing the presence of a C-Me group. The absence of any ir absorption above 1660 cm^{-1} ruled out a C_2-acetyl function like that of chelocardin. Oxidation with H_2O_2 did not produce a naphthacenequinone and reductive acetylation did not produce a pentaacetate. The uv spectrum ($\lambda^{max}_{EtOH_2}$ + 269, 292, 321, 340, 370 nm log ε 438, 4.32, 4.14, 4.14 and 4.06) is not consistent with formula <u>8</u> but would fit more closely an acetylindanone instead. Perihydroxy groups are present as boric acid increases the pKa from 7.66 to about 10. The stability of X-340 to acid and relately to base makes a β-hydroxy ketone formulation such as that assigned (<u>8</u>) unlikely. However, in the absence of more structural information proposal of alternate formulae would seem to serve no useful purpose.

The *in vitro* antimicrobial spectrum of X-340 is given in Table 9-2 from which it is evident that the drug has greater activity against Gram-positive than Gram-negative bacteria.

Table 9-2. *In vitro* antimicrobial spectrum of X-340.[9]

Culture	m.i.c.
S. aureus	0.1 -2.5 mcg/ml
B. subtilis	0.03-0.14
Str. faecalis	1.25
Str. viridans	5.0
C. diptheriae	0.01
Ps. pseudocyaneus	5.0
E. coli	125
Sh. shigae	125
S. typhosa	125
V. cholorae	170
M. tuberculosis	inactive
C. albicans	125

9.3---Chromocyclomycin and chromocycline.

In a study of aureolic acid from fermentations of *Streptomyces* LA-7017, a companion metabolite possessing little biological activity was isolated.[12] The structure of this metabolite, chromocyclomycin (9) and its aglycone (10) were subsequently determined.[13,14] The relationship to anhydrotetracyclines this reveals leads to inclusion in this section.

Complete acetic acid hydrolysis liberates chromocycline (10), whose structure interests us here, and D-olivose, D-oliose and two molecules of D-mycarose. Proof of their arrangement, as depicted in 9, is beyond the scope of this summary.[12] In the pmr spectrum of chromocycline the aromatic hydrogens are singlets at 6.71 and 6.67δ and the aromatic C-Me group occurs at 2.15δ. Three

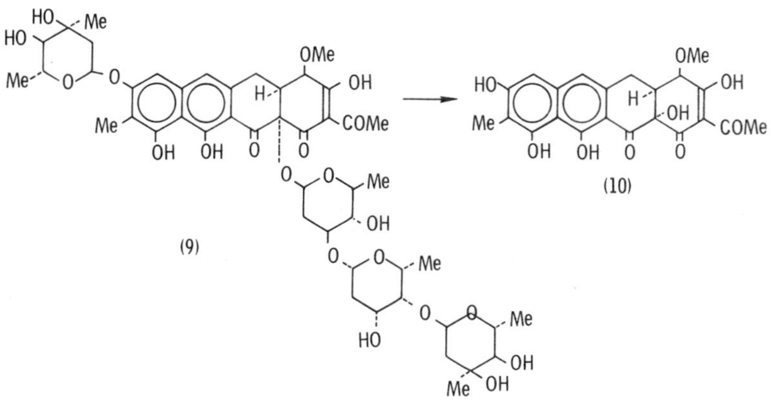

(9)

(10)

phenolic OH groups resonate at 9.20, 9.75 and 15.48δ (C_8OH, $C_{10}OH$ and $C_{11}OH$). The pKa=6.6 and is approximately the same as that of chromomycinone (11) a product of similar structure isolated from degradation of aureolic acid. The molecular weight was clear from mass spectrometry (M^+=428) and the base peak (m/e 272) is surely the retro-Diels-Alder fragment (12) by analogy with anhydrotetracyclines. Subtraction of the uv spectra of 11 from that of 10 left the 2-acetyldimedone maxima at 250 and 300 nm. This was confirmed by the presence of a 3-proton singlet at 2.51δ and the liberation of a molecule of acetic acid on dilute sulfuric acid hydrolysis. It is interesting, however, that 10 does not have the confirmatory carbonyl absorption above 1680 cm^{-1} that other acetyl tetracyclines possess. The pmr also

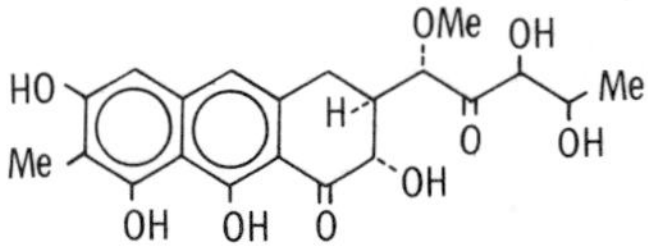

(11)

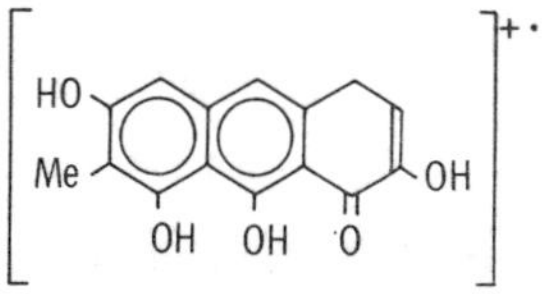

(12)

shows an $OC\underline{H}_3$ band at 3.48δ and, from the uv and mass spectra, this must be placed in ring A. Reduction of 10 with zinc and acetic acid leads to loss of the $C_{12a}OH$ and the uv shift associated with this (420 → 476 nm). On these and biogenetic grounds as well as comparison with the chemical properties of 11, structure 10 was proposed for chromocycline.

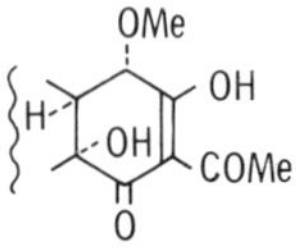

(13)

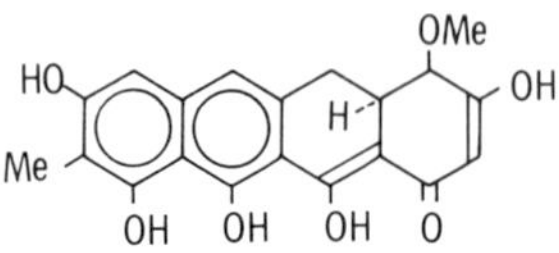

(14)

On standing in pyridine chromocycline (pmr H_4=5.05δ, J=4Hz) (10) underwent a reversible epimerization to C_4 epi chromocycline (pmr H_4=4.27δ, J=12Hz). Thus in 13, H_4 and H_{4a} must be *trans*-diaxial and 10 must be *cis*. The relative chemical shifts are also as expected for the analogous anhydrotetracycline epimers. Furthermore, in chromocycline $C_{8,10,12a}$-triacetate, the pmr shift of H_{4a} undergoes a substantial paramagnetic shift (Δ^{δ}0.75) so the $C_{12a}OH$ must be *cis* to $C_{4a}H$. The absolute configuration was established by the method of molecular rotation differences on C_4 epimerization ($\Delta[M]_D$ = + 2300°) in comparison with the epimerization of 4-epi-anhydro-tetracycline to anhydrotetracyline ($\Delta[M]_D$ = + 2340°). These considerations were confirmed by a nine-step chemical conversion of chromomycinone (11) to a degradation product (14) of chromocycline (10).

The structure that these studies revealed is a very interesting one in a comparative sense. Chromocycline possesses some precedented features -- for example, the anhydrotetracycline ring system, the C_2-acetyl group and the C_9-Me group all find analogies in other molecules, particularly with cetotetrine. On the other hand, the $C_{4\beta}$-OMe group is unique as is the C_8-OH group. In this regard, it is interesting to note that chromomycinone and chromocycline have only weak antibacterial potency against *B. subtilis*.[15]

9.4---Pillaromycin and pillaromycinone.

The antitumor antibiotic pillaromycin (15) is isolated from fermentations of *Streptomyces flavovirens* and shows mainly antitumor activity.[21,22] Detailed chemical analysis[16-22] showed a tetracycline-like structure for pillaromycin (15) and its aglycone, pillaromycinone (16). The structure was arrived at primarily *via* degradative and spectroscopic means and then confirmed in its essential details by an X-ray study. The latter also, interestingly, demonstrated *via* the anomalous dispersion technique that pillaromycin belongs to the enantiomeric series as compared to tetracyclines.

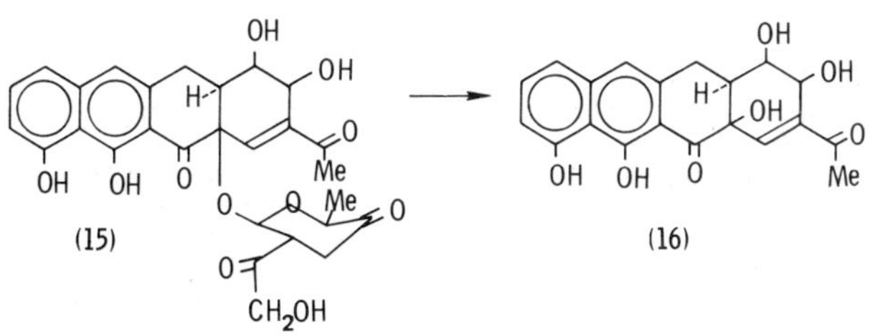

Aside from the usual ir, uv and pmr evidences and the formation, for example, of a tetraacetate, in which two phenolic and two alcoholic OH groups were esterified and an OH group remained which could be esterified under more forcing conditions; particularly revealing experiments showed that the sugar, pillarose, was removed by hydrolysis without significant affect on the uv-visible chromophore, and the product, pillaromycinone, formed normal carbonyl derivatives and a mixture of anthracenes and naphthacenes on zinc-dust distillation. Oxidation of the dimethylether of 16 gave 3-methoxyphthalic acid and 3-methoxybenzene-1, 2,4,5-tetracarboxylic acid. The uv spectrum was closely similar to that of 2-acetylnaphthalene-1,8-diol and two of the aliphatic hydroxyls were cis, forming an acetonide which showed, i.a., $J_{3,4}$=4Hz, and $J_{4,4a}$=12Hz in the pmr. Catalytic hydrogenation in MeOH over Pd-C gave three products, pillaronone (18), whose structure as an internal ketal was determined by X-ray analysis of its monobromoacetyl ester and the less abundant β-substance (17) and a further reduction product having two more hydrogens and one less oxygen than 17.

Unfortunately, no information appears to be available relative to the antibacterial potency of pillaromycinone.

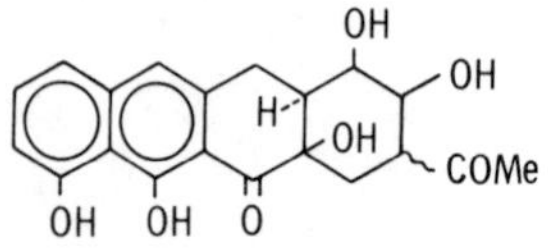

(17)

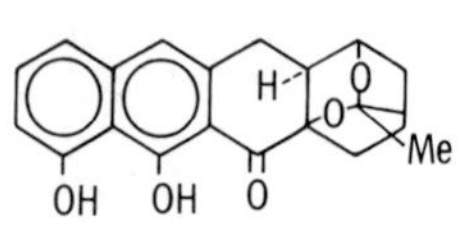

(18)

9.5---Viridicatumtoxin.

When some strains of *Penicillium viridicatum* are grown on maize meal, viridicatumtoxin, a fungal toxin, is formed.[23] The single crystal X-ray structure analysis led to structure 19. The absolute configuration is represented as that of the tetracyclines, however, the X-ray study was concluded at the relative configurational level. Unusual features of this molecule are the oxygen atoms at C_{4a} and C_8 and the isoprenyl units attached to C_6 and C_7. There are no antimicrobial data available for viridicatumtoxin. It is least like the classical tetracyclines of all the members of this group.

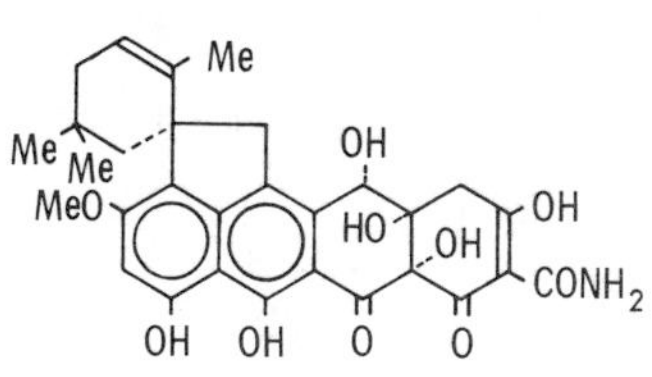

(19)

REFERENCES

1. T. J. Oliver, J. F. Prokop, R. R. Bower and R. H. Otto, *Antimicrob. Agts. Chemother.*, 583 (1962).
2. A. C. Sinclair, J. R. Schenck, G. G. Post, E. V. Cardinal, S. Burokas and H. H. Fricke, *Antimicrob. Agts. Chemother.*, 592 (1962).
3. L. A. Mitscher, J. V. Juvarkar, W. Rosenbrook, Jr., W. W. Andres, J. Schenck and R. S. Egan, *J. Am. Chem. Soc.*, 92, 6070 (1970).

4. L. A. Mitscher, W. Rosenbrook, Jr., W. W. Andres, R. S. Egan, J. Schenck and J. V. Juvarkar, Antimicrob. Agts. Chemother., 38 (1970).

5. D. T. W. Chu, D. L. Garmaise and E. Bernstein, Can. J. Chem., 53, 1434 (1975).

6. C. G. Biava and R. E. Creel, Abstr. 8th. Int. Congr. Int. Acad. Pathol., 110 (1970).

7. R. R. Bower, N. L. Shipkowitz and W. E. Grundy, Abstr. 16th Intersci. Conf. Antimicrob. Agts. Chemother., 428 (1976).

8. J. M. Stamm and R. L. Girolami, Abstr. 16th Intersci. Conf. Antimicrob. Agts. Chemother., 428 (1976).

9. L. A. Mitscher and R. Foltz, Unpublished experiments.

10. V. C. Vora, K. Shete and M. M. Dhar, J. Sci. and Ind. Res., 16C, 182 (1957).

11. V. C. Vora and M. M. Dhar, J. Sci and Ind. Res., 19B, 454 (1960).

12. Y. A. Berlin, M. N. Kolosov and I. V. Yartseva, Khimiya Prirodnykh Soedinenii, 539 (1973).

13. Y. A. Berlin, M. N. Kolosov and I. V. Severtsova, Khimiya Prirodnykh Soedinenii, 524 (1973).

14. Y. A. Berlin, M. N. Kolosov and I. V. Severtsova, Khimiya Prirodnykh Soedinenii, 532 (1973).

15. O. A. Kiseleva, N. G. Volkova, E. A. Stukacheva, M. F. Shemyakin, Y. A. Berlin and M. N. Kolosov, Mol. Biol. (Moscow), 7, 900 (1973).

16. M. Asai, Chem. Pharm. Bull., 18, 1699 (1970).

17. M. Asai, Chem. Pharm. Bull., 18, 1706 (1970).

18. M. Asai, Chem. Pharm. Bull., 18, 1713 (1970).

19. M. Asai, E. Mizuta, K. Mizuno, A. Miyake and S. Tatsuoka, Chem. Pharm. Bull., 18, 1720 (1970).

20. K. Kamiya, M. Asai, M. Nishikawa, K. Mizuno, Y. Tomiie and I. Nitta, Chem. and Pharm. Bull., 18, 1724 (1970).

21. K. Mizuno, J. Antibiotics, 16A, 22 (1963).

22. M. Shibata, M. Asai, K. Mizuno, A. Miyake and S. Tatsuoka, Proc. Japan. Acad., 40, 296 (1964).

23. C. Kabuto, J. V. Silverton, T. Akiyama, U. Sankawa, R. D. Hutchison, P. S. Steyh and R. Vleggaar, Chem. Commun., 728 (1976).

APPENDIX

UNITED STATES PATENTS DEALING WITH THE TETRACYCLINES

2,482,055 (1949). Aureomycin and Preparation of Same. B. M. Duggar (American Cyanamid)

2,516,080 (1950). Terramycin and Its Production. B. A. Sobin, A. C. Finlay and J. H. Kane (Pfizer)

2,586,766 (1952). Purifying Aureomycin by Chromatographic Adsorption. C. Pidacks and E. E. Starbird (American Cyanamid)

2,609,329 (1952). Process for Producing Aureomycin. J. G. Niedercorn (American Cyanamid)

2,649,480 (1953). Recovery of Oxytetracycline. P. P. Regna, R. A. Carboni and A. E. Timreck (Pfizer)

2,655,535 (1953). Recovery of Chlortetracycline. C. Pidacks and E. E. Starbird (American Cyanamid)

2,658,077 (1953). Crystallization of Chlortetracycline. E. R. Harms (American Cyanamid)

2,671,806 (1954). Purification of Chlortetracycline. R. Winterbottom, P. Eichler and C. Pidacks (American Cyanamid)

2,699,054 (1955). Tetracycline. L. H. Conover (Pfizer)

2,709,672 (1955). Production of Chlortetracycline. M. A. Petty, Jr. (American Cyanamid)

2,712,517 (1955). Production of Tetracycline and Substituted Tetracyclines. A. Gourevitch and J. Lein (Bristol)

2,731,497 (1956). Production of Tetracycline. J. R. D. McCormick and N. K. Smith (American Cyanamid)

2,734,018 (1956). Process for the Preparation of Tetracycline and Chlortetracycline. P. Minieri and H. Sokol (American Cyanamid)

2,739,924 (1956). Production of Tetracycline. J. Lein and A. Gourevitch (Bristol)

2,740,816 (1956). Extraction of Aureomycin. E. E. Starbird and C. Pidacks (American Cyanamid)

2,744,931 (1956). Anhydrochlortetracycline. Robert Broschard and G. Krupka (American Cyanamid)

2,744,932 (1956). Anhydrotetracycline. C. W. Waller and A. A. Goldman (American Cyanamid)

2,763,591 (1956). Tetracycline Production Using Cottonseed Endosperm Flour. A. B. Hatch and G. A. Hunt (Bristol)

2,763,681 (1956). Chlortetracycline, Purification and Alkaline Earth Salts. E. E. Starbird and C. Pidacks (American Cyanamid)

2,776,243 (1957). Process for the Production of Tetracycline and Chlortetracycline. W. J. McGhee and J. C. Megna (Bristol)

2,804,476 (1957). Process for Separating Tetracycline and Chlortetracycline. V. V. Bogert and C. J. Walsh (Pfizer)

2,847,471 (1958). Method for Purifying Tetracycline. J. Vandeputte and L. J. Heuser (Olin Mathieson)

2,866,738 (1958). Deionized Corn Steep Liquor in Production of Tetracycline. P. P. Minieri and M. C. Firman (American Cyanamid)

2,867,661 (1959). Non-hygroscopic Antibiotic Salt. J. S. Buckley, Jr. and C. R. Stephens, Jr. (Pfizer)

2,871,166 (1959). Fermentation of Oxytetracycline by Streptomyces Rimosus. J. J. Goodman (American Cyanamid)

2,871,167 (1959). Chlortetracycline Fermentation. S. A. Szumski (American Cyanamid)

2,871,264 (1959). Tetracycline Extractions. P. P. Minieri and W. M. Ziegler (American Cyanamid)

2,873,276 (1959). Antibiotic Purification and Complex Compounds. E. W. Blase (Pfizer)

2,875,247 (1959). Refining of Tetracycline Antibiotics by Direct Mash Extraction. S. M. Fox, M. S. Blicharz and R. Winterbottom (American Cyanamid)

2,878,289 (1959). 6-Demethyltetracyclines and Methods for Preparing the Same. J. R. D. McCormick, U. Hirsch, E. R. Jensen and N. O. Sjolander (American Cyanamid)

2,886,595 (1959). Tetracycline Recovery. B. Heinemann and I. R. Hooper (Bristol)

2,897,234 (1959). Antibiotic Purification. B. Heinemann and I. R. Hooper (Bristol)

2,905,714 (1959). Recrystallization of Tetracycline. H. Mendelsohn (American Cyanamid)

2,922,817 (1960). 12a-Deoxyanhydrotetracyclines. A. Green (American Cyanamid)

2,923,667 (1960). Chlorination Inhibitors in Chlortetracycline-Tetracycline Fermentations. J. J. Goodman and R. W. Young (American Cyanamid)

2,923,668 (1960). Chlorination Inhibitors in Chlortetracycline-Tetracycline Fermentations. J. J. Goodman and R. W. Young (American Cyanamid)

2,929,837 (1960). Method of Purifying Tetracycline. H. Ogawa and S. Inoue (American Cyanamid)

2,938,052 (1960). Recovery of Tetracycline. T. Yamada (American Cyanamid)

2,940,905 (1960). Tetracycline Process. F. W. Tanner (Pfizer)

2,940,906 (1960). Tetracycline Process. F. W. Tanner (Pfizer)

2,940,907 (1960). Tetracycline Process. F. W. Tanner (Pfizer)

2,940,908 (1960). Tetracycline Process. F. W. Tanner (Pfizer)

2,940,909 (1960). Tetracycline Process. F. W. Tanner (Pfizer)

2,949,406 (1960). Method for Preparing Tetracycline II. M. Arishima and Y. Sekizawa (American Cyanamid)

2,949,407 (1960). Method for Preparing Tetracycline III. M. Arishima and Y. Sekizawa (American Cyanamid)

2,952,587 (1960). Biological Transformation of Anhydro-Tetracyclines to 5a(11a)-Dehydrotetracyclines P. A. Miller and J. R. D. McCormick (American Cyanamid)

2,956,930 (1960). Antibiotic Production. L. C. Cheney and J. Lein (Bristol)

2,965,546 (1960). Biological Conversion of 5a(11a)-Dehydro-tetracyclines to Broad-Spectrum Antibiotics. J. R. D. McCormick, N. O. Sjolander and U. Hirsch (American Cyanamid)

2,970,087 (1961). Hydroxylating 12a-Deoxytetracycline with Ascomyceteae. D. Beck and G. M. Shull (Pfizer)

2,970,946 (1961). Process for the Production of Tetracycline by Fermentation. B. Chertow (Bristol)

2,970,947 (1961). Process of Producing an Antibiotic of the Tetracycline Series. J. R. D. McCormick, N. H. Arnold, U. Hirsch, P. A. Miller and N. O. Sjolander (American Cyanamid)

2,971,007 (1961). N-(9-Xanthyl) Tetracyclines. L. C. Cheney and W. J. Gottstein (Bristol)

2,972,630 (1961). Tetracycline for the Derivative and Process for Preparation. L. H. Conover and C. R. Stephens, Jr. (Pfizer)

2,976,318 (1961). Tetracycline Derivatives and Process of Producing the Same. R. K. Blackwood (Pfizer)

2,984,686 (1961). 6-Deoxy-6-Demethyl-6-Methylene-5-Oxytetracyclines. R. K. Blackwood, H. H. Rennhard, J. J. Beereboom and C. R. Stephens, Jr. (Pfizer)

2,987,449 (1961). Enhancement of 7-Chlorotetracycline Production. P. A. Miller, J. J. Goodman, N. O. Sjolander and J. R. D. McCormick (American Cyanamid)

2,997,471 (1961). Tetracycline Derivatives. L. C. Cheney and W. J. Gottstein (Bristol)

2,998,352 (1961). Production of Tetracyclines. J. R. D. McCormick, N. O. Sjolander and U. Hirsch (American Cyanamid)

2,999,111 (1961). Recovery of 6-Deoxy-6-Demethyl-Tetracycline. C. R. Stephens, Jr. (Pfizer)

3,002,021 (1961). New Derivatives of the Tetracycline-Type Antibiotics. H. H. Rennhard, L. H. Conover, P. N. Gordon and C. R. Stephens, Jr. (Pfizer)

3,005,023 (1961). Production of Tetracycline. P. A. Miller (American Cyanamid)

3,005,025 (1961). Preparation of Neutral Chlortetracycline. J. R. D. McCormick and N. T. K. Smith (American Cyanamid)

3,007,965 (1961). New Tetracyclines Produced by Streptomyces Aureofaciens. J. A. Growich and P. A. Miller (American Cyanamid)

3,009,956 (1961). 4-Epitetracycline Antibiotic Transformation Process. M. M. Noseworthy (Pfizer)

3,012,946 (1961). Production of 7-Chloro-6-Demethyl-Tetracycline. S. A. Szumski (American Cyanamid)

3,013,074 (1961). Tetracycline Purification Process. J. A. Kardys (Pfizer)

3,013,075 (1961). Bromoanhydro-12a-Bromo-12a-Deoxydedimethylaminotetracycline. J. H. Boothe and A. Green (American Cyanamid)

3,019,172 (1962). Production of 7-Chloro-6-Demethyl-Tetracycline. J. J. Goodman and M. Matrishin (American Cyanamid)

3,019,173 (1962). Method for Preparing Tetracycline. M. Arishima and Y. Sekizawa (American Cyanamid)

3,019,260 (1962). Process for the Catalytic Reduction of 6-Hydroxy Hydronaphthacenes. J. R. D. McCormick and E. R. Jensen (American Cyanamid)

3,023,148 (1962). Production of 5-Hydroxytetracycline. P. A. Miller and J. R. D. McCormick (American Cyanamid)

3,023,239 (1962). Recrystallization of Demethylchlortetracycline.

V. E. Origoni and R. Winterbottom (American Cyanamid)

3,026,354 (1962). Process for Preparing 6-Methylene-5-Oxytetracycline. R. K. Blackwood (Pfizer)

3,028,311 (1962). Process for Preparing 6-Demethyltetracyclines. D. Perlman and L. J. Heuser (Mathieson)

3,028,409 (1962). 2-Carboxamido-N-(Alkyl)-Substituted Anhydrotetracycline Compounds. C. R. Stephens, Jr. (Pfizer)

3,029,284 (1962). N-Dealkylation of Carboxamido-N-Alkyl-Tetracycline and Its Analogs. P. N. Gordon (Pfizer)

3,030,377 (1962). Process for the Manufacture of Nitriles of Tetracyclines. A. Soder and W. Siedel (Hoechst)

3,036,129 (1962). Preparation of 7-Halo-6-Deoxytetracyclines. J. J. Hlavka and J. H. Boothe (American Cyanamid)

3,037,916 (1962). Fermentation of Tetracycline. J. J. Goodman (American Cyanamid)

3,037,917 (1962). Method of Producing Tetracycline. K. Culik, M. Herold, J. Palkoska, E. Belik and J. Dasek (Spofa)

3,037,973 (1962). Tetracycline Recovery Process. G. Sarcona and J. A. Kardys (Pfizer)

3,042,716 (1962). Mannich Bases of Tetracycline Compounds and Amino Acids. R. K. Blackwood and K. J. Brunings (Pfizer)

3,043,875 (1962). Halogenated Tetracycline Derivatives and Processes for Their Preparation. J. J. Beereboom, H. H. Rennhard and C. R. Stephens, Jr. (Pfizer)

3,043,876 (1962). 4a,12a-Anhydro-4-Desdimethylaminotetracyclin and Analogs Thereof. H. H. Rennhard, L. H. Conover, P. N. Gordon and C. R. Stephens, Jr. (Pfizer)

3,043,877 (1962). Process for the 12a-Hydroxylation of 12a-Deoxytetracyclines. C. E. Holmlund and W. W. Andres (American Cyanamid)

3,047,626 (1962). 4-Desdimethylamino-6-Deoxytetracycline Derivatives. C. R. Stephens, Jr. and L. H. Conover (Pfizer)

3,050,446 (1962). Fermentation of Chlortetracycline and Demethylchlorotetracycline. J. J. Goodman (American Cyanamid)

3,050,558 (1962). Refining of Demethylchlortetracycline. L. L. Smith, T. Foell, Jr. and H. Mendelsohn (American Cyanamid)

3,053,740 (1962). Biological Conversion of Anhydrotetracyclines to Tetracyclines. P. A. Miller and J. R. D. McCormick (American Cyanamid)

3,061,522 (1962). Process for the Production of Demethyltetracyclines. S. L. Neidlman (Mathieson)

3,069,467 (1962). Hydrolysis of 2-Decarboxamido-2-Cyano-6-Deoxy-Tetracycline Derivatives. J. J. Beereboom and K. Butler (Pfizer)

3,070,514 (1962). Process for the Manufacture of 6-Demethyltetracycline. A. Virgilio and C. Hengeller (Lepetit S. P. A.)

3,081,346 (1963). Novel 12a-(O-Formyl)Tetracyclines. C. R. Stephens, Jr. and R. K. Blackwood (Pfizer)

3,092,556 (1963). Tetracycline Fermentation. J. A. Growich, Jr. and N. Deduck (American Cyanamid)

3,092,635 (1963). Process for the Preparation of Crystallized Compounds of Pyrrolidino-Methyl-Tetracycline. W. Seidel, A. Soder and W. Scheurich (Hoechst)

3,093,684 (1963). Novel N(2-Hydroxy-B-Trihaloethyl) Derivatives of Tetracyclines. A. Soder and W. Siedel (Hoechst)

3,104,240 (1963). Mannich Bases of Tetracycline Antibiotics. L. C. Cheney, W. C. Risser and W. J. Gottstein (Bristol-Myers)

3,105,016 (1963). Process of Producing Bromo-Tetracycline. A. D. Doerschuk and B. A. Bitler (American Cyanamid)

3,109,007 (1963). Derivatives of Tetracycline and Its Analogs. R. K. Blackwood, H. H. Rennhard, J. J. Beereboom and C. R. Stephens, Jr. (Pfizer)

3,113,077 (1963). Fermentative Production of Oxytetracycline by a New Species of Streptomyces. T. H. Stoudt and F. Tausig (Merck)

3,117,159 (1963). Derivatives of the Tetracycline-type Antibiotics. H. H. Rennhard, L. H. Conover, P. N. Gordon and C. R. Stephens, Jr. (Pfizer

3,121,670 (1964). Fermentative Preparation of Tetracycline and 7-Chlortetracycline. S. A. Szumski (American Cyanamid)

3,127,328 (1964). Process of Preparing 6-Demethyl-Tetracycline J. J. Goodman (American Cyanamid)

3,139,433 (1964). Bis-Tetracycline Derivatives of Piperazine. G. Kollar, L. Sipos and G. Pato (Chinoin)

3,145,154 (1964). Production of Chlortetracycline and Demethylchlortetracycline. J. J. Goodman (American Cyanamid)

3,145,228 (1964). 5-Alkoxy- and 5-Benzyloxy-Tetracycline, Derivatives and Analogues Thereof. M. S. Von Wittenau, G. Ferry and C. R. Stephens, Jr. (Pfizer)

3,146,264 (1964). Nitriles of the Tetracyclines. R. G. Wilkinson and J. H. Boothe (American Cyanamid)

3,148,212 (1964). Reductive Alkylation Process. J. H. Boothe and J. Petisi (American Cyanamid)

3,149,114 (1964). New Derivative of Tetracycline and Process for the Preparation Thereof. B. Gradnik, A. Pedrazzoli and G. Cipelletti (E. R. A. S. M. E.)

3,154,476 (1964). Process for Production of 7-Chloro-6-Demethyltetracycline. S. L. Neidleman (Olin Mathieson)

3,159,552 (1964). Process of Producing 4-Dedimethylamino-4-Methylethylamino-5-Hydroxytetracycline. P. A. Miller and H. S. Corey (American Cyanamid)

3,159,631 (1964). N-Aminomethyltetracycline Derivatives. M. Gordon, E. Park and B. M. Sutton (Smith, Kline and French)

3,159,675 (1964). Novel 4-Dedimethylamino-4-Oxo-6-Demethyltetracycline-4-Oximes and 4-Hydrazones. R. C. Esse and G. M. Sieger (American Cyanamid)

3,160,570 (1964). Method for Producing 6-Demethylchlortetracycline. E. L. Dulaney and D. Hendlin (Merck)

3,160,661 (1964). 6-Deoxytetracyclines. J. R. D. McCormick (American Cyanamid)

3,165,531 (1965). 13-Substituted-6-Deoxytetracyclines and Process Utilizing the Same. R. K. Blackwood, G. Ferry, H. H. Rennhard, J. J. Beereboom and C. R. Stephens, Jr. (Pfizer)

3,165,551 (1965). New Antibacterial Agents. R. K. Blackwood, G. Ferry, H. H. Rennhard, J. J. Beereboom and C. R. Stephens, Jr. (Pfizer)

3,172,822 (1965). Process for Preparing 6-Demethyltetracyclines. S. L. Neidleman (Olin Mathieson)

3,180,889 (1965). Preparation of Nitrotetracyclines. J. J. Hlavka and H. M. Krazinski (American Cyanamid)

3,183,267 (1965). 6-Methylenetetracycline Derivatives. R. K. Blackwood, G. Ferry, H. H. Rennhard, J. J. Beereboom and C. R. Stephens, Jr. (Pfizer)

3,188,348 (1965). 12a-Deoxytetracycline Oxidation Process. K. Butler, R. B. Woodward and P. N. Gordon (Pfizer)

3,190,810 (1965). Production of 6-Demethyltetracyclines. P. A. Miller (American Cyanamid)

3,200,149 (1965). α-6-Deoxytetracycline Derivatives and Process. R. K. Blackwood, G. Ferry, H. H. Rennhard, J. J. Beereboom and C. R. Stephens, Jr. (Pfizer)

3,201,424 (1965). Derivatives of 1,3,11,12-Tetrahydroxynaphthacene and 1,3,6,11-Tetrahydroxynaphthacene-5,12-Quinone. J. R. D. McCormick and T. Reichenthal (American Cyanamid)

3,218,335 (1965). Antibiotic Compounds. M. Scevola (Pro-Ter)

3,219,671 (1965). Substituted 6-Deoxytetracyclines and 6-Demethyl-6-Deoxytetracyclines. J. Hlavka (American Cyanamid)

3,226,305 (1965). Biological Transformation of 1,3,10,11,12-Pentahydroxynaphthacene-2-carboxamides to Tetracycline Antibiotics. J. R. D.

McCormick, N. O. Sjolander and S. J. Johnson (American Cyanamid)

3,226,434 (1965). Preparation of Neutral 6-Demethyl-7-Chlorotetracycline. P. Bitha and N. E. Rigler (American Cyanamid)

3,226,435 (1965). Novel 7,11a-Dihalotetracyclines and the Process of Preparing Them. J. R. D. McCormick, R. Winterbottom and P. Bitha (American Cyanamid)

3,226,436 (1965). 7-and-9-Alkylamino-6-Deoxytetracycline. J. Petisi and J. H. Boothe (American Cyanamid

3,226,441 (1965). 2-Decarboxamido-2-Acetyl-Tetracycline Derivatives and Process. M. W. Miller (Pfizer)

3,228,962 (1966). N-(2,2-Pentamethylene Pyrrolidino Methyl) Tetracycline and Salts. D. N. McGregor and L. C. Cheney (Bristol-Myers)

3,230,254 (1966). Process of Precipitating Tetracycline Base in Crystalline Form. G. Svanholm (Novo Terapeutisk)

3,239,499 (1966). Tetracycline Derivative. H. H. Rennhard and C. R. Stephens, Jr. (Pfizer)

3,247,226 (1966). 4-Dimethylamino and 4-Hydroxy-Tetracycloxides R. Corlyle and G. M. Sieger (American Cyanamid)

3,247,250 (1966). Carboxamido N-Substituted Tetracyclines. C. R. Tamorria (Eastman Kodak)

3,250,809 (1966). 6-Deoxy-6-Demethyl-6-Halomethylene Tetracyclines and Their 11a-Chloro and Fluoro Derivatives. R. K. Blackwood, H. H. Rennhard, J. J. Beereboom, G. Ferry and C. R. Stephens, Jr. (Pfizer)

3,250,810 (1966). 6-Hydroxy-6-Halomethyl Tetracyclines. R. K. Blackwood, G. Ferry, H. H. Rennhard, J. J. Beereboom and C. R. Stephens, Jr. (Pfizer)

3,264,348 (1966). 6-Demethyl-6-Halomethyl-5a,6-Anhydro-Tetracyclines. R. K. Blackwood, G. Ferry, H. H. Rennhard, J. J. Beereboom and C. R. Stephens, Jr. (Pfizer)

3,228,962 (1966). N-(2,2-Pentamethylene Pyrrolidino Methyl) Tetracycline and Salts. D. N. McGregor and L. C. Cheney (Bristol-Myers)

3,230,254 (1966). Process of Precipitating Tetracycline Base in Crystalline Form. G. Svanholm (Novo Terapeutisk)

3,239,499 (1966). Tetracycline Derivative, H. H. Rennhard and C. R. Stephens, Jr. (Pfizer)

3,247,226 (1966). 4-Dimethylamino and 4-Hydroxy-Tetracycloxides. R. C. Esse and G. M. Sieger (American Cyanamid)

3,247,250 (1966). Carboxamido N-Substituted Tetracyclines. C. R. Tamorria (Eastman Kodak)

3,250,809 (1966). 6-Deoxy-6-Demethyl-6-Halomethylene Tetracyclines and Their 11a-Chloro and Fluoro Derivatives. R. K. Blackwood, G. Ferry, H. H. Rennhard, J. J. Beereboom and C. R. Stephens, Jr. (Pfizer)

3,250,810 (1966). 6-Hydroxy-6-Halomethyl Tetracyclines. R. K. Blackwood, G. Ferry, H. H. Rennhard, J. J. Beereboom and C. R. Stephens, Jr. (Pfizer)

3,264,348 (1966). 6-Demethyl-6-Halomethyl-5a,6-Anhydrotetracyclines. R. K. Blackwood, G. Ferry, H. H. Rennhard, J. J. Beereboom and C. R. Stephens, Jr. (Pfizer)

3,265,732 (1966). Novel 5a,6-Anhydrotetracyclines. P. A. Miller, J. H. Martin and L. A. Mitscher (American Cyanamid)

3,269,929 (1966). Process for the Photooxygenation of Anhydrotetracyclines. M. S. Von Wittenau, G. Ferry (Pfizer)

3,272,817 (1966). N-Aminomethyltetracycline Derivatives. M. Gordon and B. M. Sutton (Smith, Kline and French)

3,272,862 (1966). Recovery of Tetracycline Antibiotics from Fermentation Broths. E. Caputo and E. Zannini (Ankerfarm)

3,275,652 (1966). Novel 2-Carboxamido-N-Imidomethyl-6-Demethyl-6-Deoxytetracyclines. M. J. Martell, Jr. and A. S. Tomcufcik (American Cyanamid)

3,277,172 (1967). Tetraphenylboron Derivatives of Tetracycline Antibiotics. J. F. Alicino (Squibb)

3,280,188 (1967). Tetracycline-N,N'-dibenzylideneethylenediamine Complexes for Use in Isolating Tetracyclines. I. Villax

3,282,779 (1967). Feed Compositions. J. M. Pensack and C. N. Huhtanen (American Cyanamid)

3,283,000 (1967). Neutral Sulfate Salts of Tetracycline. H. Mendelsohn (American Cyanamid)

3,293,133 (1967). Imparting Color to Pharmaceutical Solutions. J. A. Hill (Squibb)

3,296,073 (1967). Enhancing Tetracycline Antibiotic Blood Levels with Pyrazolidine Potentiating Agents. J. E. Fahey (Pfizer)

3,298,927 (1967). Process for Preparing 6-Demethyltetracyclines Using Ethionine Sulfoxide. S. L. Neidleman (Olin Mathieson)

3,301,899 (1967). Purification of Tetracycline. M. A. Kaplan and A. P. Granatek (Bristol-Myers)

3,304,227 (1967). Antibiotic-containing Animal Feed (With Aromatic Polycarboxylic Acids and Surface Active Agents). C. E. Loveless

3,317,403 (1967). Streptomyces Aureofaciens Fermentation Process Using Glyceride Oil and Casein. S. A. Szumski (American Cyanamid)

3,326,761 (1967). 6-Demethyl-6-deoxytetracycline Antitumor Antibiotic. R. E. Kent (Pfizer)

3,328,258 (1967). Antimicrobial Composition. L. Fontaine (LIPHA)

3,330,841 (1967). 3-(4-Carbamoyl-2,3,5-trihydroxybenzyl)-1,2,3,4-tetrahydro-4,8-dihydroxy-1-oxo-2-naphthoic Acid γ-Lactones. J. J. Hlavka and P. Bitha (American Cyanamid)

3,335,055 (1967). Tetracycline Antibiotics. J. F. Weidenheime L. Ritter and G. Sieger (American Cyanamid)

3,338,963 (1967). Tetracycline Compounds. J. Petisi and J. H. Boothe (American Cyanamid)

3,341,408 (1967). Augmenting 5-Oxytetracycline Avian Blood Levels and Feed Suppliments with Selected Cyclic Phosphates. C. Y. Shen (Monsanto)

3,341,585 (1967). Substituted 7- and/or 9-Amino-6-deoxytetracyclines. P. Bitha, J. J. Hlavka and M. J. Martel, Jr. (American Cyanamid)

3,341,586 (1967). Substituted 7- and/or 9-Amino-6-methylenetetracyclines. P. Bitha, J. J. Hlavka and M. J. Martell, Jr. (American Cyanamid)

3,345,370	(1967).	4-(N-Mono-substituted)hydrazones of 4-Dedimethylamino-4-oxo-tetracycline. R. C. Esse and G. Sieger (American Cyanamid)
3,345,379	(1967).	7-Imidomethyl-6-demethyl-6-deoxytetracyclines. M. J. Martel, Jr. and A. S. Tomcufcik (American Cyanamid)
3,345,408	(1967).	Substituted 4-Dedimethylamino-4-hydroxy-4a,12a-Anhydrotetracyclines. J. J. Hlavka and P. Bitha (American Cyanamid)
3,345,409	(1967).	A Method of Preparing 1,3,10,11,12-Pentahydroxynaphthacene-2-carboxamides. J. R. D. McCormick (American Cyanamid)
3,345,410	(1967).	Substituted 7- and/or 9-Amino Tetracyclines. R. Winterbottom, P. Bitha and H. M. Kissman (American Cyanamid)
3,349,127	(1967).	Method of Tetracycline Isolation from Fermented Media. K. Culik, J. Dasek, J. Palkoska and J. Pelzbauer (Spofa)
3,360,557	(1967).	9-Hydroxytetracyclines and a Process of Preparing Same. P. Shu (American Cyanamid)
3,360,558	(1967).	Substituted 5a,6-Anhydrotetracycline Methyl Betaines. J. J. Hlavka and P. Bitha (American Cyanamid)
3,360,559	(1967).	Substituted 1,3,4,10,11,12-Hexahydroxynaphthacene-2-carboxamides. J. R. D. McCormick and E. R. Jensen (American Cyanamid)
3,360,561	(1967).	Nitration of Tetracyclines. R. T. Zambrano (American Cyanamid)
3,338,963	(1968).	Tetracycline Compounds. J. Petisi and J. Boothe (American Cyanamid)
3,345,370	(1968).	4-(N-Monosubstituted)hydrazones of 4-Dedimethyl-amino-4-oxotetracycline. R. C. Esse and G. Sieger (American Cyanamid)
3,345,379	(1968).	7-Imidomethyl-6-demethyl-6-deoxytetracyclines. M. J. Martell, Jr. and A. S. Tomcufcik (American Cyanamid)
3,345,408	(1968).	Substituted 4-Dedimethylamino-4-hydroxy-4a,12a-anhydrotetracyclines. J. J. Hlavka and P. Bitha (American Cyanamid)
3,345,409	(1968).	1,3,10,11,12-Pentahydroxynaphthacene-2-carboxamides. J. R. D. McCormick (American Cyanamid)

3,347,861 (1968). Tetracycline Hydrochloride-piperazine Complex. S. S. M. Wang (Dow)

3,350,267 (1968). Control of Micrococcus Pyogenes (Staphyloccus aureus) with Novobiocin and Other Antibiotics H. Wallick (Merck)

3,356,571 (1968). Potentiation of Tetracyclines by Poly (Acrylic Acid) or Hydrolyzed Polyacrylonitrile. E. Takesue, J. J. Hlavka and J. H. Boothe (American Cyanamid)

3,359,160 (1968). Potentiation of Tetracycline in Blood Serum. R. S. Gordon (Monsanto)

3,360,557 (1968). 9-Hydroxytetracyclines. P. Shu (American Cyanamid)

3,360,558 (1968). Substituted 5a,6-Anhydrotetracycline Methyl Betaines. J. J. Hlavka and P. Bitha (American Cyanamid)

3,360,559 (1968). Substituted 1,3,4,10,11,12-Hexahydroxynaphthacene-2-carboxamides. J. R. D. McCormick and E. R. Jensen (American Cyanamid)

3,360,561 (1968). Nitration of Tetracyclines. R. T. Zambrano (American Cyanamid)

3,364,123 (1968). Production of 4N-Demethyl-4N-Ethyl Tetracyclines. S. L. Neidleman (Squibb)

3,364,260 (1968). 4N-Demethyl-4N-Ethyl Tetracyclines. S. L. Neidleman (Squibb)

3,372,190 (1968). Tetracycline Hydrochloride. G. Kroek, O. Lowe and J. Murray (Rachelle)

3,373,196 (1968). Production of 7- and/or 9-(Lower Alkyl)-Amino-5a,6-Anhydrotetracyclines. P. Bitha and J. J. Hlavka (American Cyanamid)

3,373,197 (1968). Substituted 6-Epitetracyclines and 5a-Epi-6-Epitetracyclines. M. J. Martell and A. S. Ross (American Cyanamid)

3,373,198 (1968). Substituted 5a,11a-Dehydro-6-Epitetracycline M. J. Martell and A. S. Ross (American Cyanamid)

3,375,276 (1968). Method for Preparing Tetracycline Products. S. L. Neidleman, R. W. Kinney and F. L. Weisenborn (Squibb)

3,385,765 (1968). Novel Process of Producing 1,3,4,10,11,12-Hexahydroxy-6-Methylnaphthacene-2-carboxamide. J. R. D. McCormick, U. Joachim, E. R. Jensen and N. O. Sjolander (American Cyanamid)

3,388,161 (1968). Aminomethyl Derivatives of Tetracycline. G. Lancini and P. Sensi (Lepetit)

3,388,162 (1968). Production of 7- and/or 9-Nitro or Amino Tetracyclines. R. Winterbottom, P. Bitha and H. M. Kissman (American Cyanamid)

3,389,174 (1968). Stable Tetracycline Solutions. R. A. Nash and B. E. Haeger (American Cyanamid)

3,389,175 (1968). Stable Tetracycline N,N-dimethyllauramide Solutions. R. A. Nash and B. E. Haeger (American Cyanamid)

3,390,005 (1968). Fermentative Production of N-Ethyl-oxytetracycline. E. L. Dulaney and I. Putter (Merck)

3,394,178 (1968). N-Ethyloxytetracycline. E. L. Dulaney and I. Putter (Merck)

3,397,230 (1968). Nitration of Tetracyclines. R. Winterbottom, P. Bitha and H. M. Kissman (American Cyanamid)

3,397,231 (1968). Refining of α-6-Deoxy-5-Oxytetracycline. J. J. Korst (Pfizer)

3,398,057 (1968). Process for Producing Tetracycline. E. Zannini, E. Piacenza and G. Fabbri (Ankerfarm)

3,400,050 (1968). Preparation and Isolation of Tetracyclines with the Aid of Tetracycline Complexes. I. Villax (International Rectifier)

3,401,088 (1968). Process of Fermentation of Chlortetracycline and Tetracycline Antibiotics. I. Villax (International Rectifier)

3,403,179 (1968). Novel 7-(1,2-Bis-Substituted-Hydrazino)-Tetracyclines and Methods of Preparing the Same. R. T. Zambrano (American Cyanamid)

3,408,258 (1968). Process for Producing Oxytetracycline Antibiotic. A. Grein, G. Canevazzi and R. Barchielli (Societa Farmaceutici Italia)

3,409,616 (1969). α-Amino-4-oxo-10-hydroxy-1,2,3,4-tetrahydro-2-anthraceneacetate Esters. L. H. Conover (Pfizer)

3,423,457 (1969). 7-Chloro-6-demethyl-9-nitrotetracycline. R. Winterbottom and M. L. Sassiver (American Cyanamid)

3,424,839 (1969). Tetracycline and Enteric-Coated Chymotrypsin Oral Tablets and Therapy. J. Montandraud (Societe Generale de Recherches et d'Applications Scientifiques Sogeros)

3,425,911 (1969). Method of Producing Tetracycline. M. Vondracek, J. Slezak, M. Herold and K. Culik (Spofa)

3,429,780 (1969). Fermentation Process for the Production of Tetracycline. K. Culik, J. Palkoska, M. Vondracek, J. Skoda and Milos Herold (Spofa)

3,429,781 (1969). Process for the Production of Tetracycline. K. Culik, M. Herold, J. Palkoska, B. Sikyta and J. Slezak (Czeckloslavakia)

3,431,303 (1969). 6,11-Dihydro-11-oxo-6-methyl-3,6,10,12-tetrahydroxynaphthacene-1,4-quinone-2-carboxamide, An Intermediate in the Fermentation of Tetracycline. J. R. D. McCormick, U. Joachim, E. R. Johnston and N. O. Sjolander (American Cyanamid)

3,432,394 (1969). Fermentative Production of Tetracycline. I. Villax (International Rectifier)

3,433,709 (1969). Biological Transformation of α-6-Deoxy-Tetracyclines to Tetracyclines. J. R. D. McCormick and N. O. Sjolander (American Cyanamid)

3,433,710 (1969). Process for the Preparation of 7-Chloro-5-Hydroxytetracyclines. J. R. D. McCormick, S. J. Johnson and N. O. Sjolander (American Cyanamid)

3,433,834 (1969). 7- and (or) 9-Nitrotetracyclines by Nitration of 11a-Chlorotetracyclines. R. Winterbottom and H. M. Kissman (American Cyanamid)

3,434,844 (1969). Stabilization of Animal and Poultry Feeds Containing Tetracycline. I. Klothen, R. B. Fortenbaugh and A. Abbey (American Cyanamid)

3,434,930 (1969). Method of Producing Tetracycline. F. Paleckova, Z. Hostalek and Z. Rehacek (Spofa)

3,442,943 (1969). Process for Preparing 6-Deoxytetracyclines. M. J. Martell, Jr. and A. S. Ross (American Cyanamid)

3,444,198 (1969). Process for Producing α-6-Deoxy-tetracyclines. J. J. Korst (Pfizer)

3,446,841 (1969). Isolation of 5-Hydroxy-7-Chlorotetracycline. L. A. Mitscher and J. H. E. J. Martin (American Cyanamid)

3,454,639 (1969). Tetracycline Recovery. C. O. Putnam (Pfizer)

3,455,800 (1969). Process of Preparing 4-Dedimethyl-Amino-tetracyclines. J. J. Hlavka and P. Bitha (American Cyanamid)

3,456,007 (1969). Carboxymethyl Derivatives of Tetracycline Antibiotics. J. Rondelet (R. I. T.)

3,458,572 (1969). Tetracycline Recovery Process. A. J. O'Donnell (Pfizer)

3,459,554 (1969). Ripening Siages. S. Hashimoto (Kaken)

3,462,487 (1970). Tetracycline Derivatives. R. W. Kinney, S. L. Neidleman, F. L. Weisenborn and J. S. P. Schwarz (Squibb)

3,463,791 (1969). 7-Chloro-4-dedimethylamino-12,12α-seco-tetracycline-12-carboxylic Acid 6,12 Lactones. S. L. Neidleman, R. W. Kinney and F. L. Weisenborn (Squibb)

3,483,199 (1970). Water Soluble Derivatives of Tetracylines. D. Silva and J. R. F. Joao (CIPAN)

3,483,251 (1970). Antibacterial (Alkylamino) Tetracyclines. R. T. Zambrano (American Cyanamid)

3,485,914 (1970). Pharmaceutical Antibiotic Preparation Having Delayed Therapeutic Action. M. E. Corn (Chemical and Pharmaceutical Patent Holding Ltd.)

3,491,187 (1970). Iron Salt-Antibiotic Compositions. C. M. Ely (Diamond Shamrock)

3,492,398 (1970). Aminopolyamide Resin Coating for Biologically Active Substances. G. J. Marco, E. J. Prill and E. J. Jaworski (Monsanto)

3,499,959 (1970). Tetracycline Preparation with Delayed Therapeutic Action. M. E. Corn (Chemical and Pharmaceutical Patent Holding Ltd.)

3,502,660 (1970). Antibiotic 6-Deoxy-6-demethyltetracyclines. K. Butler, L. H. Conover and R. B. Woodward (Pfizer)

3,502,696 (1970). Antibiotic 6-Deoxy-6-demethyltetracyclines. L. H. Conover (Pfizer)

3,505,450 (1970). Treating Coccidiosis in Poultry with 6-Chloropurine and a Tetracycline Antibiotic. M. W. Miller, H. L. Howes, Jr. (Pfizer)

3,509,184 (1970). Anthracyclidene-acetic Acid Derivatives as Antibiotics. L. H. Conover and R. B. Woodward (Pfizer)

3,514,477 (1970). 2(Cyanoaminomethyl)-4,10-dioxo-1,2,3,4,4a,9,9a,10-octahydroanthracenes. L. H. Conover (Pfizer)

3,515,713 (1970). Antibacterial Tetracyclines. L. H. Conover (Pfizer)

3,515,717 (1970). Isolation of Antibiotics. D. Y. Cha, H. K. Jahnke (Upjohn)

3,516,909 (1970). Biosynthesis of Tetracycline Antibiotics. H. Bishop (American Cyanamid)

3,518,306 (1970). Antibacterial 7- and/or 9-(N-nitrosoalkylamino)-6-demethyl-6-deoxytetracyclines. M. J. Martell, Jr. and A. S. Ross (American Cyanamid)

3,524,862 (1970). (Isoxazolyl)(Amino)-methyl-tetrahydroanthracenes. L. H. Conover (Pfizer)

3,526,629 (1970). 4-(β-Hydroxyethyl)piperazinocarboxymethyl-7-dimethylamino-6-deoxy-6-demethyltetracycline and Its Antibacterial Activity. M. J. Martell, Jr. and J. H. Boothe (American Cyanamid)

3,532,791 (1970). Antibiotic N,N'-ethylenebis[2-(o-hydroxyphenyl)-glycine]. C. Johnston (Dow)

3,531,563 (1971). Urea Particles Coated with Tetracycline Antibiotics, For Use in Animal Feed. I. Klothen and A. W. Brahm (American Cyanamid)

3,538,215 (1971). Stabilized Antibiotic in Liquid Ruminant Feed Supplement. F. M. Snyder and S. L. Hallows (Allied)

3,546,339 (1971). Stable Dimethyl Sulfoxide Solutions of Tetracycline Antibiotics for Parenteral Use. L. J. Leeson, R. A. Nash and L. Ritter (American Cyanamid)

3,549,663 (1971). 3,4,10-Tioxo-1,2,3,4,4a,9,9a,10-octahydroanthracenes; Antimicrobial and Complexing Agents and Intermediates for Preparation of Tetracycline. L. H. Conover and J. D. Johnston (Pfizer)

3,579,564 (1971). 5-Hydroxytetracycline Esters. R. K. Blackwood and M. S. Von Wittenau (Pfizer)

3,579,579 (1971). Substituted 7- and (or) 9-Amino-6-demethyl-6-deoxytetracyclines. J. J. Hlavka, P. Bitha, A. S. Ross and M. J. Martell (American Cyanamid)

3,536,759 (1972). Antibiotic Tetracycline Sulfamate and Its Derivatives. A. Jurado and J. M. Puigmarti (Hosbon)

3,586,483 (1971). Test for Detecting the Presence of Tetracycline Antibiotics in Biological Fluids. J. G. Heider and R. G. Kelly (American Cyanamid)

3,616,239 (1972). 7-Chloro-6-demethyltetracycline Fermentation. J. A. Growich, Jr. (American Cyanamid)

3,616,240 (1972). 7-Chloro-6-demethyltetracycline Fermentation. J. A. Growich, Jr. (American Cyanamid)

3,616,241 (1972). Microbiological Production of 7-Chloro-5a,11a-Dehydrotetracycline. J. A. Growich, Jr. (American Cyanamid)

3,622,627 (1972). Antimicrobial 4-(dedimethylamino)tetracyclines and Their 5a,6-Anhydro Derivatives. R. K. Blackwood and C. R. Stephens, Jr. (Pfizer)

3,632,647 (1972). Purifying Chlortetracycline Hydrochloride and Chlortetracycline Neutral Base. S. B. Greenbaum, R. Griffith and H. C. Klein (Diamond Shamrock)

3,634,500 (1972). 2-(1,8-Dimethoxy-4-methyl-2-naphthoyl)-3,5-dialkoxyterephthalamic Acids. J. R. D. McCormick and N. H. Arnold (American Cyanamid)

3,636,063 (1972). 6-Methyl-1,3,10,11-tetrahydroxynaphthacene-2-carboxamide-5,12 Quinone. J. R. D. McCormick and N. H. Arnold (American Cyanamid)

3,636,081 (1972). 2-Formyl-3,5-disubstituted Terephthalate Esters. J. R. D. McCormick and N. H. Arnold (American Cyanamid)

3,636,202 (1972). Compositions for Treating Rheumatoid Arthritis and Related Diseases. L. A. Klein.

3,637,463 (1972). Production of Oxytetracycline Using Streptomyces alboflavus. I. Villax (International Rectifier)

3,639,214 (1972). Fermentative Production of 6-Demethyltetracycline Using Streptomyces aureofaciens C. K. Mercer and G. P. Wilkin (Upjohn)

3,642,987 (1972). Antibiotic Lincomycin-tetracycline Compositions. M. E. Bergy, R. R. Herr and D. J. Mason

3,651,208 (1972). Dentifrice for Peridontia Purposes. E. L. Lauster (Lafant)

3,658,989 (1972). Antibacterial Compositions Containing Tetracycline Sulfamate and Its Derivatives. A. Jurado-Soler and J. M. Puigmarti-Codina (Hosbon)

3,660,558 (1972). Determination of Capacitation of Sperm Employing a Fluorescent Form of Tetracycline. R. J. Ericsson (Upjohn)

3,689,646 (1972). Antimutagenic Treatment of Bacteria. M. G. Sevag (University of Pennsylvania)

3,696,189 (1972). Stabilized Antibiotic and Method. F. M. Snyder

3,697,552 (1973). Anthracyclidine-acetic Acid Derivatives. L. H. Conover and R. B. Woodward (Pfizer)

3,699,117 (1973). 2-[5-(3- and 4-Substituted Isoxazolyl) aminomethyl]3,4,10-trioxo-1,2,3,4,4a,9,9a,10-octa-hydroanthracenes and Related Compounds. K. Butler, L. H. Conover and R. B. Woodward (Pfizer)

3,743,727 (1973). Enhancing Tissue Penetration of Antimicrobial Agents with Dimethyl Sulfoxide. R. J. Herschler (Crown Zellerbach)

3,754,986 (1973). Organic Semiconductors. E. A. Perez-Albuerne (Eastman Kodak)

3,809,751 (1974). Antibiotic-stable Liquid Protein Supplements Containing Non-protein Nitrogen, Phosphorus and a Tetracycline Antibiotic. A. Abbey (American Cyanamid)

3,812,188 (1974). Purification of 7-Chlorotetracycline. W. M. Ziegler (American Cyanamid)

3,824,285 (1974). 4-Oxo-4-(dedimethylamino)tetracycline 4,6-Hemiketals. R. K. Blackwood and C. R. Stephens, Jr. (Pfizer)

3,835,190 (1975). N,N'-Dibenzylethylenediaminodimethylditetracycline. E. N. Lazareva, O. P. Belozerova, T. I. Efimova, L. V. Sitnikova and A. P. Kryuchkova.

3,846,486 (1975). Water Soluble Tetracycline Sodium 4-(Methyleneamino)salicylate Complexes. I. Marcus

3,863,009 (1975). Glycine Derivatives as Potentiators for Tetracyclines. C. Johnston (Dow)

3,879,456 (1975). Chlortetracycline Neutral Base. K. H. Schaaf (Diamond Shamrock)

3,906,043 (1975). Water Soluble Tetracycline Complexes with Sodium p-(methyleneamino)salicylate. I. Marcus

3,907,889 (1975). Chelocardin Derivatives. M. Inaba, E. Bernstein and D. L. Garmaise (Abbott)

3,907,890 (1975). α-6-Deoxy-5-hydroxytetracycline. C. J. V. Sconio (Pfizer)

AUTHOR INDEX

Numbers in parentheses are rererence numbers and indicate that an author's work is referred to although his or her name is not given in the text. Underlined numbers give the page on which the complete reference is listed.

SUBJECT INDEX